Nutrition in Infancy and Childhood

Nutrition in Infancy and Childhood

PEGGY L. PIPES, R.D., M.P.H.

Assistant Chief, Nutrition Section, Clinical Training Unit,
Child Development and Mental Retardation Center;
Lecturer, Parent and Child Nursing, School of Nursing,
University of Washington, Seattle, Washington

Fourth Edition

with new illustrations

TIMES MIRROR/MOSBY College Publishing

St. Louis • Toronto • Boston • Los Altos   1989

Editor: Pat Coryell
Editorial Assistant: Shannon Ruyle
Production Editor: Kathy Lumpkin
Designer: Rey Umali

Fourth Edition

Copyright © 1989 by Times Mirror/Mosby College Publishing

A division of The C.V. Mosby Company
11830 Westline Industrial Drive, St. Louis, Missouri 63146

Library of Congress Cataloging in Publication Data

Pipes, Peggy L.
    Nutrition in infancy and childhood.

    Includes bibliographies and index.
    1. Children—Nutrition.   2. Infants—Nutrition.
I. Title.   [DNLM: 1. Child Nutrition.   2. Infant
Nutrition.   3. Nutrition—in adolescence.   WS 115 P665n]
RJ206.P56   1989   613.2'088054   88-39774
ISBN 0-8016-3823-2

PS/RRD/RRD 9 8 7 6 5 4 3 2 1

Contributors

JUDITH BUMBALO, M.S.
Doctoral student, Wayne State University, Detroit

MIRIAM E. LOWENBERG, Ph.D.
Professor Emerita, Pennsylvania State University, University Park,
Pennsylvania; Consultant, Seattle

BETTY LUCAS, M.P.H.
Lecturer, Parent and Child Nursing, School of Nursing; Nutritionist,
Child Development and Mental Retardation Center, University of Washington,
Seattle

L. KATHLEEN MAHAN, M.S., R.D.
Nutrition Consultant, Private Practice

MARY J. O'LEARY, M.S.
Perinatal-Pediatric Nutritionist
Department of Pediatrics, School of Medicine,
University of Washington, Seattle

SALLY M. O'NEIL, Ph.D.
Behavioral Psychologist, Private Practice

ROBIN PRITKIN GLASS, M.S., O.T.R.
Occupational Therapist, Children's Orthopedic Hospital, Seattle

JANE MITCHELL REES, M.S.
Teaching Associate, Department of Pediatrics, School of Medicine; Nutritionist,
Adolescent Clinic, Child Development and Mental Retardation Center, University
of Washington, Seattle

CRISTINE M. TRAHMS, M.S.
Teaching Associate, Department of Pediatrics, School of Medicine; Nutritionist, Child Development and Mental Retardation Center, University of Washington, Seattle

BONNIE WORTHINGTON-ROBERTS, Ph.D.
Professor of Nutrition, Department of Epidemiology/Pediatrics; Chief, Nutrition Section, Child Development and Mental Retardation Center, University of Washington, Seattle

To Miriam E. Lowenberg,
A pioneer in the study of children's
food behavior, my mentor and friend

Preface

Nutrition in Infancy and Childhood has been prepared to provide students with information necessary for the clinical application of nutrition for infants and children. Because the effective delivery of these services requires insight into development and behavioral patterns, as well as growth and nutrient needs, these topics have been integrated into the discussion.

AUDIENCE

The text is appropriate for a variety of students preparing to enter service professions, including pediatric, nutrition/dietetic, occupational and physical therapy, and maternal-child nursing students. Emphasis on education for handicapped infants and children from birth through the school years and the need for health and nutrition services mandated by PL99-457 should make the chapters on infants and children with developmental and related problems useful for not only potential health professionals, but for students preparing to enter special education as well.

The usefulness of the text is not limited to students. Many practitioners, including those employed by WIC programs, by Maternal and Child Programs in Health Departments, by pediatric hospital units, and by diagnostic and evaluation centers for the developmentally delayed, will find practical approaches to the provision of appropriate nutrient intakes for the population they serve.

IN THIS EDITION

1. A new chapter on the formation of food patterns (Chapter 7) has been added for two reasons. Behavioral issues influence food intake at all ages in childhood, and it seemed important to organize them in one chapter rather than find them repeated at each age. Also, information is added on taste and relevant issues contributing to the reader's understanding of factors that influence children's food intake.
2. Chapter 6, prepared by Dr. Lowenberg, remains intact since it is a compilation of a pioneer's studies of child feeding.
3. The behavior modification chapter (Chapter 15), remains intact to provide a tool for the resolution of many nutrition problems.
4. Much new information has been accumulated since the third edition, especially in regard to the premature infant. This section, Chapter 12, has experienced a major revision.
5. All chapters have been revised and updated to reflect current approaches to feeding infants and children.

PEDAGOGY

To aid the student in the use of this text, learning objectives and learning activities are included in each chapter. The glossary has been expanded to provide a more comprehensive list of unfamiliar words.

AUTHOR'S NOTE

Recommended dietary allowances are being revised and are to be published in the first half of 1989. Because the publication date for this book preceded the planned publication of the RDAs, the recommended quantities have not been included in the text. It seems advisable for anyone interested in the nutrition of infants and children to obtain this text and to integrate the RDA information into Chapter 2, "Nutrient Needs of Infants and Children."

ACKNOWLEDGEMENTS

As with the previous editions, many people have contributed to this edition of *Nutrition in Infancy and Childhood*. Every contributor wrote and produced with very busy work schedules under considerable stress. The faculty and students at the Child Development and Mental Retardation Center provided many worthwhile suggestions and much needed understanding and support. Our clients provided the basis by which we developed the philosophy of infant and child nutrition described in the text.

The public health nurses with whom I have worked in Clallam and Whatcom Counties have also had an input on the clinical approach to nutrition intervention described in the text by making me aware of nutrition problems in the community. The questions they have raised and the home visits they planned to children at "high risk" took the practice of nutrition from the "Ivory Tower" to the real world. They showed me children who have symptoms of nutritional deficiency and confirmed the fact that in this affluent country there are malnourished and hungry children.

The reviewers provided many helpful suggestions for reorganization of the text, in chapter sequences and in the information on behavioral and interpersonal effects on food intakes. My personal thanks go to the following people:

Dr. Miriam Alexander
Cornell University

Dr. Sally Hunt
Northwestern University

Dr. Elsa McMullen
Bowling Green State University

Dr. Anne Smith
University of Utah

Professor Beth Zimmer
University of Tennessee

To Ruth Boyd, who has typed all four editions, I am extremely grateful, not only for having typed the manuscript and helped me meet deadlines, but for having maintained her composure and tact during the process.

Finally, to the professors and students who have maintained the market for the first three editions so that this fourth edition is a reality, I express my thanks.

Peggy L. Pipes, MPH, R.D.

1, 2, 4, 11, 12

Contents

1

Nutrition: Growth and Development

Peggy L. Pipes

OBJECTIVES

After studying this chapter, the student should:

1. Understand the effect of nutrition on physical growth and development.
2. Understand characteristics of cell growth and the concept of critical stages of development.
3. Recognize appropriate equipment necessary to secure accurate measurments of height, weight, and fatfolds.
4. Recognize if anthropometric measurements are secured in a manner that provides accurate data.
5. Be able to interpret growth data on individual children in relation to norms.

A normal, healthy child grows at a genetically predetermined rate that can be compromised or accelerated by undernutrition, imbalanced nutrient intake, or overnutrition. Progress in physical growth is one of the criteria used to assess the nutritional status of populations and of individual children. It is therefore important that persons concerned with nutrition and feeding of infants and children be familiar with the process and parameters of growth, as well as the charts and grids used to measure it.

Although every aspect and component of growth is thought to be influenced by nutrition, this discussion focuses on those parameters dealt with by persons concerned with a child's food intake: increases in linear growth and weight, changes in body composition, how to secure accurate measurements of growth, and how to intrepret physical growth patterns of normal children. Patterns of catch-up growth after an episode of wasting (when there is a greater deficit in weight than length) and stunting (when a deficit of both height and weight are present) are discussed.

NUTRITION AND PHYSICAL GROWTH

Children who suffer from undernutrition are shorter and weigh less than their well-nourished peers. The rate of gain in weight is more affected than is the rate of gain in height, but if the nutritional deficit is severe enough and continues long enough, linear growth will be retarded or may cease and/or pubertal maturation and **epiphyseal closure** will be delayed. Linear growth is delayed when energy intake is adequate but protein intake is deficient. Weight is affected when energy intake is deficient, and linear growth will eventually be retarded. Overnutrition results in taller, heavier, more mature children.

Children from low-income families consume less food and therefore less energy and total nutrients than children from families with greater financial resources. Nutritional status studies have shown that children from these families are shorter and weigh less than children whose families are more affluent. Differences in stature are greater than those in weight. In fact, several studies have found that children who live under conditions of marginal food supplies are shorter yet appear fatter than those who have an abundant supply of food available.[1, 2] Results of studies to determine the effect of nutritional supplementation during the third trimester of pregnancy through the third year of life on impoverished children in Colombia, South America, who were at risk for malnutrition show that children who received supplements were taller and heavier than those in nonsupplemented control group at 18 and 36 months of age. They, however, remained smaller than Colombian children from higher socioeconomic families who probably had more food available.[3] Infants and children at nutritional risk who have received the Women's, Infants', and Children's supplemental food packages that include iron-fortified cereal, iron-fortified infant formula, or milk, cheese, eggs, and fruit and vegetable juices have experienced increased rates of growth in height and weight.

Growth patterns of children of racial groups whose members have been believed genetically small have been found to increase under conditions of improved nutrition. Especially striking is the change in the growth pattern of Japanese children born since World War II. In 1962 boys at 14 years of age were found to be 7.6 **cm** taller and girls at 11 years of age 6.6 cm taller than prewar children of the same ages. The change in growth patterns has been credited to an increase in the intake of animal protein.[5] A 1960 survey of children in Japanese orphanages whose food budgets were limited found heights to be significantly less than those of the national averages for children of the same age and sex. Adolescents were shorter as compared with their age-group average than were younger children. During the subsequent 10 years the provision of 180 gm milk and one egg daily and increases in food budgets resulted in improvements in the quality and quantity of protein, as well as in the amount of total nutrients consumed. Increases in average stature were greater than expected. A 1970 survey found that only teenage boys were significantly below the national averages for height.[6]

CHARACTERISTICS OF GROWTH

Growth may be defined as an increase in the physical size of the body as a whole or as an increase in any of its parts associated with an increase in cell number or cell size. Development is defined as the acquisition of function associated with **cell differentiation** and **maturation** of individual organ systems or as a change from a lower to a more advanced stage of complexity for greater facility in functioning. Growth and development are affected by genetic, hormonal, environmental, and behavioral factors that interact to determine an individual's growth pattern.

Individual children have their own genetically predetermined growth patterns. Growth and development, however, proceed in an orderly and predictable sequence. Each organ and organ system has its own period of rapid growth marked by rapid cell differentiation, changes in form, and susceptibility to physical and environmental influences. Growth is the composite of many tissues that are growing at different rates. Skeletal muscle growth approximates whole body growth. The brain, lymphoid, adrenal, and reproductive tissue follow different patterns as shown in Figure 1-1.

The head reaches 90% of its adult size by 6 years of age, whereas growth of the reproductive system proceeds slowly until puberty, when sexual maturation occurs. The lymph tissue grows rapidly until puberty and then reduces in size.

CRITICAL PERIODS OF GROWTH

Increases in physical size are achieved by increases in both the number and size of cells. Cell growth in any organ proceeds in three stages: **hyperplasia**, in which an increase occurs in cell number; **hypertrophy** and hyperplasia, in which increases occur in both the size and number of cells; and hypertrophy, in which only the size of the cells increases. Growth in both the number and size of cells can be assessed by calculation of the rates of weight to deoxyribonucleic acid (DNA) or of protein to DNA.

Enesco and Leblond[7] determined the number of cells in each organ of the rat at different ages throughout growth by measuring the DNA content of the organ. Knowing the weight of the organ, they then estimated the size of the cells. Winick and Noble,[8] using the same method for rat studies, found that there is a time when cell division stops before the organ attains its final size. There is a phase when cell number is not increasing but cell size is. Some tissues like the brain reach a full adult complement of DNA sometime in the second year,

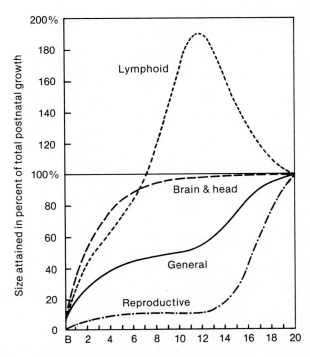

Figure 1-1 Growth of four types of body tissue as percent of adult size. (From Scammon, R.E.: Measurement of the Body in Childhood. In: The Measurement of Man. Minneapolis, 1930, University of Minnesota Press.)

whereas other tissues, such as muscle, continue to increase in DNA throughout adolescence.

Winick and Noble[9] found that rats malnourished by restriction of total food intake during the period of increase in cell number but given normal diets during later growth had a reduction in the number of brain cells, whereas those malnourished in later life and rehabilitated had normal numbers and sizes of cells. Elliott and Cheek,[10] in studies of muscle and liver cells of rats, found that restriction of calories resulted in fewer cells, whereas restriction of protein and calories resulted in both a decrease in cell size and number. Winick and Nobel[11] have also found that overnutrition during a period of hyperplasia resulted in larger animals with a larger number of cells in the organs. The period of hyperplasia, the time when cell numbers are increasing, is the time the organ is most vulnerable to compromised nutrition and can be considered critical to an individual's acquistion of a normal complement of cells.

GROWTH IN HEIGHT AND WEIGHT

The birth weight is determined by the mother's prepregnancy weight and weight gain during pregnancy. The average weight of the normal full-term newborn is approximately 3500 gm. However, about 7% of infants born in the United States are low birth weight (LBW) and weight less than 2500 gm or are very low birth weight (VLBW) infants and weigh less than 1500 gm.[12]

Infants may be low birth weight because of a premature delivery or because of a retarded rate of growth in utero. A small for gestational age infant whose intrauterine weight gain was poor but whose linear and head growth are appropriate for gestational age has experienced **asymmetric** intrauterine growth retardation. A small for gestational age infant whose length and head circumference are also below the 10th percentile is said to be symmetrically growth retarded. The second type of growth retardation reflecting early and prolonged intrauterine nutritional deficit is more detrimental to later growth and development.

After birth, genetic influences are target seeking. A period of catch-up or lag-down growth may occur. The majority of infants who are genetically determined to be longer shift channels of growth during the first 3 to 6 months. However, many infants born at or below the 10th percentile who are determined to be of average height may not achieve a new channel until 1 year of age. Larger infants whose genotypes are for smaller sizes grow at their fetal rates for several months before the lag-down in growth becomes evident. Often a new channel is not apparent until the child is 13 months of age.[13]

Immediately after birth there is a weight loss resulting from a loss of fluid and some catabolism of tissue. It averages 6% of body weight but occasionally exceeds 10%. Thereafter, weight gain in infancy proceeds at a rapid but decelerating rate. Average weight gains for the first 4 months of age are 20 to 25 gm/day, during the last 8 months, 15 gm/day.

By 4 months of age most infants have doubled their birth weights, and by 12 months of age their birth weights have usually tripled. Males double their birth weight earlier than do females, and smaller newborns double their birth weights sooner than do heavier infants. The weight increment during the second year is slightly less than the birth weight. The normal newborn infant who weighs 3.5 **kg** at birth, for example, can be expected to weigh 7 kg at 4 to 6 months, 10.5 kg at 1 year, and 13 kg at 2 years of age. Thereafter, the yearly increments in weight proceed at a slower but constant rate averaging 2.3 kg/year until the ninth or tenth year, when the rate of gain shows a steady increase. This rate continues until adolescence, when a rapid increase in rate of gain occurs.

Height, as weight, increases at a rapid but decelerating rate until adolescence when the adolescent growth spurt occurs (Figure 1-2). Infants usually increase their lengths by 50% by 1 year of age, double them by 4 years of age, and triple them by 13 years of age. The average birth length of 50 cm increases to 74 to 76 cm at 1 year of age, 100 to 105 cm at 4 years of age, and 150 to 155 cm in the preadolescent years. Between 6 years of age and puberty sex differences can be noted. At age 6 years boys are taller and heavier than girls. By 9 years of age the height of the average girl is the same as the 9-year-old male and her weight is greater.

The growth spurt in adolescence is closely related to the stages of sexual maturation (Figure 1-3 and Table 1-1).

In males the height growth spurt follows about 1 year after testicular enlargement is first noted. Peak height velocity occurs approximately 1 year later when the penis is at its maximal rate of growth and pubic hair is at stage 3 and 4.

In females, a growth spurt in height preceeds the appearance of breast buds, the first stage of puberty. **Menarche** occurs after the height velocity has reached its peak during the period of decelerating growth. Acceleration of growth generally occurs 2 years later in males than in females and is more intense. Males take 4 to 6 years to complete the growth spurt compared to 3 years for females. Growth continues after adolescence but at a very slow rate until the epiphyses close and linear growth ceases.

Racial differences have been noted in rates of growth. American black infants are smaller than American white infants at birth. They grow more rapidly during the first 2 years and from that age through adolescence are taller than American white boys and girls of the same age groups. Asian children tend to be smaller than black children and white children.[14]

CHANGES IN BODY PROPORTIONS

Increases in height and weight are accompanied by changes in body proportions. The head at birth accounts for approximately one fourth of the total body length; however, the

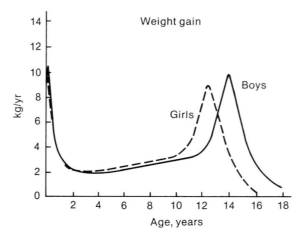

Figure 1-2 Mean weight gain for age of males and females between infancy and 18 years of age. (From: Hamill, P.V.V, Johnston, F.E., and Lemeshow, S., Heights and Weights of Youths 12-17 Years, United States, 1966-1970. Vital and Health Statistics, Series II, No. 124. DHEW Publication No. (HSM) 73-1606, Washington, D.C., 1973, Government Printing Office.)

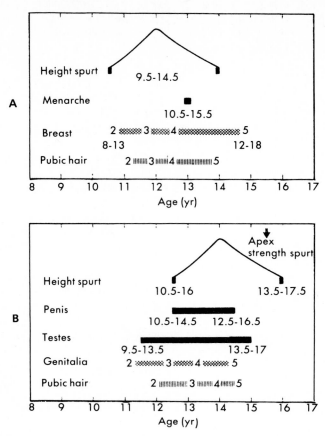

Figure 1-3 Diagram of sequence of events at puberty in **A,** girls and **B,** boys. (Reprinted by permission of The New England Journal of Medicine. Marshall, W.A., and Tanner, J.M.: Arch. Dis. Child. **45:**13, 1970.)

head is one eighth of body length by the time growth has ceased. Brain growth is 75% complete by the end of the second year, and the brain is 100% of adult size by age 6 to 10 years. Leg length increases from approximately three eighths to one half of total body length between birth and adulthood (Figure 1-4).

BODY COMPOSITION

Changes occur not only in height and weight during growth but also in the compo-

nents of the tissues. Increases in height and weight and skeletal maturation are accompanied by changes in body composition—in adiposity, lean body mass, and hydration. Estimates of the changes in body composition have been made from chemical analysis of human bodies and of individual tissues, from indirect measurements of water and electrolyte levels, from excreations of **creatinine** and **hydroxyproline,** and from estimates of fatness. Indirect measurements of body fat have

Table 1-1 Stages of sexual maturation

Boys	Pubic Hair	Genitalia
Stage 1	None	No change from childhood
Stage 2	Small amount at outer edges of pubis; slight darkening	Beginning penile enlargement; teste enlarged to 5 ml volume; scrotum reddened and changed in texture
Stage 3	Covers pubis	Longer penis; testes 8-10 ml; scrotum further enlarged
Stage 4	Adult type; does not extend to thighs	Larger, wider, and longer penis; testes 12 ml; scrotal skin darker
Stage 5	Adult type; now spread to thighs	Adult penis; testes 15 ml

Girls	Pubic Hair	Breasts
Stage 1	None	No change from childhood
Stage 2	Small amount; downy on labia majora	Breast bud
Stage 3	Increased; darker and curly	Larger; no separation of nipple and areola
Stage 4	More abundant; coarse texture	Increased size; areola and nipple form secondary mound
Stage 5	Adult type; now spread to thighs	Adult distribution of breast tissue; continuous outline

Modified from Tanner, J.M.: Growth at adolescence, ed. 2, Oxford, 1962, Blackwell Scientific Publications, Ltd.

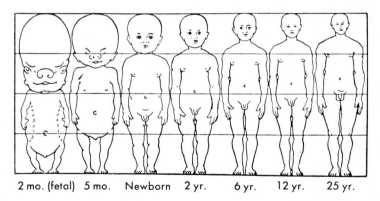

2 mo. (fetal)   5 mo.   Newborn   2 yr.   6 yr.   12 yr.   25 yr.

Figure 1-4 Changes in body proportions from second fetal month to adulthood. (From Robbins, W.J., and others: Growth, New Haven, Conn., 1928, Yale University Press.)

been attempted by several methods, including measurement of the density of the whole body, measurements of total body weight minus lean body mass, use of fat-soluble gases, measurement of the thickness of fat by **roentgeno-graphic studies,** and measurements of subcutaneous fat layers. Although there is much yet to be learned about body composition, there is an important body of data that can be related to physical growth and nutrient needs.

Determinations of total body water alone or in combination with other measurements such as density or potassium have been used as a basis for estimations of lean body mass. Total body water as a percentage of body weight decreases throughout infancy from approximately 70% at birth to 60% at 1 year of age. Reduction of body water is almost entirely extracellular. Extracellular water decreases from 42% of body weight at birth to 32% of body weight at 1 year of age. This change results from decreases in the water content of adipose tissue, increases in adipose tissue, and relative increases in lean body mass.[15] The percentage of weight of water in lean body mass at any age is relatively stable. In other words, there is a direct relationship between total body water and lean body mass. Water is estimated to be responsible for 80% of the weight of fat-free mass at birth and 72% to 73% of the weight of fat-free mass of an adult. Fomon and others[15] estimated the percentage of water in fat-free mass of the male reference as 77.9% at 4 months, 79.0% at 12 months, 77.5% at 3 years, and 75.1% at 10 years of age. They estimated the percentage of water in fat-free mass of the reference female to be 79.7% at 4 months, 78.8% at 12 months, 77.9% at 3 years, and 76.9% at 10 years of age. Adipose tissue contains about 15% water.

Since potassium is found predominantly within the cells of lean tissue and ^{40}K in a fixed relationship to total body potassium, measurements of ^{40}K give an estimate of lean body mass in older children and adults. The concentration of potassium in lean body mass of newborn infants is less than in the adult, and it increases during infancy and early childhood. Because of these changes ^{40}K is not currently considered a reliable indicator of lean body mass in young children. It is considered, however, to be a valid measure of lean body mass in the older child and adolescent.

Anderson and Langham[16] found that the potassium concentration (gm/kg of body weight) increases from the first year of life, reaches a maximum at 8 or 9 years of age, and then declines sharply. After this, sex differences become apparent. The decline continues in females, but an increase is noted in males between 14 and 16 years of age, followed by another decline.

Using data on total body water and total body potassium, knowledge of the concentration of potassium in extracellular and cellular water, and the mineral content of the body, Fomon and others[15] have estimated the body composition of children between birth and 10 years of age.

Forbes,[17] in studies of persons 7.5 to 10.5 years of age, with a ^{40}K counter, found a linear relationship between height and lean body mass at any age and an exponential relationship between lean body mass, height, and age groups. Sex differences in lean body mass and height ratios were noted in the earlier years, although they were not great enough to be significant. Males had greater amounts of lean body mass per cm of height than did females. After 12.5 years of age the lean body mass: height ratio increased rapidly in the male, whereas the increase was more gradual in the female. The female's lean body mass: height ratio maximum, which was about two thirds that of the male maximum value, appeared to be attained at 16 years of age, 3 years earlier than in the male. At 20 years of age males had one and a half times more lean body mass per cm of height than did females.

Fat is found in adipose tissue, in sites in the bone marrow, in phospholipids in the brains and the nervous system, and as a part of cells. It is the component of the body in which the greatest differences between children, age groups, and sexes are seen. The fat content of the body increases slowly during early fetal development, then increases rapidly in the last trimester. Widdowson and Spray found total body fat of the newborn infant to have a mean value of 16%.[18] Fat accumulates rapidly during infancy until approximately 9 months of age.

Between 2 and 6 months of age the increase in adipose tissue is more than twice as great as the increase in the volume of muscle. Sex-related differences appear in infancy, the female depositing a greater percentage of weight as fat than the male.

During childhood the yearly increments for fat show a steady decrease. In many children there is a prepubertal fat spurt occurring before the true growth spurt. When growth proceeds most rapidly in height, adipose tissue increases least rapidly in the female. In the male there is an actual decrease and loss of fat during high velocity periods of growth.

EXAMPLES OF GROWTH IN SPECIAL SYSTEMS

Brain and adipose cellular development have been intensively studied in relation to nutrition and nutrient intake. Although the long-term physiological and behavioral effects have yet to be clarified, events during early growth of these two systems are thought by many investigators to be important to an individual's growth and development.

Brain Growth

The most rapid and critical period of brain growth in humans begins 9 months before birth and continues into the second year. During this time there is rapid cell multiplication and increasing differentiation. Thereafter, there is an increase only in cell size, with a resulting increase in mass. A study comparing brain growth of marasmic and normal infants who died in the first year of life demonstrated significant reductions in wet weight, dry weight, total protein content, and total DNA in the **cerebrum**, cerebellum, and brainstems of marasmic infants compared to normal infants. The

brainstem was less affected.[19] Brains of children thought to be adequately fed in the first year of life but malnourished at an older age have been found to have a normal complement of DNA but reduced brain weight. This indicates a normal cell number but reduced cell size, further defining the critical period of increase in cell number of the brain.[20]

Dobbing and Sands[21] believe that there are two periods of rapid growth of total DNA in the brain: one at approximately 18 weeks gestation, thought to represent **neuronal** multiplication, and one at 3 months after birth, thought to be glial replication.

Brasel and Gruen[22] have concluded that most neuronal cell division, at least in the cerebrum, occurs prenatally during the second trimester. They believe that glial cell division is a postnatal event that peaks at 3 months of age. Growth in DNA in the total brain and its two major regions continues into the second year of postnatal life, probably reaching a plateau at approximately 18 months of age.

The rapid increase in brain mass is accompanied by rapid increases in head circumference. The head grows rapidly prenatally and during the first year of life. Head circumference achieves two thirds of its postnatal growth by 24 months of age. Head circumferences of malnourished children have been found to be smaller than those of their well-nourished peers. Early studies found that children malnourished in early infancy, even when they had been nurtitionally rehabilitated, performed less well on a variety of intelligence tests than did normal controls.[23] However, subsequent studies recognizing that environments that produce malnourished infants and children are depressed and unstimulating have suggested social and environmental factors as more important variables. Children subjected to malnutrition prenatally because of war-induced famine or during infancy because of disease or anomalies and who have been discharged to families that provided sufficient food and stimulation have been able to make up any nutritionally induced deficit.[24, 25] Malnourished children adopted by middle-class families have been able to catch-up in mental development.[26]

Current research has focused on the mental development of the symmetrically versus the asymmetrically growth-retarded infant. The symmetrically growth-retarded infant presents a uniform retardation in body size with reduction in all organs. The asymmetrically growth retarded infant has a lower body weight than length with a normal size head for gestational age. Most deficits are related to cell size rather than number. One study from a community in Guatemala in which chronic undernutrition is endemic found 3-year-old symmetrically growth-retarded children received lower scores on tests evaluating perceptual performance, problem solving performance, memory facility, and verbal facility than did asymmetrically growth-retarded infants, who performed as well as normal controls. Differences in performance were not noted until 24 months and at that age were not yet significant.[27]

POSTNATAL GROWTH AND COGNITION

Data from populations in which malnutrition is endemic indicate a relationship between growth retardation of infants and young children and low performance on tests of mental development. Of special interest is the follow-up study of all children in Barbados who were diagnosed as having **marasmus** during the first of life as compared to a matched group of adequately nourished children.[28] Those children who were malnourished in infancy and tested at 5 to 11 years of age performed less well academically than did well-nourished controls, and effect mediated by deficits in classroom behavior (for instance, lack of attention, poor memory, poor motivation, and easy distractibility). At 8 to 15 years of age the same

children performed less well on the Purdue Pegboard test than did controls, an effect thought to be mediated by a lower I.Q.[29]

In the United States two large scale studies disclosed small but significant relationships between anthropometric measurements and cognitive performance. Investigators associated with the Collaborative Perinatal Project of the National Institute of Neurological Diseases and Blindness[30] followed 37,945 children from before birth until amost 10 years of age. Anthropometric variables (e.g., weight and head circumference) explained a small but statistically significant portion of the variance in I.Q. at 4 years of age for both black and white males and females, when other prenatal and postnatal variables were considered. The United States National Health Survey of 7119 noninstitutionalized children aged 6 to 11 years demonstrated a positive and statistically significant correlation between height and test scores.[31]

Adipose Cell Size and Number

The study of the development of adiposity has suffered for several reasons. The number and size of fat cells is estimated by biopsy of surgical specimens. Cell size is estimated by microscopic examination of tissue sections or after collagenase digestion, precipitation of stromal tissue, and osmium fixation of free adipose cells. Cell number is defined by determining the weight of lipid in the average cell and estimating how many cells are in the weight of the body.

Adipose tissue is distributed throughout the body. However, cell size varies within a site and the range of cell size varies from one site to another. Estimates of fat, number, or size of cells based on a single biopsy may not be representative of body fat. The method of Hirsch and Gillian requires a given amount of lipid in the cell to make it float. Only cells with that amount of lipid can be identified. Those that are depleted cannot be identified and counted.

Studies of obesity in adults have shown that obesity may be associated with an increase in both adipose cell number and cell size or with only an increase in the size of the cell. Weight reduction in adults results only in a decrease in the size of adipose cells, not a reduction in the number of adipose cells. Studies of 21-year-old obese subjects who had a history of childhood obesity before and after weight reduction showed a larger number of adipose cells as compared with nonobese adults. Reduction in weight of the subjects was associated with a reduction only in cell size, not in cell number.[32]

Brook[33] found that the number of adipose cells of children who became obese in the first year of life was higher than the number of adipose cells of children who became obese in later childhood. He also found that those children who were light for their age and who suffered an insult to growth in infancy had a profound deficit in adipose cell number.

In spite of the limitations of methodology, a body of comparable data from a number of researchers leads some to believe that there are periods when the development of adiposity may have implications in the development and prognosis of future obesity. These periods are thought to be from birth to 2 years of age and during preadolescent and adolescent growth spurt.

Knittle[34] has studied children throughout growth and reports data on children and adolescents 2 to 16 years of age. He found that obese children had significantly more fat cells at 2 years of age than nonobese children and that this persisted through all ages studied. Obese children showed increases in cell number at all ages. Nonobese children experience no change in cell number between 2 and 10 years of age but a significant increase after 10 years of age.

Obese children had significantly larger fat cells than nonobese children of the same age between 2 and 10 years of age. After that, age differences in fat cell size were not significant. Nonobese children experienced an increase in the size of their cells between 10 and 16 years of age that was not experienced by obese children.

Brook[33] noted in older nonobese children little change in cell size during chilhood and hypothesized that the increase in body fat during childhood must be a result of a gradual increase in number of adipose cells and that variations in body fatness must be caused by differences in cell size. He believes that the adipose organ grows by increases in both cell size and number during childhood and that increases in cell number do not occur after puberty.

The results of a study of 18 grossly obese girls 8.4 ± 1.2 years of age compared with nonobese control subjects show that the obese girls have an increase in cell number and size. This increase in cell numbers remained after more or less successful weight reduction but was unchanged in the nonobese group. No difference was noted in fat cell number between those who had early-onset or late-onset obesity.[35]

Whether an increased adipose cell number at any age predisposes a child to later obesity and has an influence on the prognosis for weight reduction and maintenance of normal weight remains hypothetical. There is, however, evidence that obesity in school-age years is likely to continue into adolescence and adulthood and that early onset obesity is much more resistant to therapy than onset of obesity in later life.[36] The accumulation of excessive numbers of adipose cells or larger cells is to be discouraged at any age.

METHODS OF ASSESSMENT

It is important that persons concerned with a child's nutrient intake be aware of how growth progresses. Assessments are made by periodic determinations of height, weight, and head circumference. The measurements must be determined accurately, and they must be interpreted in relation to the child's current stage of growth. Individual children whose growth does not appear to be proceeding normally may require additional methods of assessment, such as bone-age and fatfold measurements.

Growth Standards

Growth standards for height, weight, and head circumference make it possible to visualize how a child's growth is proceeding. Standards for bone age permit an estimate of physiological maturity. Fatfold and arm circumference standards provide a basis for determining whether a child is lean, normal, overweight with greater than average muscle and average fat, or obese.

Height, weight, and head circumference

Standards for growth have been devised from studies in which large numbers of healthy, normal children of the same race and socioeconomic group were carefully measured at various ages and the data ranked in percentiles, the number in the percentile indicating the position that a measurement would hold in a series of 100.[37] Data from these studies have been presented in tables, charts, and graphs. Growth curves and grids have been designed to measure how far the child has grown (distance curves) or how fast the child has grown (velocity curves). These growth grids are used in health **evaluation** to give some indication of how a child is growing, and are often used in the assessment of nutritional status.

The grids are prepared so that age values lie along the axis, whereas height or weight values or changes in height or weight values are plotted along the abscissa. Height and weight values plotted for one age give information as to how children rank in size in relation to other children of the same sex, age, and ethnic background, and information as to the relationship of weight to height as compared with other children. Several measurements of height and weight at different ages plotted on

the grids enable one to visualize if the child's growth is progressing as might be expected. Most children stay in approximately the same percentile during growth. Growth, however, does not proceed in a smooth curve as the charts might indicate. Children grow in spurts, and changes may not adhere to the normal curve. A child may have no gain one month but considerable gain the next. During adolescence the growth patterns of many individuals change in percentile, the early maturer moving to a higher percentile and the later maturer to a lower percentile. Both patterns usually return to the original percentiles by the time growth is complete. It is for this reason that the maturational stages become important in adolescence.

Velocity grids give an indication of how fast a child is growing.[38] Children tend not to stay at a given velocity percentile nearly as closely as they do to a distance percentile. However, change does signal an important acceleration or deceleration. These grids are particularly useful in adolescence when children and parents often become concerned about height and weight in relation to peers and about final stature.

The most commonly used growth grids in North America are those prepared by an expert committee for the National Center for Health Statistics (NCHS).[37] Data from the Fels Research Institute was used to determine the standards for children from birth to 36 months of age. The committee used data from the Health Examination Surveys and the Health Nutrition Examination Survey to prepare grids for children from 2 to 18 years of age.

Tanner has prepared both distance and velocity growth grids from the same data for children from 2 to 19 years of age.[38] The distance linear growth grid for adolescent males is shown in Figure 1-5. Note that percentile standards for sexual maturity are graphed on the bottom of the chart.

If the clinician is concerned about the physical growth of a child whose parents are very

Figure 1-5   Height attained for American boys. *Red lines*, 50th centile *(solid)* and 95th centile *(dashed)* for boys 2 SD of tempo early; *green lines;* 50th centile *(solid)* and 5th centile *(dashed)* for boys 2 SD of tempo late.

short or very tall, a correction using mid-parent height can be made utilizing data collected at the Fels Institute.[39]

In addition to graphs that reflect gains in weight and height, the committee constructed body weight for length or stature graphs that are appropriate for plotting values for pre-pubescent boys and girls.

Appropriate use of these charts requires that mesurements be made in the same manner in which the reference data were secured. Weight values for the child less than 36 months of age should be obtained while the child is nude, using calibrated beam balance scales. Length values should be of recumbent length, not of upright height (Figure 1-6). The charts for children between 2 and 18 years of age use measurements of children in stocking feet and standard examination clothing (Figure 1-7).

Figure 1-8 shows the effect of undernutrition on a female infant subjected to inadequate calorie intake because of a dilute formula. The mother of this infant was concerned because the baby was spitting up. A neighbor suggested that she add additional water. When the baby continued to spit up, the mother diluted the formula even more. When a nutritional evaluation was requested at 10 weeks of age, it was found that the child had gained only 460 gm since birth. Her weight was increasing at a very slow rate, dropping from the 10th to the 3rd percentile. Her linear growth continued in the 50th percentile. She was consuming an incredible amount of formula but only 190 to 225 kcal/day, approximately 50 kcal/kg. A change to a concentrated formula that provided 24 kcal/oz resulted in a gain of 500 gm the first week and 240 gm the second week. The rapid rate of gain continued until she reached the 25th percentile, where she has remained.

Figures 1-9 and 1-10 show the effect of a restriction in food intake on the growth of a preschool boy because of a sudden change in income and the parents' inability to buy the quantity of food they had previously provided. Catch-up occurred when the family applied for and received food stamps and the child was given his normal ration of food.

Growth grids for premature and low birth weight infants have been prepared by Gairdner and Pearson[40] (Figure 1-11). These grids use the concept of conceptual age, that is, chronological age as corrected to the expected date of delivery.

Measurements of head circumference are made in health examinations by passing a metal, cloth, or paper tape measure over the most prominent part of the **occiput** and just above the **supraorbital** ridges (Figure 1-12.)

The NCHS growth grids include data on changes in head circumference from birth to 36 months of age in percentiles. Nellhaus prepared a graph of head circumference measurements from birth to 18 years of age. His graph reflects weighted averages of variance from records of fourteen reports in the world's literature and shows standard deviations.

Most clinics use the NCHS head circumference grid for children less than 36 months of age and the Nellhaus grid for children over 3 years of age. Sequential mesurements plotted on these grids can be used to identify children whose cranial growth is deviating from normal. A rapid increase in the rate of growth may indicate hydrocephalus. A slowdown or arrest in the rate of growth may indicate a condition that can cause developmental delays. Such slowdowns and arrests have been noted in children who were subjected to severe undernutrition.

Skeletal maturation

Fusion of the epiphyses and the appearance of ossification centers occur first in one bone and then in others in a predictable order. As a result, skeletal maturation can be assessed by observation of the various centers of ossification and the fusion of the epiphy-

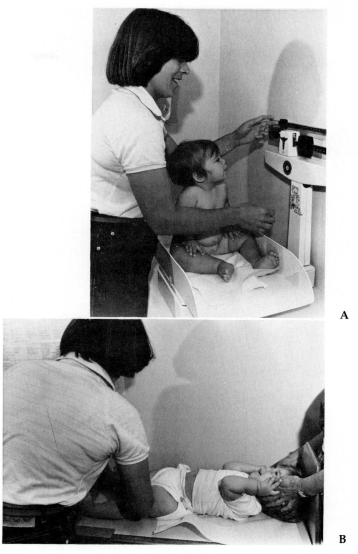

Figure 1-6 **A,** Infant is weighed nude on calibrated-beam balance scale. **B,** Recumbent length is measured with a suitable measuring board.

ses on roentgenographic studies. Standards of bone age have been devised from longitudinal roentgenographic studies of hands and wrists of children. The most commonly used stan- dards are those of Greulich and Pyle, which were based on 100 hand films of children who were examined periodically from birth to 18 years of age.[42]

Figure 1-7 **A,** Four-year-old is weighed on beam scale. **B,** The child is measured with heels, buttocks, shoulders, and head touching the wall.

Bone age is often used to assess the physiological maturity of a child whose linear growth appears to be proceeding at a very slow or very rapid rate. It is an especially useful tool in adolescence when parents and/or children become concerned about late and early maturation. Bone age correlates with secondary sex characteristics and with mature height.

Undernutrition retards skeletal ossification. Insufficient calorie intakes slow bone growth and delay calcification of the ossification centers. Also, the bone appears normal but often is thinner. Protein malnutrition, caused by an insufficient intake of protein, an intake of poor quality protein, or both, results not only in a reduction in bone growth but also in delays in the appearance of ossification centers and possible alterations in the sequence of ossification.[42] Obese children have been found to have advanced skeletal ages.

Fatfold thickness

Since approximately half of the total body fat is deposited in subcutaneous adipose tissue, the fatness of an individual can be estimated by measuring the thickness of the fatfold at selected sites with special calipers that have been calibrated to provide a constant tension. It is important that proper calipers be used. Plastic calipers are generally not adequate.[43] In general, one truncal (subscapular) measurement and one limb (triceps) measurement are

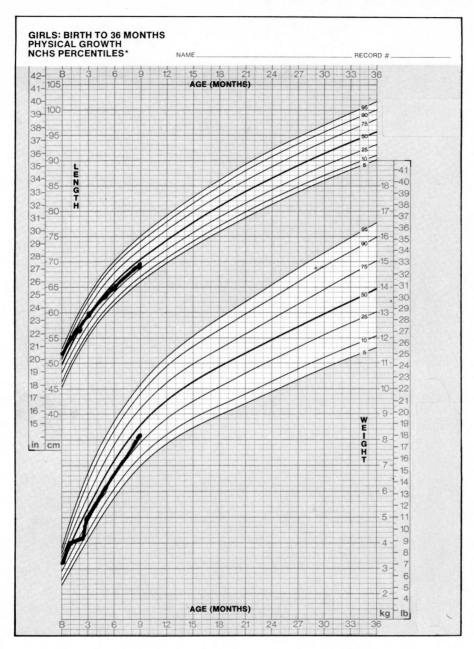

Figure 1-8   Growth chart for infant girls. (Courtesy Ross Laboratories.)

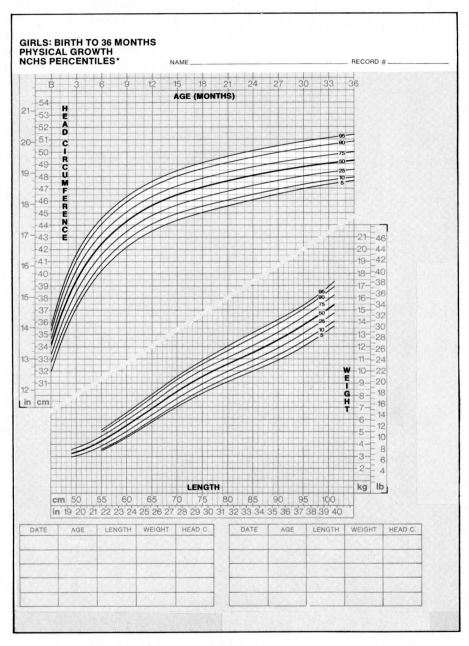

Figure 1-8, cont'd.   For legend see p. 17. (Courtesy Ross Laboratories.)

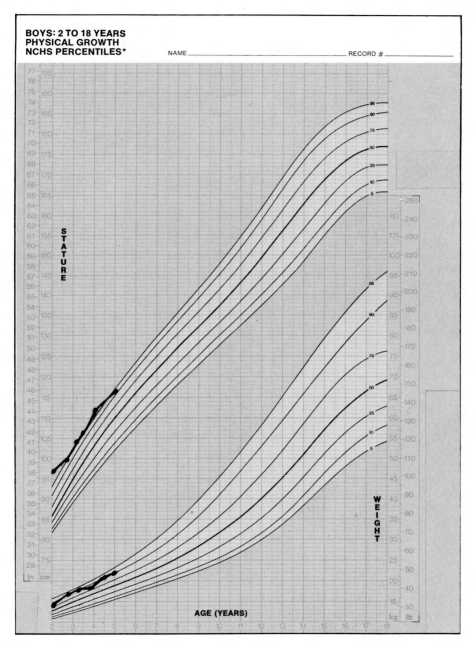

Figure 1-9   Growth chart for boys aged 2 to 18 years. (Courtesy Ross Laboratories.)

Figure 1-10   Growth chart for boys aged 2 to 18 years.

Figure 1-11 Heights and weights of a male infant born at 34 week's gestation. ⊗ denotes plottings when corrected for gestational age. ⊙ denotes plottings by chronologic age. The infant caught up to the 95th percentile by age 24 months. (From Gairdner, D., and Pearson, J.: A growth chart for premature and other infants, Arch. Dis. Child. **46**:783, 1971. Copyright Castlemead Publications.)

advised. If only one measurement is to be used, measurement of the triceps is preferred. The triceps is the easiest site to measure and is representative of body fatness (Figure 1-13).

The triceps measurement is taken midway between the acromion and olecranon processes. The client stands with the back to the measurer,

arm relaxed with palm facing the lateral thigh. The tips of the acromial process and olecranon are palpated, and a point halfway between is marked on the skin. The skinfold is picked up over the posterior surface on the triceps muscle 1 cm above the mark on the vertical line, and the jaws of the caliper are applied to the

Figure 1-12 Head circumference is measured over the most prominent part of the occiput and just above the supraorbital ridges.

Figure 1-13 Triceps fatfold measurements are taken midway between the acromon and olecranion processes.

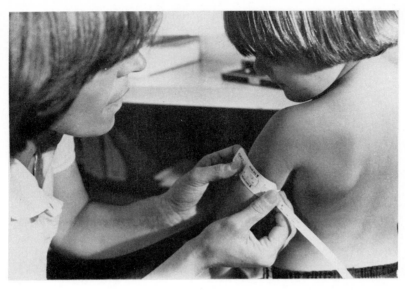

Figure 1-14 Mid–upper arm circumference is measured with paper insertion tape that touches skin but does not compress the tissue.

marked level.[44] The jaws of the caliper are permitted to exert full pressure as the trigger level of the caliper is released. The dial is read to the nearest 0.5 mm. Measurement error can be minimized by averaging three measurements.

Standards for triceps fatfold measurement have been published.[45] Triceps fatfold measurement have been compiled from a cross-sectional study of white subjects from 1 to 75 years of age and are included in the Health and Nutrition Examination Survey I (1971-1974) (Table 1-2). Such measurements are very useful as a complement to standard growth charts in the evaluation of children's growth and in the decision as to the necessity to modify calorie or nutrient intake. Athletic, muscular children may appear overweight with greater than average muscle and average fat or obese if only height and weight are used as criteria for judgment. On the other hand, handicapped children with poor muscle tone often plot in a lower percentile for weight than height even though they have an adequate amount of adipose tissue.

It must be noted that all data in these norms are derived from white children. Racial differences have been noted in measured fat thickness. Puerto Ricans have greater fat measurements than do North American whites and blacks. Black children have a greater deposition of adipose tissue from infancy through 4 years of age than do their white peers. After 4 years of age, the differences are reversed.[46] Group norms and genetic differences must be considered in interpreting fatfold measurements.

Mid–upper arm circumference

Measurement of mid–upper arm circumference combined with triceps fatfold is one method used to estimate muscle and fat bulk. The measurement, as the triceps fatfold, is made at the midpoint of the upper part of the left arm. A paper insertion tape is used most often (Figure 1-14). The subject is positioned with the left arm completely relaxed and extended by the side. A mark is drawn on the lateral side of the arm midway between the acromion and the olecranon. The tape is passed

Table 1-2   Percentiles for triceps skinfold (mm^2) for whites of the United States: Health and Nutrition Examination Survey I of 1971 to 1974

Age group	Males								Females							
	n	5	10	25	50	75	90	95	n	5	10	25	50	75	90	95
1-1.9	228	6	7	8	10	12	14	16	204	6	7	8	10	12	14	16
2-2.9	223	6	7	8	10	12	14	15	208	6	8	9	10	12	15	16
3-3.9	220	6	7	8	10	11	14	15	208	7	8	9	11	12	14	15
4-4.9	230	6	6	8	9	11	12	14	208	7	8	8	10	12	14	16
5-5.9	214	6	6	8	9	11	14	15	219	6	7	8	10	12	15	18
6-6.9	117	5	6	7	8	10	13	16	118	6	6	8	10	12	14	16
7-7.9	122	5	6	7	9	12	15	17	126	6	7	9	11	13	16	18
8-8.9	117	5	6	7	8	10	13	16	118	6	8	9	12	15	18	24
9-9.9	121	6	6	7	10	13	17	18	125	8	8	10	13	16	20	22
10-10.9	146	6	6	8	10	14	18	21	152	7	8	10	12	17	23	27
11-11.9	122	6	6	8	11	16	20	24	117	7	8	10	13	18	24	28
12-12.9	153	6	6	8	11	14	22	28	129	8	9	11	14	18	23	27
13-13.9	134	5	5	7	10	14	22	26	151	8	8	12	15	21	26	30
14-14.9	131	4	5	7	9	14	21	24	141	9	10	13	16	21	26	28
15-15.9	128	4	5	6	8	11	18	24	117	8	10	12	17	21	25	32
16-16.9	131	4	5	6	8	12	16	22	142	10	12	15	18	22	26	31
17-17.9	133	5	5	6	8	12	16	19	114	10	12	13	19	24	30	37
18-18.9	91	4	5	6	9	13	20	24	109	10	12	15	18	22	26	30
19-24.9	531	4	5	7	10	15	20	22	1060	10	11	14	18	24	30	34

From Frisancho, A.R.: Am. J. Clin. Nutr. **34**:2540, 1981 ©Am. J. Clin. Nutr. American Society for Clinical Nutrition.

around the arm so that it is touching the skin but not compressing the tissue. It is important to ensure that the tape is in a plane perpendicular to the long axis of the arm.[44] Arm circumference is measured to the nearest 0.1 cm. Arm muscle diameter may be estimated by the following formula:

$$\text{Arm muscle diameter (mm)} =$$
$$\frac{\text{Arm circumference (mm)} - \text{triceps fatfold (mm)}}{\pi}$$

Standards for arm muscle diameter and arm circumference have been derived from the Health and Nutrition Examination Survey I.[45]

Some researchers have developed weight-height indexes of relative body weight. Several that are reliable for adults are not applicable for children. Durant and Linder[47] found that the weight-length index calculated by the following formula was the most appropriate for children:

$$\text{WLI} = \frac{\text{A}}{\text{B}} \times 100$$

$$\text{A} = \frac{\text{actual weight (kg)}}{\text{actual height (cm)}}$$

$$\text{B} = \frac{\text{50th percentile expected weight (kg) for age}}{\text{50th percentile expected height (cm) for age}}$$

The normal range for children is between 90 and 109. Those who score below 89 can be considered lean; those over 110, overweight; and those over 120, obese. The method does classify muscular children as overweight. However, fatfold measures can validate or negate the assumption.

Potassium 40

Research centers may be equipped to estimate body composition by measuring the amount of ^{40}K emitted from an individual by radioactive counting. The gamma rays of ^{40}K are counted by using NaI crystals as detectors or in a liquid scintillation chamber. Both of these instruments that mesure ^{40}K must be accurately calibrated, are relatively expensive, and are rarely available for clinical evaluation of individual children. Neither instrument offers the potential for any hazard or trauma to the individual other than claustrophobia, which may be experienced in the steel chamber that is used when ^{40}K radiaion is measured with NaI. The length of time the individual must remain in the counter ranges from several minutes to several hours.

When the ^{40}K content of the body has been determined, the fat-free or lean body mass is calculated by dividing the total ^{40}K content of the body by the known ^{40}K content of lean body mass.

$$LBW = \frac{^{40}K \ (gm)}{gm \ of \ ^{40}K/kg \ of \ lean \ body \ weight}$$

Forbes and Lewis[48] estimated that there are 2.66 gm of ^{40}K/kg of lean body weight. Behnke and Wilmore[49] calculated the ^{40}K content of lean body weight to be 2.46 gm/kg for males and 2.28 gm/kg for females.

FAILURE TO THRIVE

If any infant or child fails to grow at the expected rate over a period of several months, a diagnosis of failure to thrive will be made. In one fourth to one third of such children, the growth delay is caused by nonorganic environmental factors, including nutrition.[50] The children may be offered inadequate food because of poverty and lack of food, poor feeding techniques, or child neglect. Abnormal mother-child interactions may lead to a child who refuses to eat sufficient food or a mother who does not offer appropriate foods. This often results from inadequate bonding or psychosocial deprivation.

The first step in the evaluation of children with failure to thrive is to evaluate the adequacy of nutrients and energy provided by the food offered and of the food consumed. Observations of a feeding time during the evaluation can give important information when appropriate foods are offered but not consumed (see Chapter 3). If failure to thrive is suspected to result from neurological problems, observations of oral motor skills to assess the child's ability to suck, chew with rotary movements, and self feed will give information needed to plan intervention. (See Chapters 3 and 13).

If a disturbance of mother-child interaction is suspected, the mother's feelings about her child and her expections about appropriate feeding patterns for the child need to be explored. Such children are often viewed as having had feeding problems in infancy and difficulty in accepting semisolid foods. They frequently consume more food when it is offered by their fathers rather than their mothers. When placed in an environment that provides adequate mothering and stimulation, such as a foster home, they consume large quantities of food; they catch-up. Therapy for this failure to thrive must be directed to correction of the psychosocial difficulties that caused the disturbed mother-child relationship.

CATCH-UP GROWTH

During recovery from malnutrition of illness that has ceased or depressed growth, a child grows at a rate above that expected for his or her age. As the more rapid growth proceeds, the child catches up with his or her growth curve. Gain in weight proceeds very rapidly until the child reaches the correct weight for height, then proceeds at a slower rate as height and weight increase together. During the second phase, growth proceeds at a height-expected rather than age-expected rate.

The range and magnitude of growth deficits vary with the condition and severity of the disorder that caused it. Catch-up is, however, possible in all situations, even when growth retardation has been severe and prolonged, provided the epiphyses have not closed and the condition that caused the deficit has been remedied.

It is not unusual for children recovering from malnutrition who were both wasted and stunted to gain weight at rates 20 times faster than those of normal healthy age group peers until their weight is appropriate for their length; then, the rate of gain approximates that of children who were only wasted. The average catch-up rates of weight gain for children who are only stunted is approximately three times faster than would be expected for chronological age.[51]

Children who have experienced growth retardation because of malnutrition and continue to live with marginal or insufficient food may have little opportunity for catch-up. For these children, pubertal development is delayed. In some cases catch-up occurs because of prolongation of the growth period. In other instances children severely malnourished in early childhood who continue to live with a marginal food intake do not catch-up even though pubertal development may be delayed 2 years.[51]

Summary

Children grow at their individual predictable rates; the range of growth rates at any age is large. When plotted on growth grids, measurements of growth provide information as to whether children are expressing their genetic potential for growth. Fatfold measurements taken with calibrated instruments provide important information when children are suspected to be undernourished or overfat. If children are not growing as expected, the adequacy of their energy and nutrient intake should be investigated.

As physical growth proceeds, changes in body compostion occur. During adolescence the deposition of lean body mass per inch of height is greater in the male than female. At maturity, males have one and a half times the lean body mass as females.

There are critical stages of development during cell growth when the number of cells in an organism in increasing and an organ is most vulnerable to deprivation. Even so, catch-up growth appears possible if rehabilitation occurs and if sufficient foods and stimulation are provided.

SUGGESTED LEARNING ACTIVITES

1. Obtain heights and weights of a child over several years from a school health record or medical chart, plot them on a growth grid, and interpret the curves on the grid.
2. Describe how one would interpret to a schoolage boy and his parents the physical growth of a child growing at the 10th percentile whose neighbor of the same age and sex is growing at the 95th percentile.
3. Calculate the weight-height index of a child suspected to be a growth failure.
4. Describe measuring devices and scales that provide valid information.
5. Demonstrate how to correctly measure mid–upper arm circumference and triceps fatfold thickness.

REFERENCES

1. Committe to Review the Ten-State Nutrition Survey. American Academy of Pediatrics: The ten-state survey: a pediatric perspective, Pediatrics 51:1095, 1973.

2. Adrianzen, T.B., Baertl, J.M., and Grahm, G. G.: Growth of children from extremely poor families, Am. J. Clin. Nutr. 26:926, 1973.

3. Mora, J.O., and others: The effects of nutritional supplementation on physical growth of children at risk of malnutrition, Am. J. Clin. Nutr. 34:1885, 1981.

4. Edozien, J.C., Switzer, B.R., and Bryan R.B.: Medical evaluation of the special supplemental food programs for women, infants, and children, Am. J. Clin. Nutr. 32:677, 1979.

5. Mitchell, H. S.: Nutrition in relation to stature, J. Am. Diet. Assoc. 40:521, 1962.

6. Mitchell, H. S., and Santo, S.: Nutritional improvement in Nokkaido orphanage children—1960–1970, J. Am. Diet. Assoc. 72:506, 1978.

7. Enesco, M., and Leblond, C. P.: Increase in cell numbers as a factor in the growth of the organs of the young male rat, J. Embryol. Exp. Morphol. 10:530, 1962.

8. Winick, M., and Noble, A.: Quantitative changes in DNA, RNA, and protein during prenatal and postnatal growth in the rat, Dev. Biol. 12:451, 1965.

9. Winick, M., and Noble, A.: Cellular growth in rats during malnutrition at various ages, J. Nutr. 89:300, 1966.

10. Elliot, D. A., and Cheek, D. B.: Muscle and liver cell growth in rats with hypoxia and reduced nutrition. In Cheek, D. B., editor: Human growth, body compostion, cell growth, energy, and intelligence, Philadelphia, 1968, Lea & Febiger.

11. Winick, M., and Noble, A.: Cellular response with increased feeding in neonatal rats, J. Nutr. 91:179, 1967.

12. Johnson, K., Rosenbaum, S., and Simons, J.: The Data Book: the nation, states and cities, Washington, D. C., 1985, Children's Defense Fund.

13. Smith, D., and others: Shifting linear growth during infancy: illustration of genetic factors in growth from fetal life through infancy, J. Pediatr. 89:225, 1976.

14. Smith, D. W.: Growth and its disorders, Philadelphia, 1977, W. B. Saunders Co.

15. Fomon, S. F., and others: Body composition of reference children from birth to 10 years, Am. J. Clin. Nutr. 35:1169, 1982.

16. Anderson, E. C., and Langham, W. H.: Average potassium concentration of the human body as a function of age, Science 130:713, 1959.

17. Forbes, G. B.: Relation of lean body mass to height in children and adolescents, Pediatr. Res. 6:32, 1972.

18. Widdowson, E. M., and Spray, C. M.: Chemical development in utero, Arch. Dis. Child. 26:205, 1951.

19. Winick, M., Rosso, P., and Waterlow, J.: Cellular growth of cerebrum, cerebellum, and brain stem in normal and marasmic children, Exp. Neurol. 26:393, 1970.

20. Winick, M.: Nutrition and nerve cell growth, Fed. Proc. 29:1510, 1970.

21. Dodding, J., and Sands, J.: Quantitative growth and development of the human brain, Arch. Dis. Child. 48:757, 1973.

22. Brasel, J. A., and Gruen, R. K.: Cellular growth, brain, liver, muscle, and lung. In Falkner, F., and Tanner, J. M., editors: Human growth, vol. 2, New York, 1978, Plenum Publishing Corp.

23. Stoch, M. B., and Smythe, P. M.: The effect of undernutrition during infancy on subsequent brain growth and intellectual development, S. Afr. Med. J. 41:1027, 1967.

24. Stein, Z., and others: Nutrition and mental performance, Science 178:708, 1972.

25. Beardslee, W. R. and others: The effect of infantile malnutrition on behavioral development, a follow-up study, Am. J. Clin. Nutr. 35:1437, 1982.

26. Graham, G. G. and Adrianzen, T. B.: Late "catch-up" growth after severe infantile malnutrition, Johns Hopkins Med. J. 131:204, 1972.

27. Villar, J. and others: Heterogenous growth and mental development of intrauterine growth-retarded infants during the first three years of life, Pediatrics 74:783, 1984.

28. Galler, J. R., Ramsey, F., Solimano, G.: The influence of early malnutrition on subsequent development. III. Learning disabilities as a sequel to malnutrition, Pediatr. Res. 18:309, 1984.

29. Galler, J. R., Ramsey, F., Solemano, G.: A follow-up study of the effects of early malnutrition on subsequent development. II. Fine motor skills in adolescence, Pediatr. Res. 19:524, 1985.

30. Bromsan, S. H., Nichols, P. L. and Kennedy, W. A.: Preschool I. Q.: prenatal and early developmental correlates, New York, 1975, John Wiley and Son.

31. Edwards, L. N., and Grossman, M.: The relationship between children's health and intellectual development in health: what is it worth? In Muskin, S. editor: Measures of health benefits, New York, 1980, Pergamm Press.

32. Brook, C. G. D.: Cellular growth: adipose tissue. In Falkner, F., and Tanner, J. M., editors: Human growth, vol. 2, New York, 1978, Plenum Publishing Corp.

33. Brook, C. G. D.: Cell growth in man, Am. Heart J. 86:571, 1973.

34. Knittle, J. L.: Obesity in childhood: a problem in adipose tissue cellular development, J. Pediatr. 81:1048, 1972.

35. Hager, A., and others: Adipose tissue cellularity in obese school girls, before and after dietary treatment, Am. J. Clin. Nutr. 31: 68, 1978.

36. Committe on Nutrition, American Academy of Pediatrics: Nutritional aspects of obesity infancy and childhood, Pediatrics 68:880 1981.

37. National Center for Health Statistics: NCHS growth charts, 1976, Monthly vital statistics report, vol. 25, no. 3, Suppl (HRA)76-1120, Rockville, Md., 1976, Health Resources Administration.

38. Tanner, J. M., and Davies, P. S. W.: Clinical longitudinal standards for height and height velocity for North American children, Pediatrics 107:317, 1985.

39. Himes, J. H., and others: Parent-specific adjustments for evaluation of recumbent length and stature of children, Pediatrics 75:304, 1985.

40. Gairdner, D., and Pearson, J.: A growth chart for premature and other infants, Arch. Dis. Child. 46:783, 1971.

41. Nellhaus, G.: Head circumference from birth to 18 years, Pediatrics 41:106, 1968.

42. Greulich, W. W., and Pyle, S. I.: Radiographic atlas of skeletal development of the hand and wrist, Stanford, Calif., 1959, Stanford University Press.

43. Gray, G. E., and Gray, L. K.: Anthropometric measurements and their interpretation: principles, practices, and problems, J. Am. Diet. Assoc. 77:534, 1980.

44. Cameron, N.: The methods of auxological anthropometry. In Falkner, F., and Tanner, J. M., editors: Human growth, vol. 2, New York, 1978, Plenum Publishing Corp.

45. Frisancho, A. R.: New norms of upper limb fat and muscle areas for assessment of nutritional status, Am. J. Clin. Nutr. 34:2540, 1981.

46. Garn, S. M., Clark, D. C., and Guire, K. E.: Growth, body composition, and development of obese and lean children. In Winick, M., editor: Childhood obesity, New York, 1975, John Wiley & Sons, Inc.

47. Durant, R. N., and Linder C. W.: An evaluation of five indexes of relative body weight for use with children, J. Am. Diet. Assoc. 78:35, 1981.

48. Forbes, G. B., and Lewis, A. M.: Total sodium, potassium, and chloride in adult man, J. Clin. Invest. 35:596, 1956.

49. Behnke, A. R., and Wilmore, J. H.: Evaluation and regualtion of body build and composition, Englewood Cliffs, N. J., 1974, Prentice-Hall, Inc.

50. Rallison, M. L.: Growth Disorders in Infants, Children and Adolescents, New York, 1986, John Wiley Medical Publications.

51. Ashworth, A. and Millward, D. J.: Catch-up growth in children, Nutr. Rev. 44:157, 1986.

2

Nutrient Needs of Infants and Children

Peggy L. Pipes

OBJECTIVES

After studying this chapter, the student should:

1. Understand the rationale for recommended intakes of nutrients and energy in infancy and childhood.

2. Recognize appropriate foods as sources of nutrients and energy for infants and children.

3. Be aware of the reasons for the wide range of acceptable energy intakes in infancy and childhood.

4. Be able to make appropriate recommendations for the use of nutrient supplements in infancy and childhood.

5. Understand factors that affect the bioavailability of nutrients.

Children must consume sufficient high-quality protein, vitamins, minerals, and energy if acceptable growth is to occur. Energy generated from the metabolism of fats, carbohydrates, and proteins provides the fuel that supports the maintenance of bodily functions and provides for activity and growth. Protein provides amino acids for the synthesis of new tissues and nitrogen for the maturation of existing tissues in early childhood.

Vitamins function in a variety of metabolic processes that make protein synthesis and energy metabolism possible. Their requirements are therefore determined by intakes of energy, protein, and other nutrients. Minerals are essential components of body tissue. Their requirements are influenced by rates of growth and the interrelationships they share with other nutrients.

A wide range of opinions exists as to optimal intakes of nutrients for individuals at all ages. In fact, such a diversity of opinions exists that the standards proposed by the original 10th expert committee for changes in the Recommended Dietary Allowances (RDA) were not accepted when reviewed. A second panel was appointed to make recommendations acceptable to all parties. Specific recommendations will be found in the document prepared by this group and published in 1989.

It is important to remember that the RDAs are standards for planning food supplies to meet the needs of populations and for designing public programs. They are not designed to define individual requirements or to assess the adequacy of an individual's intake. If, however, one is knowledgeable about the data used to establish the guidelines and the safety factors added, one can use this knowledge to identify children at risk and to plan diets for children. Combined with growth data and a knowledge of foods as sources of nutrients, such information can be used to identify a need for change in the dietary intake of an individual infant or child.

NUTRIENT NEEDS

Many factors determine a child's needs for nutrients, including body size, rate of growth, physical activity, basal energy expenditure, and reserves acquired in utero by the fetus or from dietary intake by the infant and older child.

Energy

Total energy requirements reflect that expended for basal metabolism, specific dynamic action, activity and growth. Because of wide variations in all of the parameters at any age, ranges of recommended intake have been suggested.[1]

The energy requirement is very high per unit of body size in a child's first few months of life but declines as the rate of growth decreases. A higher basal metabolic demand in infancy is thought to be caused by a larger loss of heat because of a relatively greater body surface and by a larger proportion of metabolic tissue. Males expend greater amounts of basal energy than do females. The differences are small during the preadolescent years but become pronounced during adolescence.

Maintenance requirements approximate 1.5 the basal metabolic expenditure, since some movement occurs even during sleep, and the specific dynamic action is estimated to be 6% of ingested energy. Energy costs of growth have been estimated to approximate 4.4 to 5.7 kcal/gm of tissue gained.[2] Decreasing rates of growth result in decreasing requirements for energy per unit of size (kcal/kg). In other words, as children grow older they need greater numbers of calories because of larger body sizes, but their need for energy per unit of size decreases.

The contribution of physical activity to total energy expenditure is variable among children and in individual children from day to day. At all ages, activity patterns among children show wide ranges both in the time spent in the various activities and the intensity of the activities. Some infants, for example, may be quiet, cuddly, and satisfied to explore their environment with their eyes, but others may expend more energy in crying, kicking, and physical movement to see the world around them. Some older children engage in such sedentary activities as looking at books or watching television, whereas their peers may be engaged in physical activities that demand running, jumping, and general body movements.

Spady estimated the energy expenditure of activity of fourth and fifth grade schoolchildren to be 31.2% and 25.3% of total energy expenditure for males and females, respectively.[3]

Energy requirements, which are greatest per unit of size in infancy, decline until adolescent growth is complete. During adolescence the energy expenditure is a reflection of the adolescent growth spurt. Since adolescents enter the growth spurt at different ages, standards established for a given age must be applied with caution.

During a period of catch-up growth, the requirement for energy and nutrients is greatly increased. Intakes of 150 to 250 kcal/kg of body weight have been recommended for children of preschool age. An intake of 200 kcal/kg/day should produce a weight gain of 20 gm/kg/day.[2]

The energy needs of individual children of the same size, age, and sex vary. Reasons for these differences remain unexplained. Differences in physical activity, in the metabolic cost of minimal and excessive protein intakes at equivalent levels of energy intake, and in the efficiency with which individuals utilize energy have all been hypothesized to exert an influence. Recent studies suggest that infants and children are consuming less energy than recommended. Butte found intakes of exclusively breast-fed infants declined from 110 ± 24 kcal/day at 1 month of age to 71 ± 17 kcal/day at 4 months of age. Adair found the intake of a formula-fed infant during the first year was never more than 90% of the 1980 dietary allowances.[5] Six to eleven-year-old children have been reported to consume more than 20% less than the suggested intake.[6] Spady found that although the total energy expenditures of fourth and fifth grade boys approximated the recommended allowances, girls expended only 80% of the 1974 recommended allowances.[3]

In 1930 an expert committee, after reviewing energy intake data in relation to physical parameters, stated that height appeared to be the most appropriate criterion on which to base studies of energy needs.[7] The observation was never used. In estimating energy needs of children, body surface or weight has continued to be used as a reference for suggested energy intakes of children. Energy per centimeter of height has proved clinically, however, to be a useful reference in estimating energy needs and designing diets for individual children. It is an especially useful reference for children who are genetically short. For example, preschool children with **Prader-Willi syndrome** maintain their weight in the growth channel by consuming 10 to 11 kcal/cm of height as compared with 14.7

to 15.4 kcal/cm of height, the 50th percentile of intake of normal males, and 12.9 to 13.8 kcal/cm of height, the 50th percentile of intake of normal females of the same age.

The best evaluation of the adequacy of infant's and children's energy intake is the adequacy of their growth rates in length and weight. If changes in weight percentiles occur without changes in length percentiles, undernutrition or overnutrition should be suspected.

Food Sources

Energy values of foods commonly consumed in infancy and childhood are given in Tables 2-1 and 2-2. To demonstrate food intakes that support appropriate energy intakes for several age-groups, data for 2-month-old, 10-month-old, and 4-year-old children are given in Table 2-3.

Protein and Amino Acid Requirements

Protein provides calories but also serves a more important and complex function. Protein is the basic component of the protoplasm in cells; therefore an adequate intake of protein is essential if normal growth is to occur. Increases in body protein average 3.5 gm/day for the first 4 months and 3.1 gm/day for the next 8 months, with the body protein increasing from 11.0% to 14.6% in the first year.

Amino acid requirements of infants have been estimated by Holt and Snyderman from studies in which pure amino acids were supplied in proportions of amino acids of human milk.[8] The requirement of an amino acid was defined as the least amount required to maintain satisfactory nitrogen retention and weight gain when nitrogen levels and other amino acids were held constant. Fomon and others, and Fomon and Filer have estimated amino acid requirements from intakes of infants between 8 and 112 days of age who were fed whole protein in cow's milk formulas and soy formulas.[9, 10] Satisfactory linear growth and weight gain, nitrogen balance, and serum con-

Table 2-1 Selected foods as sources of energy for infants

Food	Energy	
	kcal/oz	kcal/tbsp
Milk		
Human milk	24	12
Commercially available infant formula	20	10
Whole cow's milk	20	10
Commercially available infant foods (average value)		
Dry infant cereals	105	9
Strained and junior fruits	16	8
Strained and junior vegetables	11	5
Strained and junior meats	32	16
Strained egg yolks	58	29
Strained and junior dinners		
Vegetables with meat	15	7.5
High meat dinners	24	12
Strained and junior desserts	22	10

Adapted from Gebhardt, S.E., Cutrufelli, R., and Matthews, R.H.: Composition of foods, baby food, raw, processed, prepared, Agriculture Handbook No. 8-3, Washington, D.C., 1978, U.S. Department of Agriculture.

centrations of albumin equivalent to those of normal breast-fed infants were used as criteria of adequacy.

The FAO/WHO expert committee has suggested that a composite of the lower estimates of the data from the studies of Holt and Snyderman and from Fomon and Filer provide estimates of the upper range of the requirement for infants up to 6 months of age.[11] (Table 2-4).

Estimates of amino acid requirements of 10- to 12-year-old preadolescents based on studies by Nakagawa and others are given in Table 2-5. These investigators found amino acid requirements for 10- to 12-year-old children to be two to three times greater than those for adults. Requirements of males in all cases exceeded those of females.[12] Histidine is essential in infancy but not in the older child.

Protein needs for growth (expressed as percentages of requirement) decrease as rates of growth decline. Fifty percent of the protein requirement is used for growth in the first 2 months of life. This declines to 11% at 2 to 3 years of age and is gradually reduced to 0% after an increase during the adolescent growth spurt. Amino acids required for growth differ from those required for maintenance. Factorial calculations based on patterns of growth indicate that the suggested amino acid requirements after infancy have been overestimated.[13]

Recommended intakes

The recommendations for daily protein intakes for infants and children have been assumed an adequate intake of energy. These

Table 2-2   Selected foods as sources of energy for children

Food	Portion Size	Average kcal
2% milk with 2% nonfat milk solids	$\frac{1}{2}$ cup	72
Meat, poultry, or fish	1 oz	80
Egg	1 medium	80
Peanut butter	1 tbsp	94
Cheese	$\frac{1}{2}$ oz	57
Legumes, cooked	$\frac{1}{4}$ cup	90
Enriched bread	$\frac{1}{2}$ slice	35
Ready-to-eat cereals (not sugar coated)	$\frac{3}{4}$ cup	70
Cooked cereal	$\frac{1}{2}$ cup	55
Saltine crackers	1	12
Rice, macaroni, spaghetti, cooked	$\frac{1}{4}$ cup	50
Potato (boiled)	$\frac{1}{2}$ medium	45
Potato chips	5	55
Green beans	$\frac{1}{4}$ cup	6
Carrots		
Cooked	$\frac{1}{4}$ cup	15
Raw	2 medium sticks	14
Apple	1 small	80
Banana	1 small	80
Orange	1 small	50
Orange juice	$\frac{1}{2}$ cup	60
Sugar	1 tsp	16
Jam or jelly	1 tsp	20
Butter, margarine, oil, mayonnaise	1 tsp	35
Cookies, assorted	1	40-50
Ice cream	$\frac{1}{4}$ cup	70

Adapted from Adams, C.F.: Nutritive value of American foods in common units, Agriculture Handbook No. 456, Washington D.C., 1975, U.S. Department of Agriculture.

recommendations are based on ingestion of milk protein in infancy and a mixed diet that provides protein that has an efficiency of utilization of 75% in older children.[1]

Based on nitrogen balance studies, Abernathy and Ritchey conclude that an appropriate protein allowance for 7- to 10-year-old children would be 45 gm or more per day.[14] Reported protein intakes of children in the United States have shown actual protein intakes to be 10% to 15% of kilocalories consumed. During periods of catch-up growth, protein requirements increase. Intakes of 3.2 gm of milk protein/kg when energy intakes are adequate have been suggested.[2]

Fomon and others have suggested that during infancy, amino acid and protein requirements expressed per unit of calories consumed (reflecting both size and rate of growth) are more meaningful than expressions of requirements on the basis of body weight alone. They estimate the protein requirement to be 1.6

Table 2-3 Foods that provide appropriate energy for various age groups

Age	Weight (kg)	Intake (kcal) Needs	Examples of Foods that Provide Appropriate Energy Intakes
2 months	5	575	28-32 oz human milk or infant formula
10 months	9.5	1000	24 oz homogenized milk or infant formula
			8 tbsp dry infant cereal
			14 tbsp junior fruit
			8 tbsp junior vegetable
			4 tbsp junior meat
			$\frac{1}{2}$ slice toast
			1 oz chopped chicken
			1 tbsp mashed green beans
			1 small banana
			2 tbsp ice cream
			2 arrowroot biscuits
4 years	18	1530	24 oz milk
			6-8 oz fruit juice
			3 slices bread
			$\frac{1}{2}$ to $\frac{3}{4}$ cup dry cereal
			2 tbsp peanut butter
			1 tsp jelly
			1 frankfurter
			$\frac{1}{4}$ cup macaroni and cheese
			$\frac{1}{4}$ cup green beans
			$\frac{1}{3}$ cup ice cream
			1 graham cracker
			1 medium apple
			1 small banana

gm/100 kcal for children 1 to 4 months of age and 1.4 gm/100 kcal for children 8 to 12 months of age.[10]

The Committee on Nutrition of the American Academy of Pediatrics has set minimum standards for infant formula of 1.8 gm/100 kcal with a protein efficiency ratio to that of casein.[15]

The protein requirement for any child depends on the rate of growth and the quality of protein in the diet. This implies that evaluation of a child's protein intake must be approached on the basis of the adequacy of the rate of growth, the quality of protein in the foods ingested, the combinations of foods that provide amino acids consumed together, and the adequacy of those nutrients (minerals and vitamins) and energy that are necessary for protein synthesis.

Food sources

Protein of high quality is available to most infants in developed countries as human milk and modified cow's milk formula. Infants whose parents are unwilling to feed them cow's milk formulas or infants who have allergic reactions to cow's milk are often fed formulas prepared form water-soluble soy isolates.

Table 2-4   Estimated amino acid requirements of infants

Amino Acid	Estimated Requirements		Composite of Lower Values (mg/kg/day)‡
	Holt and Snyderman[8] (mg/kg/day)*	Foman and Filer[9] (mg/kg/day)†	
Histidine	34	28	28
Isoleucine	119	70	70
Leucine	229	161	161
Lysine	103	161	103
Methionine plus cystine	45 plus cys	58§	58
Phenylalanine plus tyrosine	90 plus tyr	125§	125
Threonine	87	116	87
Trytophan	22	17	17
Valine	105	93	93

From Energy and Protein Requirements, Report of a Joint FAO/WHO Ad Hoc Committe, World health Organization Technical Report Series No. 522, FAO Nutr. Meet. Rep. No. 52, Geneva, 1973, World Health Orgainization.
*Requirements estimated when amino acids were fed or incorporated in basal formulas. The values represent estimates of maximal individual requirements to achieve normal growth.
†Calculated intakes of amino acids when formulas were fed in amounts sufficient to maintain good growth in all the infants studied; the amino acids were not varied independently.
‡Based on a safe level of 2 gm grotein/kg/day, the average of suggested levels for the period 0 to 6 months of age .
§The values for cystine and tyrosine were estimated on the basis of the methionine: cystine and phenylalanine: tyrosine ratios in human milk.

As discussed in Chapter 4, commercially prepared formulas are made up so that all nutrients are provided in the appropriate amounts. Home preparation of soy formulas should be discouraged because parents may not be careful to heat the milk sufficiently to achieve inactivation of the trypsin inhibitor and may discard the residue of soy material from which the milk was made. In so doing, much of the protein and many of the other essential nutrients are discarded.

Table 2-6 lists foods commonly consumed in infancy that contribute protein.

As children grow older and accept table food, they receive additional foods that provide high-quality protein. Examples of foods acceptable to preschoolers that provide high-quality protein are given in Table 2-7.

Examples of combinations of foods that meet the recommended intakes for protein for 2-month-old, 10-month-old, and 4-year-old children are given in Table 2-8. The examples given include much less protein than most children consume. In fact, it would be difficult to provide sufficient energy in the diet if protein intakes were restricted to only the recommended amounts and milk and small amounts of other animal protein were included in the diet. For example, 4-year-old children who consume the food listed receive approximately 500 kcal/day from these sources, leaving 1000 kcal that need to be met totally from vegetables, fruits, fat, and sweets, without protein from meats, breads, nuts, other cereal grains, or cheese (Table 2-8).

The protein intakes of some children are a matter of concern. **Kwashiorkor** (severe protein deficiency) has been reported in infants whose

Table 2-5 Estimated amino acid requirements of schoolchildren 10 to 12 years of age

Amino acid	Observed Requirement* (mg/kg/day)
Histidine	0
Isoleucine	30
Leucine	45
Lysine	60
Methionine plus cystine	27
Phenylalanine plus tyrosine	27
Threonine	35
Tryptophan	4
Valine	33

From Energy and Protein Requirements, Report of a Joint FAO/WHO Ad Hoc Committee, World Health Organization Technical Report Series No. 522, FAO Nutr. Meet. Rep. No. 52, Geneva, 1973, World Health Organization.
*Based on Nakagawa, I., and others: The values represent estimates of the upper range of individual requirements for the achievement of positive nitrogen balance in boys.

Table 2-6 Approximate protein contents of various milks and foods fed to infants

Food	Protein (gm/oz)
Human milk	0.3
Commercial formulas	0.5
Homogenized milk	1.1
Evaporated milk prepared	1.1
Infant cereals, high protein, dry	10.2
Infant cereals, rice	2.0
Strained chicken noodle dinners	0.6
Strained split pea, vegetable, and ham or bacon dinners	1.1
Strained beef and vegetable dinners	1.6
Strained turkey and vegetable dinners	1.6
Strained egg yolk	2.8
Strained beef	3.9
Strained veal	3.8

From Gebhardt, S.E., Cutrufelli, R., and Matthews, R.H.: Composition of foods, baby foods, raw, processed, prepared Agriculture Handbook No. 8-3, Washington D.C., 1978, U.S. Department of Agriculture.

Table 2-7 Selected foods as sources of protein for preschool children

Food	Portion Size	Protein (gm)
Yogurt, made from whole milk	$\frac{1}{2}$ cup	3.7
Cheddar cheese	1 oz	7.1
Hamburger patty	2 oz	15.4
Chicken drumstick	1	12.2
Peanut butter	1 tbsp	4.0
Egg	1 medium	5.7
Liverwurst	1 oz	4.6
Tuna	$\frac{1}{4}$ cup	11.5
Frankfurter, 5" by $\frac{3}{4}$"	1	5.6
Nonfat milk solids, dry	1 tbsp	1.52

From Adams, C.F.: Nutritive value of American foods in common units, Agricultural Handbook No. 456, Washington D.C., 1975, U.S. Department of Agriculture.

Table 2-8 Foods that provide appropriate protein intakes for children

Age	Weight (kg)	Protein Intake (gm)	Examples of Foods that Meet Protein Needs
2 months	5	11	33 oz human milk *or*
			22 oz commercially manufactured infant formula
10 months	9.5	19	18 oz homogenized milk
4 years	18	27	16 oz milk
			1 tbsp peanut butter
			1 medium egg

parents purposely withheld milk after episodes of vomiting or diarrhea treated with clear liquids and in children from families who live in extreme poverty where there was marked restriction of protein intake.[16,17] Children with multiple allergies who have learned to control parents by refusing all protein-rich foods have been known to experience catch-up growth when their parents learned to reinforce their acceptance of the meats and soy milk to which they had no allergic reactions. Children who are hypersensitive in the oral area frequently refuse all meat and eggs and consume very limited amounts of milk and dairy products if unlimited amounts of carbohydrates such as starches and sugars are available to them. Limited financial resources restrict the amounts of high-quality protein parents can purchase for their children. Without careful planning the quality of a child's protein intake may be compromised. However, peanut butter and whole wheat bread, beans, rice, eggs, and powdered milk provide inexpensive high-quality protein.

Fat

Fat, the most calorically concentrated nutrient, supplies between 40% and 50% of the energy consumed in infancy and approximately 40% of the energy consumed after infancy by individuals in developed countries. Because it is calorically concentrated, it may be very important in the diet of children who are lean and physically active and have a small appetite or in the diet of children with oral motor problems who can consume only a limited volume of food. However, chunky, passive children should limit the quantity of fat they consume to keep from gaining weight too rapidly.

Essential fatty acids

Polyunsaturated **linoleic acid** has been conclusively proven to be an essential nutrient for both children and adults. Although arachidonic acid performs some of the same functions, it is not essential because it can be synthesized from linoleic acid.

Some investigators consider linolenic acid also essential although no specific deficiency of linolenic acid has been reported in humans.

One of the earliest manifestations of fatty acid deficiency recognized in animals was an increased basal metabolic rate. Infants who are fed formulas low in the essential fatty acid consume greater numbers of calories than do those who consume adequate quantities of linoleic acid to maintain normal growth. Caloric utilization has been reported to vary with intakes of linoleate up to 4% to 5% of total calories. It has been suggested that the ratio of triene:tetraene fatty acids in the blood serum can be used in assessing nutritional status of linoleic acid. A triene:tetraene ratio of 0.4 or less is considered indicative of normal fatty acid status, and a ratio greater than 0.4 is indicative of an insufficient intake of essential fatty acid.[18] Such biochemical evidence of deficiency appears when linoleic acid is less than 1% of the total calories. On this basis the minimal requirements for linoleic acid are considered to be approximately 1% of the calories consumed, and an optimal intake is thought to be 4% to 5% of the calories consumed.

Recommended intakes

If less than 30% of energy intakes are derived from fat, a dry and unpalatable diet may result.

Fomon[19] suggests that diets that provide less than 30% of total calories or greater than 50% of total calories as fat should be avoided.

Food sources

Human milk, cow's milk, and commercially available infant formulas provide approximately 50% of calories as fat. Approximately 4% of the total calories in human milk and 1% of the calories in cow's milk are provided by linoleic acid. Commercially available infant formulas contain blends of vegetable oils and contribute greater amounts of linoleic acid.

The Committee on Nutrition of the American Academy of Pediatrics[15] has recommended that infant formulas contain a minimum of 300 mg of 18:2 fatty acids/100 kcal (1.7% of the energy content).

Prepared infant foods are relatively low in fat as compared with foods consumed by older children. Tables 2-9 and 2-10 list the amounts of fat provided by foods commonly consumed by infants and children.

CARBOHYDRATES

Carbohydrates supply between 40% and 50% of the energy consumed by most infants and children in North America.

Table 2-9   Foods as sources of fat for infants

Food	Fat (gm/oz)
Infant cereal, dry (11-13 tbsp/oz)	0.8-2.2
Vegetable and meat dinners	0.1-1.1
Meat and vegetable dinners	0.6-1.6
Strained and junior meats	1.1-2.7
Strained egg yolks	4.9

From Gebhardt, S.E., Cutrufelli, R., and Matthews, R.H.: Composition of foods, baby foods, raw, processed, prepared Agriculture Handbook No. 8-3, Washington D.C., 1978, U.S. Department of Agriculture.

Recommended Intakes

Since glucose can be synthesized from amino acids and the glycerol moiety of fat, no specific recommendations for intake have been made. The Food and Nutrition Board of the

Table 2-10   Foods as sources of fat for preschool children

Food	Portion Size	Fat (gm)
Cooking fat	1 tbsp	12.5
Mayonnaise	1 tbsp	11.2
Butter	1 tsp	3.8
Cheddar cheese	1 oz	7.1
Peanut butter	1 tbsp	8.1
Frankfurter, 5" by ¾"	1	11.5
Broiled hamburger patty	2 oz	15.4
Chicken drumstick	1	12.2
Egg	1 medium	5.1
Tuna, drained	¼ cup	3.3
Ice cream	¼ cup	3.5
Potato chips	10	8.0

From Adams, C.F.: Nutritive value of American foods in common units, Agriculture Handbook No. 456, Washington D.C., 1975, U.S. Department of Agriculture.

National Research Council suggests minimum intakes of 50 to 100 gm/day.

Current interest in dietary fiber as a means to prevent diverticular disease, cancer of the colon, coronary heart disease, obesity, and irritable bowel syndrome in later life has caused many professionals to recommend a high-fiber diet. The Committee on Nutrition of the American Academy of Pediatrics has stated that more work must be done on the effect of a high-fiber diet on mineral status before firm recommendations can be made. However, the committee recommends a substantial amount of fiber to ensure normal laxation.[20] The inclusion of whole grain cereals, breads, fruits, and vegetables in the diet of preschool, school-age, and adolescent children is important.

Food Sources

The predominant carbohydrate in the young infant's diet is lactose, found in human milk and cow's milk. It has become a common practice for parents to add starch (in the form of prepared cereals and ingredients of commercially prepared infant foods) and sucrose (which they add to fruits and vegetables) to the infant's diet at 4 to 6 months of age (Table 2-11).

Some foods contain carbohydrate and few other nutrients, whereas others contribute carbohydrate and other essential nutrients. Candy, cookies, and potato chips, for example, provide primarily calories, whereas cereal grains are important sources of the B vitamins; potatoes contribute vitamin C; and legumes offer amino acids, iron, and B vitamins as well as carbohydrates. Therefore careful attention to the nutrients carried by the carbohydrate-containing foods is important in planning diets for children.

Most children prefer sweet foods. In fact, infants at birth appear to distinguish sugar water from plain water. They accept larger quantities of sugar-sweetened solutions than unsweetened mixtures (Table 2-11). Indis-

Table 2-11 Carbohydrates in foods for infants

Food	Carbohydrate (gm/oz)
Human milk	2.9
Prepared infant formulas	2.1
Homogenized milk	1.5
Infant cereals, dry	16.4-22.8
Strained and junior desserts	3.7-6.1
Strained and junior vegetable and meat dinners	1.9-3.2
Strained and junior meat and vegetable dinners	1.2-5.3
Strained and junior fruit	2.9-6.1
Strained and junior vegetables	1.6-4.6

From Gebhardt, S.E., Cutrufelli, R., and Matthews, R.H.: Composition of foods, baby foods, raw, processed, prepared, Agriculture Handbook No. 8-3, Washington D.C., 1978, U.S. Department of Agriculture.

criminate consumption of candy, cookies, carbonated beverages and other sweetened drinks dulls the appetite for other foods and should be discouraged. The impact of these sucrose-containing foods on the incidence of dental caries is discussed in Chapter 10.

WATER

Even more essential to the body than food is water. It functions as an essential component of body structure and as a solvent for minerals and other physiologically important compounds. It transports nutrients to and waste products from the cells and helps to regulate body temperature.

The percentage of body weight provided by water decreases from approximately 75% at birth to 60% at 1 year of age (see Chapter 1). After 1 year of age intracellular water accounts for approximately 60% and extracellular water for 40% of total body water.

Recommended Intakes

Water is lost by evaporation through the skin and respiratory tract (**insensible water loss**), through perspiration when the environmental temperature is elevated, and by elimination in the feces and the urine. During growth a positive water balance is necessary since additional water is obligated as a constituent of tissue and for increases in the volume of body fluids. The amount of water required for growth, however, is very small at all ages.

Water lost by evaporation in infancy and early childhood accounts for more than 60% of that needed to maintain homeostasis, as compared with 40% to 50% in the adult. At all ages approximately 24% of the basal heat loss is by evaporation of water through the skin and respiratory tract.[22] This amounts to 45 ml of insensible water loss per 100 kcal expended. Fomon[19] estimates evaporative water loss at 1 month of age to average 210 ml/day and at 1 year of age, 500 ml/day. Adult losses by evaporation average 800 to 1050 ml/day under ordinary circumstances. Evaporative losses increase with fever and higher environmental temperature. Increases in humidity decrease respiratory loss. Loss of water in the feces averages 10 ml/kg/day in infancy.[49]

The volume of urine in general reflects fluid intake. It includes both water required to concentrate the solutes presented to the kidney for excretion and water in excess of baby's need. The renal water requirement is determined by the diet and by the concentrating power of the kidney.

Ziegler and Fomon have developed a method for estimating the renal **solute** load by calculating the amount of dietary sodium, chloride, potassium, and urea (estimated to be 4mOsm/gm of protein). The urinary water requirement can then be estimated from the sum of these values. An intake of 1.0 ml/kcal/day for the adult has been suggested. Balance studies of 5-year-old children showed intakes of 1100 ml/day; metabolic water contributed an additional 200 ml/day. Water intakes averaged 0.7 ml/kcal/day.[24] Ranges of average water requirements of infants and children are given in Table 2-12.

Food Sources

Fluid in liquids and food consumed are the primary source of water. In addition, metabolic water is created from the metabolism of protein, fat, and carbohydrate: 1 gm protein produces 4.1 ml water, 1 gm carbohydrate produces 5.5 ml water, and 1 gm fat produces 1.07 ml water. Table 2-13 gives the water content of representative foods consumed in infancy and early childhood. When milk is boiled the liquid evaporates and protein and electrolytes are concentrated. Boiled milk is an inappropriate food for infants.

Because of a relatively greater demand for insensible water and a renal concentrating capacity that may be less than that of the adult, the infant is vulnerable to water imbalance. Under normal environmental conditions infants do not need additional water.

Table 2-12 Water requirements of infants and children

Age	Water Requirement (ml/kg/day)
10 days	125-150
3 months	140-160
6 months	130-155
1 year	120-135
2 years	115-125
6 years	90-100
10 years	70-85
14 years	50-60

From Barness, L.A.: Nutrition and nutritional disorders. In Berman, R.E., and Vaughan, V.C.: Nelson textbook of Pediatrics, ed. 13. Philadelphia, 1987, W.B. Saunders Co.

Table 2-13 Percentage of water in selected foods

Food	Water (%)	Food	Water (%)
Human milk	85.2	Strained carrots	92.3
Cow's milk	87.4	Hamburger patty	68.3
Infant cereals, high protein	6.1	Chicken, cooked, dark meat	64.4
Infant cereals, rice	6.7	Egg, hard boiled	73.7
Strained macaroni and cheese	87.1	Oatmeal, cooked	83.6
Strained chicken with vegetables	90.0	Bread, white, enriched	35.6
Strained beef with vegetables	85.4	Carrots, cooked	91.2
Strained applesauce	88.6	Peas, canned	81.5
Strained peaches	80.1	Banana	75.7
Strained beef	80.6	Pears, canned	91.1
Strained peas	87.5		

From Gebhardt, S.E., Cutrufelli, R., and Matthews, R.H.: Composition of foods, baby foods, raw processed, prepared, Agriculture Handbook No. 8-3, Washington D.C., 1978, U.S. Department of Agriculture.

Difficulties arise when formulas are improperly prepared (see Chapter 4), when infants ingest limited volumes of milk during illness, and when extrarenal losses are greater than usual, such as during episodes of vomiting and diarrhea.[19] To ensure adequate water intakes, infant formula should not be concentrated to more than 100 kcal/100 ml.

As children grow older the concentrating power of the kidney increases. Children learn to communicate and ask for water when they become thirsty. Difficulties in achieving water balance are unlikely in the absence of vomiting or diarrhea.

MINERALS

Although minerals contribute only 3% to 4% of body weight, they play important roles in the regulation of body fluids, acid base balance, and metabolic processes.

Calcium and Phosphorus

Calcium and phosphorus occur in three systems in the body. Bone contains 99% of body calcium; the remaining 1% is found in body fluids and striated muscle. Bone contains 80% of body phosphorus; the remaining 20% is found in striated muscle and blood serum. Plasma calcium and phosphorus levels are higher in children than in adults. Serum concentrations of the minerals are highest during early childhood, then decrease, paralleling decreases in the parathyroid hormone. The levels stabilize between 6 and 12 years of age and decline to adult values during adolescence.[25]

The calcium content of the body reflects both sex and stature. The body of the adult female contains approximately three fourths as much calcium as the body of the adult male. The skeletons of blacks tend to be larger than those of whites. The amount of calcium accumulated during growth depends on the rate of growth and final stature attained. It has been estimated that the fetus acquires an average of 97 mg of calcium/day.[26] Shaw estimates the placental transfer at term to be 150 mg/kg/day.[27] The body of the full-term newborn infant has been estimated to contain approximately 27 gm of calcium, that of the adult female 770 to 920 gm of calcium, and that of the adult male 950 to 1290 gm of calcium.

Skeletal requirements for calcium and phosphorus depend on body size and rates of growth. Requirements are greatest for taller, more rapidly growing children at any age.

Garn has estimated gains in skeletal weight and amounts of calcium and phosphorus retained in bone from longitudinal and cross-sectional roentgenographic studies of the second metacarpal.[28] Christiansen, Rödbro, and Neilsen have measured **bone density** of school-age children at different ages by **photon absorption**.[29] Other investigators have analyzed skeletal weights and percentages of skeletal ash of individuals from infancy to adulthood.[30] Leitch and Aitken have estimated skeletal calcium requirements from analysis both of the calcium content of analyzed bodies and of rates of growth.[31]

Garn estimates an average skeletal retention in males of 90 mg of calcium/day and 43 mg of phosphorus/day in the first year of life. Leitch and Aitken suggest skeletal calcium increments during the same period to average 150 mg/day. Both investigators estimate a decline in skeletal retentions of the minerals between the first and fourth years, after which the skeletal retentions gradually increase. Garn estimates that during the adolescent growth spurt males retain an average of 275 mg of calcium and 132 mg of phosphorus/day. Leitch and Aitken suggest that between 15 and 17 years of age, skeletal requirements for calcium average 375 to 400 mg/day. The Committee on Nutrition of the American Academy of Pediatrics estimates a retention of 290 to 400 mg of calcium/day in males and 210 to 240 mg of calcium/day in females during their peak growth spurts.[26] Skeletal retentions of the two minerals are less in females than in males except between the tenth and twelfth years, when rates of growth of females are greater than those of males.

Recommended intakes

Attempts to establish recommended intakes of calcium have caused considerable controversy for many years. Populations that have adapted to intakes of 200 to 400 mg/day without adverse effects have been identified. However, rickets has been reported in one full-term infant who for 10 months consumed a lamb-base formula deficient in calcium but adequate in vitamins.[32] **Osteomalacia**, which improved rapidly with calcium supplements, has been identified in three black children: a 4-year-old girl, and 6- and 13-year-old boys in South Africa.[33] Most recommended intakes have been planned to meet the needs of formula-fed infants who retain 25% to 30% of the calcium consumed in cow's milk. Although breast-fed infants ingest less calcium, they retain approximately two thirds of intake. Children may need two to four times as much calcium as adults since they are growing. The need for higher intakes during the preadolescent years and puberty should provide for maximum calcium retention.[1]

Food sources

Milk and dairy products are the richest sources of calcium in the North American diet. Table 2-14 shows the contribution of selected milk and dairy products. Egg yolks and most dark green leafy vegetables also contribute appreciable amounts of calcium. Absorption of calcium fluctuates from 30% to 60% of intake. Lactase increased absorption. Phytic and oxalic acid reduce absorption. Calcium absorption from carbonate, acetate, gluconate, and citrate salts of calcium and from whole milk are similar.[34]

Phosphorus is found in combination with calcium in dairy products but also occurs in foods that contain little calcium. It occurs in most protein-rich foods such as meats, eggs, nuts, and legumes and is also found in grains. Phosphate-containing additives are ingredients of many carbonated beverages, pro-

Table 2-14   Calcium in milk and dairy products

Food	Household Measure	Calcium (mg)
Human milk	4 oz	40
Cow's milk	4 oz	144
Powdered milk, nonfat, instant dry	$\frac{1}{3}$ cup	293
Cheddar cheese	1 oz	213
Yogurt	$\frac{1}{2}$ cup	147
Custard, baked	$\frac{1}{2}$ cup	148
Chocolate pudding, cooked with milk	$\frac{1}{2}$ cup	133
Chocolate pudding, instant	$\frac{1}{2}$ cup	187
Ice cream	$\frac{1}{2}$ cup	97

From Adams, C.F.: Nutritive value of American foods in common units, Agriculture Handbook No. 456, Washington D.C., 1975, U.S. Department of Agriculture.

cessed meats, cheese, and refrigerated bakery goods.

Neonatal hypocalcemia

Plasma concentrations of calcium and phosphorus are greater in cord blood than in maternal blood. During the first 2 to 3 days of life the levels of calcium fall significantly.[35] The decline is greatest in premature infants, infants of abnormal pregnancies and deliveries, infants with asphyxia, and infants of diabetic mothers. In normal, full-term infants the decline is greatest in those who are formula-fed and least in those who receive human milk. The fall in plasma calcium levels is accompanied by a rise in plasma inorganic phosphorus levels.

After the initial decline, plasma calcium levels stabilize and tend to rise by the tenth day of life, the level being dependent on the phosphorus content or the calcium: phosphorus ratio of milk. Serum calcium concentrations in breast-fed infants are greater than those in formula-fed infants. Serum concentrations of phosphorus reflect the phosphorus content of the milk consumed, being significantly less in breast-fed infants than in formula-fed infants. Breast-fed infants generally show an increase in serum

calcium concentration by 5 to 7 days of age. Snodgrass and others[36] noted no increase in levels of plasma calcium in formula-fed infants between the first and sixth to eighth day of life. They noted a fall in serum calcium concentrations in one third of formula-fed infants during the first week of life; in 9% of infants the levels fell below 7.5 mg/100 ml, a level at which **hypocalcemia** is defined by many and at which the infant is at risk of **tetany**.

There are two periods when hypocalcemia is detected in the neonate. Early **neonatal** hypocalcemia occurs in the first 24 to 48 hours and is thought to be the result of depressed levels of parathyroid hormone as a result of transient functional hypoparathyroidism.[37] It occurs most frequently in infants of diabetic mothers, infants who have experienced asphyxia, and low birth weight infants. Some investigators have suggested that a continuous prophylactic infusion or oral supplements of calcium and magnesium lactate be given to all low birth weight infants.[38] Late neonatal hypocalcemia occurs in association with hyperphosphatemia in otherwise normal, full-term infants between the fifth and eighth day of life. It is rarely seen in breast-fed infants but occurs more often in infants who receive a high dietary intake of phosphorus. Phosphorus consumed in excess of that which can be excreted by the kidney elevates serum phosphate levels. It has been hypothesized that elevated serum phosphorus levels depress serum calcium levels by causing deposition of calcium in bone. A normal response would be an increased output of parathroid hormone, causing solubilization of bone mineral, phosphate diuresis, and blockage of tubular resorption. The neonatal infant with an immature parathyroid gland may not be able to respond with the normal homeostatic mechanism, and his serum calcium levels may fall. Irritability and convulsions often, although not inevitably, occur when serum levels fall below 7 mg/100 ml.

One of the striking differences between human milk and cow's milk is the content of calcium and phosphorus. Cow's milk contains more than three times as much calcium and six times as much phosphorus as does human milk. There is less calcium relative to phosphorus in cow's milk than in human milk. In 1951 Gittleman and Pincus found that newborn infants who were given a high-phosphate diet as represented by evaporated milk or whole cow's milk mixtures responded with hyperphosphatemia and a tendency toward hypocalcemia.[39] In 1952 Gardner suggested that excess dietary phosphorus in the face of limited kidney function has profound effects on the renal tissue as well as on the parathyroid gland, causing hypertrophy of the parathyroid gland and renal lesions.[40]

Manufacturers of infant formulas have reduced the quantity of phosphorus in cow's milk formulas. Isolated cases of neonatal hypocalcemic tetany, however, continue to be reported. Pierson and Crawford reported two cases of neonatal hypocalcemia, resulting in tentany, that occurred on the eighth and ninth days of life.[41] One infant received a high-phosphate load from a soybean formula preparation, the other from the addition of cereal to the formula. Monitoring the amount of phosphorus consumed by infants in the early neonatal period continues to be important.

Magnesium

Magnesium is the fourth most abundant mineral in the body and the second most abundant intercellular cation. Approximately 50% of the body's magnesium is deposited with calcium and phosphorus in bone, 25% is in muscle, and the remainder is found in soft tissue.

Recommended intakes

Harris and Wilkinson state that the newborn infant needs to retain 10.2 mg/day of magnesium to satisfy the requirement for growth.[42] Fomon estimates the requirement to be 16.5 mg/day during the first 4 months and suggests an intake of 25 mg/day. Barness suggests intakes of 40 to 70 mg/day for infants, 100 to 150 mg/day for children 1 to 3 years of age, 200 to 300 mg/day for children 3 to 12 years of age, and 350 to 400 mg/day for adolescents 12 to 18 years of age.[43]

Food sources

Magnesium is found in many foods. Nuts, soybeans, whole grains, legumes, and shellfish are excellent sources. Magnesium also exists in all green plants as a component of chlorophyll. Human milk contains approximately 4 mg of magnesium/100 ml and cow's milk contains 12 mg of magnesium/100 ml.

Iron

Iron is the most abundant trace mineral in the body, accounting for approximately 75 mg/kg of the full-term newborn infant, 50 mg/kg of the adult male, and 35 mg/kg of the adult female.

The concentration of **hemoglobin** at birth averages 17 to 19 gm/100 ml of blood. During the first 6 to 8 weeks of life it decreases to approximately 10 to 11 gm/100 ml because of a shortened life span of the fetal cell and decreased **erythropoiesis**. After this age there is a gradual increase in hemoglobin concentration to 13 gm/100 ml at 2 years of age. During adolescence a sharp increase occurs in males at the time of the growth spurt. Infants, children, and adolescents need iron not only to maintain hemoglobin but also to increase the iron mass related to growth increases in body size.

Iron deficiency is the most common nutritional deficiency in North America. It occurs most frequently in 12- to 36-month-old children, in adolescent males, and in females during their childbearing years.[44] It may result from inadequate iron intakes, impaired absorption, a large hemorrhage, or repeated small hemorrhages.

Iron is accumulated in utero in proportion to body size. Premature and low birth weight infants have limited reserves at birth that are quickly depleted during rapid growth. Even with the advantage of full-term iron stores, the rapidly growing infant is at risk of iron deficiency.

Iron deficiency

Iron deficiency results when body iron is diminished. There are three stages of depletion. The first is a decrease in iron status represented by a drop in plasma **ferritin**. The second is normocytic-iron deficient erythropoiesis, when red cell protoporphyran is elevated and transferrin saturation is reduced. The third stage is iron-deficiency anemia, when red cells are **microcytic** and hypochromic and hemoglobin levels are reduced. Iron deficiency is diagnosed when **transferrin** saturation falls below 16%; anemia is diagnosed when hemoglobin concentrations fall below 11.0 gm/100 ml and **hematocrits** fall below 33%.

Recommended intakes

Iron requirements of individual children vary with rates of growth, increasing blood volumes, iron stores, variations in menstrual losses of iron of adolescent females, and the timing of growth spurts of adolescents. Larger, more rapidly growing children have the greatest requirement for iron at any age.

Because of stored iron the normal newborn can maintain satisfactory hemoglobin levels solely from human milk for 3 months, but beginning at age 3 months and continuing to age 3 years, a daily intake of 1 mg/kg to a maximum of 15 mg/day is usually considered appropriate. Iron loss during menstruation varies widely among females but is consistent from month to month in individuals. Average losses of blood of 15-year-old girls in a Swedish study were 33.8 ml/period, equivalent to an iron loss of approximately 0.5 mg of iron/day.[46] To attain stores of 500 mg for both sexes by age 20 to 25 years, an intake of 10 mg/day is recommended for children. An additional 2 mg/day intake is recommended for males during the pubertal growth spurt and 5 mg/day for females starting with the pubertal growth spurt and menstruation and continuing through the menstrual years.[45]

Food sources

Diets in North America have been estimated to provide 6 mg of iron/1000 kcal. Organ meats, shellfish, and muscle meats provide the richest and most usable sources. Other food sources include nuts, green vegetables, whole wheat flour, and bread.

Of the iron in pork, liver, and fish, 30% to 40% is in the form of heme iron, and of the iron in beef, lamb, and chicken, 50% to 60% is in the form of heme iron. These foods are sources of nonheme iron also, as are greens, vegetables, grains, legumes, and eggs. Human milk and cow's milk contain 0.5 to 1.0 mg of iron/L. During infancy, iron-fortified formulas and cereals fortified with reduced iron are primary food sources. Table 2-15 lists representative sources of iron for infants and children.

Iron absorption from food

The percentage of iron absorbed from food depends on the presence of heme iron or nonheme iron, the combinations of food consumed together, and the iron reserves of the

Table 2-15 Selected food sources of iron

Food	Household Measure	Iron (mg)
Iron-fortified formula	8 oz	3.0
Infant cereals, high protein	1 tbsp	1.8
Infant cereals, rice	1 tbsp	1.8
Strained split peas with ham	1 oz	0.1
Strained chicken with vegetables	1 oz	0.1
Strained beef with vegetables	1 oz	0.1
Strained beef	1 oz	1.0
Strained liver	1 oz	1.5
Hamburger, cooked	2 oz	1.8
Chicken, dark meat	1 oz	0.5
Liver, beef	1 oz	2.5
Liver, chicken	1 liver	2.1
Liverwurst	1 oz	1.7
Frankfurter, 5" by $\frac{3}{4}$"	1	0.9
Egg	1 medium	1.0
Pork and beans	$\frac{1}{4}$ cup	1.5
Peanut butter	1 tbsp	0.3
Bread, enriched white	1 slice	0.7
Macaroni, enriched, cooked	$\frac{1}{4}$ cup	0.4
Carrots, cooked	$\frac{1}{4}$ cup	0.2
Orange	1 medium	0.6
Canned pears	$\frac{1}{4}$ cup	0.1

From Adams, C.F.: Nutritive value of American foods in common units, Agriculture Handbook No. 456, Agriculture Research Service, Washington D.C., 1975, U.S. Department of Agriculture; and Gebhardt, S.E., Cutrufelli, R., and Matthews, R.H.: Composition of foods, baby foods, raw, processed, prepared, Agriculture Handbook No. 8-3, Washington, D.C., 1978, U.S. Department of Agriculture.

individual. Individuals with inadequate iron stores absorb approximately 35%; those with adequate iron stores absorb 25% of heme iron consumed. Individuals with deficient iron reserves may absorb as much as 20% of nonheme iron, whereas iron-replete individuals may absorb as little as 2%. The presence of meat, which offers heme iron and ascorbic acid, increases the absorption of nonheme iron. Absorption is decreased by the inclusion of dairy products, eggs, calcium phosphate salts, or tea in the foods consumed at the same time. Overall, 49% of the iron in human milk, 19% of the iron in cow's milk, and 3% of the iron in iron-fortified formula is absorbed.[48] The addition of strained vegetables to the infant's diet significantly reduces the availability of iron from human milk.[48]

Many foods are fortified with iron salts. Of particular importance to persons concerned with the iron intakes of infants and children are those iron salts used to fortify the commercially prepared infant formulas, cereal grains, and cereals consumed so abundantly by children. Iron-fortified formulas contain 12 mg of iron as ferrous sulfate. Cereals and baked products may be fortified with reduced iron, sodium iron pyrophosphate, or ferric orthophosphate.

Ferrous sulfate is the most available of the iron salts, but it is seldom used to fortify food because of difficulties in manufacturing. The percentage of absorption of reduced iron will depend on the particle size, surface area, and porosity of the salts, which in turn determines the extent to which the particles dissolve in the acid of the stomach. One study in humans indicated absorption is about 5% of that of ferrous sulfate. Fomon feels this iron salt is not a reliable source of iron for infants.[44]

Some pediatricians believe it may be advantageous for infants over 6 months of age to receive one feeding that includes not milk but iron-fortified cereal, vegetables, and fruit or fruit juice containing vitamin C.

A desirable iron status can be compromised by a low-calorie diet, poor selection of foods, or any dietary extremes. Assuming that a well-chosen diet contains approximately 6 mg of iron/1000 kcal, adolescents dieting to lose weight will be receiving minimal iron intakes. In addition to this, the common practice of choosing foods such as yogurt and cottage cheese as primary protein foods in a reducing diet results in an even lower dietary iron intake.

Ideally, regular monitoring of iron status should be provided for infants and adolescents, expecially those with limited high-iron foods or those practicing various dietary extremes or restrictions.

Iodine

Of the iodine in the human adult, 70% to 80% is concentrated in the thyroid gland, which synthesizes its only functional compounds, thyroxine and triiodothyronine. The remaining iodine in the body is distributed in the blood, skin, and other tissues.

Recommended intakes

The breast-fed infant receives 10 to 20 μg of iodine/100 kcal from an adequately fed lactating mother. It has been suggested that requirements for 8- to 16-year-old children

may not be much greater than 56 μg/day.[19] Average intakes of iodine in the United States are five to ten times the recommended amounts. However, wide variations in iodine intakes may be experienced by individuals, depending on sources of food and geographical locations.

Food sources

Iodized salt, bread made with iodate as a dough conditioner, milk, and seafood are excellent sources of dietary iodine. The fact that the iodine content of food is determined by the soil in which it is grown is no longer significant in the etiology of iodine deficiency. Food consumed in one area is often transported from another. The iodine content of milk and dairy products depends on whether the cattle have been given iodine-supplemented feed or iodized salt blocks. Milk iodine may be as high as 450 μg/L.

The amounts of iodine absorbed from environments polluted by the combustion of fossil fuels and organic matter can be significant. Many therapeutic drugs also contain large amounts of iodine.[49]

Zinc

Zinc is distributed throughout all cells and tissues. The fetus contains approximately 20 mg/kg, whereas the adult has 30 mg/kg of fat-free tissue.[50] It leaves the hair only when the hair is shed. During infancy, serum zinc levels are determined primarily by the zinc content of the milk consumed.[51]

Hambidge and others reported low concentrations of zinc in hair in 10 of 132 children over 4 years of age from middle-income and upper-income families that were studied in Denver, Colorado. The children had histories of poor appetite, consumed small amounts of meat, and had diminished taste acuity. Nine of the ten children had heights that plotted at or below the 10th percentile. Supplements of zinc sulfate providing 0.2 mg zinc/kg resulted in improvements in growth, taste, and appetite.[52]

It appears that many preschool and school-age children from low-income and middle-income families may be ingesting inadequate amounts of zinc. Studies in Denver of Headstart children 3.5 to 6 years of age whose heights were less than the 3rd percentile revealed that 40% had low concentrations of hair zinc and 69% had low plasma and hair zinc concentrations.[53]

A Canadian study found 4- to 5-year-old boys who had low hair zinc had lower mean height for age percentiles than those with average hair levels of zinc.[54]

Recommended intakes

Recommendations for intake have been made from studies of zinc intakes of apparently well-nourished individuals and from studies of zinc balance. Growth velocity is the main determinant of the zinc requirement in childhood. The infant is born without zinc stores and rapidly becomes dependent on an adequate supply of biologically available zinc.

Normal breast-fed infants have been noted to be in negative balance at 1 week of age. One study comparing hair zinc concentration of breast-fed and formula-fed babies during the first 6 months found that only male formula-fed infants experienced a significant decline in hair zinc concentrations.[55]

Variations in plasma zinc concentrations during growth reflect the continual utilization and depletion of body stores of zinc. Declines occur during periods of most rapid growth. Calculations indicated that the requirement at 4 to 6 months of age is 50% less than at 1 month.[51] The steepest decline appears to occur at 10 to 11 years of age in the female and at 12 to 13 years of age in the male.[56]

Breast-fed infants receive 0.7 to 5 mg/day, approximately 0.2 to 1.2 mg/kg.[57] Intakes of children 1 to 3 years of age have been estimated to average 5 mg/day; those of children 3 to 5 years of age, 5 to 7 mg/day; and those of adolescents, 13 mg/day.[58] Balance studies of

Engel, Miller, and Price suggest that 6mg/day is adequate for preadolescent children.[59] Studies by Tribble and Scoular indicate that 12 mg/day is adequate for college students.[60]

Food sources

Seafoods and meats are rich sources of available zinc. Cereals and legumes also contain significant amounts. The bioavailability ranges from 20% to 30%. Estimates of zinc in human milk and cow's milk range from 3 to 5mg/L. Picciano and Guthrie found ranges of 0.14 to 3.95 mg/L in milk of 50 lactating women.[61] Colostrum contains 20 mg/L, three to five times as much as later milk. Levels of zinc in human milk decline after 2 months of lactation and may fall below 1 mg/L. Infant formulas are supplemented and contain 3 to 4 mg of zinc/L. Animal studies suggest a bioavailability of 59.2% of zinc in human milk, 43% to 53.9% of zinc in cow's milk, and 26.8% to 39.5% of zinc in infant

Table 2-16   Selected food sources of zinc

Food	Household Measure	Zinc (mg)
Cow's milk	4 oz	0.5
Ground beef, cooked	2 oz	2.5
Chicken drumstick	1	1.4
Liver, beef, cooked	2 oz	2.9
Liverwurst	1 oz	0.8
Frankfurter	1	0.9
Egg	1 medium	0.5
Oatmeal, cooked	$\frac{1}{2}$ cup	0.6
Bread, white	1 slice	0.2
Bread, whole wheat	1 slice	0.5
Green beans, canned	$\frac{1}{4}$ cup	0.2
Spinach	$\frac{1}{2}$ cup	0.6
Banana	$\frac{1}{2}$ medium	0.2
Orange	1 medium	0.3

Adapted from Murphy, E.W., Willis, B.W., and Watt, B.K.: J. Am. Diet Assoc. 66:345, 1975.

formula.[62] Table 2-16 gives the zinc content of representative foods consumed by infants and children.

Fluoride

Fluoride in the body is concentrated in the bones and teeth. The concentration in bones increases linearly with increased intakes.

The role of fluoride as an essential trace mineral lies in its ability to reduce the incidence of dental caries. It has not been proved essential to survival. Epidemiological studies have repeatedly proved that there is a close relationship between tooth decay and the amount of fluoride ingested during tooth development.[63] When the fluoride content of community drinking water has been adjusted to a level of 1 ppm (1 mg/L), the incidence of dental caries has been reduced 40% to 60%. Although the effect is especially important during tooth development, fluoride has also been shown to be beneficial to adults.

Recommended intakes

The Committee on Nutrition of the American Academy of Pediatrics[64] recommends that supplemental fluoride dosages be adjusted to the fluoride content of the water supply (Table 2-17). In communities with less than 0.3 ppm

Table 2-17 Supplemental fluoride dosage schedule (mg/day)*

Age	Concentration of Fluoride in Drinking Water (ppm)		
	< 0.3	0.3 - 0.7	> 0.7
2 weeks to 2 years	0.25	0	0
2 to 3 years	0.50	0.25	0
3 to 16 years	1.00	0.50	0

From Committee on Nutrition: Pediatrics 63:150, 1979. Copyright American Academy of Pediatrics 1979.
*2.2 mg of sodium fluoride contains 1 mg of fluoride.

of fluoride in the water supply, supplements of 0.25 mg of fluoride/day are recommended from 2 weeks to 2 years of age, 0.5 mg/day between 2 and 3 years of age, and 1 mg/day after 3 years of age. It is suggested that children whose drinking water contains between 0.3 and 0.7 mg of fluoride ppm receive 0.25 mg between 2 and 3 years of age and 0.5 mg between 3 and 16 years of age.

Food sources

All foods and water contain very small amounts of fluoride. Seafood and tea are exceptions and contain greater amounts. Food produced and prepared in areas in which the water is fluoridated reflect the fluoride content of the water. Cow's milk contains 0.03 to 0.1 μg of fluoride/L, human milk contains less than 0.05 mg/L. Average intakes of 15- to 19-year-old males are estimated to be 1.85 mg/day in areas with fluoridated water supplies and 86 mg/day in those with nonfluoridated water. Beverages and water contributed approximately 75% of intake.[66]

There is an increasing concentration of fluoride in the food chain. Processing food with fluoridated water significantly increases its fluoride content. The fluoride content of ready-to-drink fruit juices increases five to twenty times when fluoridated water is used in processing. The fluoride content of infant cereals is influenced by the fluoride content of the water in which they were produced. Mechanically deboning meat increases the fluride content of the end products, because bone chips are incorporated during processing. Infant formula is no longer manufactured with fluoridated water.

Mottling and fluorosis of tooth enamel

When the fluoride concentrations of drinking water increase above 2 ppm, mottling (a brown stain on the teeth) during tooth development occurs. The incidence and severity of the manifestation increases as the fluoride content of the water increases. At levels of 8 ppm almost all individuals who consumed the water during tooth development have extensively mottled teeth.[67] In areas with a high natural concentration of fluoride, it has become a practice to dilute fluoride in water supply to no more than 1.2 ppm. In warmer climates and during periods of elevated environmental temperatures when the intakes of water are increased, suggested levels for fluoridation of water are 0.6 to 0.7 ppm.[68]

Fluorosis, usually manifested as opaque spots or streaks on the enamel of permanent teeth and not discernable by the layman, has been noted in 63% of children by the time they were 7 to 12 years of age in a community without fluoridated water when the use of fluoride supplements was common.[67] Leverett suggests that the definition of the optimum concentration of fluoride in community water supplies needs to be reassessed.

Remaining Trace Elements

The fact that only safe and adequate intakes have been recommended for the remaining trace minerals—copper, manganese, chromium, selenium, and molybdenum—indicates the lack of information necessary to define needs during the life cycle.

Less than adequate intake during infancy and childhood may occur in cases of generalized malnutrition or in infants maintained on low copper formulas. Infants and children who consume a variety of foods are likely to consume appropriate quantities of these nutrients.

VITAMINS

The function of vitamins in metabolic processes makes the requirement determined by intakes of energy, protein, and saturated fats. Exact needs are difficult to define.

Most vitamins cross the placenta and accumulate in the fetus at greater concentrations than in the mother. Maternal hypovitaminemia will be reflected in the fetus.

Vitamins A, E, and beta-carotene concentrations are lower in the newborn infant's blood than in the mother's. The concentration of water-soluble vitamins in the blood of the neonate is higher than in that of the mother.[69]

Fat-soluble vitamins in excess of need are not excreted but are stored. Reserves can be accumulated. The **toxicity** of excessive intakes of vitamins A and D is well documented.

In contrast to vitamins A, D, E, and K, the water-soluble vitamins are stored in small amounts and deficiencies can be expected to occur in a relatively short period if the nutrient is absent from dietary intake.

Fat Soluble Vitamins

Recommendations for intakes of vitamin A are interpolated from infant and adult needs.[70] Although 100 international units (IU) per day of vitamin D prevents rickets and ensures adequate absorption of calcium and normal mineralization of bone in the infant, better calcium absorption and some increase in growth has been noted with intakes of 400 IU/day. Vitamin D can be formed by the action of sunlight on the skin. The amount formed depends on several variables, and amounts formed cannot be readily measured.

Defining appropriate intakes for vitamin E is complicated by large variations in the susceptibility to peroxidation of fatty acids in the diet and tissues. Also, large losses occur in producing products that provide vitamin E.[71] Requirements are related to the polyunsaturated fatty acid content of cellular structures. An assumption is made that requirements increase with body weight until maturity. An intake of 5 IU at 9 kg increasing to 12 IU at 40 kg of body weight should be satisfactory in diets providing 4% to 7% of kilocalories as linoleic acid.

Newborns have low stores of vitamin E. If an adequate supply is not provided, a deficiency characterized by hemolytic anemia will occur. Their diets should include 1 mg of tocopherol per gram of polyunsaturated fatty acids.[71]

Water Soluble Vitamins

Requirements for thiamine and riboflavin are related to energy intake. Studies suggest that the minimum requirement of thiamine of infants is approximately 0.27 mg/1000 kcal.[72] One study indicated that 3 mg/1000 kcal was adequate for preadolescent children.[73] Another study of 14- to 17-year-old males indicated that 0.38 ± 0.059 mg/1000 kcal[74] meets their minimum requirement. An intake of 0.4 mg/1000 kcal has been suggested with the provision that no less than 0.89 mg/day be consumed by adolescent males.[71]

Urinary excretion of riboflavin is low in adults and in children maintained on diets containing up to 0.5 mg/1000 kcal; it increases as riboflavin intakes increase up to 0.75 mg/1000 kcal.[75] The minimum requirement is thought to be 0.85 mg/day.[71]

The fact that tryptophan is converted to niacin makes basic requirements for niacin difficult to determine. Minimum requirements appear to be 4.4 mg/1000 kcal.[71]

The recommended intake of vitamin B_6 for infants is based on experience with proprietary formulas. An intake of 1.4 gm of B_6 with an intake of 60 gm of protein should be adequate. Two gram/day is considered a generous intake for adolescents.[71]

The requirement for folacin in infancy has been estimated to be 5 μg/kg of body weight.[76] For older children and adults, folacin needs are extrapolated from those of infants. Herbert believes 3.6 μg/kg an adequate intake from birth to 1.9 years, and 3 μg/kg is adequate for older children and adolescents.[76]

The B_{12} allowance for infants is based on that in the milk of a lactating woman with adequate serum B_{12} and a margin of safety. For formula-fed infants, the Committee on Nutrition of the American Academy of Pediatrics[76b] recommends an intake of 0.15 μg/100 kcal.

Herbert recommends an intake of 0.3-0.5 μg/day in infancy with gradual increases based on body size to 2 μg/day in adolescents.[77]

An intake of 10mg/day of vitamin C is adequate to prevent and cure scurvy in humans. It does not, however, provide for acceptable reserves. Newborn infants consuming 7 to 12 mg of vitamin C have been protected from scurvy. An intake of 25 mg/day, 10 mg less than the 1980 RDA, should provide an adequate margin of safety.[78] In relation to body weight, the vitamin C requirement of older children is higher than that of adults. The recommended intake increases after age 18 to 30 mg/day for females, 40 mg/day for males.[78]

Food Sources

Vitamins reported to be most often consumed in less than appropriate amounts by preschool and school-age children are vitamins A, C, B_6, and riboflavin. Food sources of these vitamins are given in Tables 2-18 through 2-21. Because goat's milk is folate deficient, attention must be given to that vitamin if infants are fed goat's milk.

Vitamin Supplements

A prophylactic intramuscular dose of 0.5 to 1 mg of vitamin K or an oral dose of 1 to 2.1 mg of vitamin K is usually given to infants at birth as a protection against hemorrhagic disease of the newborn.[79] After receiving this dose, human beings are able to synthesize vitamin K from the bacteria in their gut. Vitamin K supplement is needed only for children who malabsorb fat.

The importance of appropriate vitamin supplementation of breast-fed infants is discussed in Chapter 4. After infancy, the percentage of children who are given vitamin supplements declines; however, over half of preschool and school-age children receive multi-vitamin-mineral preparations.[80]

Because Cook and Payne[80] found the use of vitamin supplements significantly increased the

Table 2-18   Selected foods as sources of vitamin A

Food	Household Measure	Vitamin A (IU)
Cow's milk	8 oz	350
Human milk	8 oz	560
Cheddar cheese	1 oz	370
Egg	1 medium	520
Liver, beef	1 oz	15,112
Liver, chicken	1 liver	3080
Liverwurst	1 slice, $\frac{1}{3}$ oz	650
Butter	1 tsp	160
Apricots, canned	$\frac{1}{4}$ cup	1125
Orange	1 medium	280
Peach	1 medium	1330
Watermelon	$\frac{1}{2}$ cup diced	470
Carrots	$\frac{1}{4}$ cup	3808
Acorn squash	$\frac{1}{4}$ baked and mashed	718
Sweet potatoes, mashed	$\frac{1}{4}$ cup	5038
Green peas	$\frac{1}{4}$ cup	280
Spinach	$\frac{1}{4}$ cup cooked	3645
Tomatoes, canned	$\frac{1}{4}$ cup	542

From Adams, C.F.: Nutritive value of American foods in common units, Agriculture Handbook No. 456, Washington D.C., 1975, U.S. Department of Agriculture.

Table 2-19   Selected food sources of vitamin C

Food	Household Measure	Vitamin C (mg)
Human milk	8 oz	16
Cow's milk	8 oz	2
Broccoli	1 spear	22
Brussels sprouts	$\frac{1}{4}$ cup	31
Cabbage, raw, chopped	$\frac{1}{4}$ cup	11
Cabbage, cooked, wedge	$\frac{1}{4}$ cup	10
Cantaloupe, diced	$\frac{1}{2}$ cup	27
Grapefruit	$\frac{1}{2}$	37
Orange	1 medium	66
Orange juice	$\frac{1}{2}$ cup	62
Potato, boiled ($2\frac{1}{2}$ inch)	$\frac{1}{2}$	11
Strawberries	1 cup	88
Tomato, raw, ($2\frac{1}{8}$ inch)	1	42
Tomatoes, canned	$\frac{1}{2}$ cup	20
Tomato juice	$\frac{1}{2}$ cup	20

From Adams, C.F.: Nutritive value of American foods in common units, Agriculture Handbook No. 456, Washington D.C., 1975, U.S. Department of Agriculture.

Table 2-20 Foods as sources of riboflavin

Food	Household Measure	Riboflavin (mg)
Human milk	8 oz	0.08
Cow's milk	8 oz	0.41
Prepared infant formula	8 oz	1.48-2.80
Cheddar cheese	1 oz	0.13
Infant cereals, high protein	1 tbsp	0.06
Infant cereals, rice	1 tbsp	0.06
Farina	$\frac{1}{2}$ cup	0.035
Oatmeal	$\frac{1}{2}$ cup	0.025
Macaroni, enriched	$\frac{1}{4}$ cup	0.03
Liver, beef	1 oz	1.18
Liver, chicken	1 liver	0.67
Broccoli	1 spear	0.03
Green peas	$\frac{1}{4}$ cup	0.03
Spinach	$\frac{1}{4}$ cup	0.06

From Adams, C.F.: Nutritive value of American foods in common units, Agriculture Handbook No. 456, Washington D.C., 1975, U.S. Department of Agriculture.

percentage of second and sixth grade children who meet 67% of the RDA compared with nonsupplemented children, they consider vitamin supplementation advisable.

Farris and others studied 158 10- to 13-year-old children and found that 0.5% to 0.75% of the children had never taken vitamin supplements. At age 13 years, 12% of the children were taking supplements. Children who could benefit most from supplements were not taking them. Those taking supplements often had dietary intakes that met the RDA from food alone.[81] Breskin noted no significant differences in biochemical indices with the exception of RBC folate of children who consumed supplements compared with those who did not, even though mean intakes of vitamin B_6 of the nonsupplemented group were 30% below the RDA. Many of the nonsupplemented children did not ingest two thirds of the RDA of folate. All values were in the normal range of accepted standards.[82]

The Committee on Nutrition of the American Academy of Pediatrics[79] has defined four groups of children who are at particular risk and for whom vitamin supplementation may be appropriate: children from deprived families, especially those who suffer from parental neglect or abuse; children who have **anorexia**, poor and capricious appetites, poor eating habits, and who are on regimens to manage obesity; pregnant teenagers; and children who consume **vegan** diets.

Vitamin supplementation of diets of older children should be recommended only after careful evaluation of food intake. Diets of children who restrict their intake of milk because of real or imagined allergies, lactose intolerance, or for psychosocial reasons should be monitored for riboflavin and vitamin D. Diets of infants and children receiving goat's milk should be carefully monitored for food sources of folacin. Diets of children who consume limited amounts of fruits and vegetables should be checked for sources of vitamins A and C.

Vitamin supplements, especially those that are colored and sugar coated, should be stored in places inaccessible to young children.

Table 2-21   Selected food sources of vitamin B$_6$

Food	Household Measure	Vitamin B$_6$ (mg)
Cow's milk	1 cup	0.1
Human milk	1 cup	0.02
Infant cereals, high protein	1 tbsp	0.01
Infant cereals, rice	1 tbsp	0.007
Infant dinners, split peas and bacon	1 oz	0.014
Infant dinners, vegetables and liver	1 oz	0.036
Strained beef	1 oz	0.056
Strained liver	1 oz	0.227
Beef liver, uncooked	$3\frac{1}{2}$ oz	0.84
Chicken liver, uncooked	$3\frac{1}{2}$ oz	0.75
Beef, uncooked	$3\frac{1}{2}$ oz	0.33
Chicken canned	1 oz	0.084
Peanut butter	1 tbsp	0.053
Egg	1 medium	0.055
Whole wheat bread	1 slice	0.05
White bread	1 slice	0.011
Green peas, canned	$\frac{1}{4}$ cup	0.008
Tomatoes, canned	$\frac{1}{4}$ cup	0.054
Squash, frozen	$\frac{1}{4}$ cup	0.055
Banana	1 small	0.71
Orange juice	$\frac{1}{2}$ cup	0.05
Strawberries	$\frac{1}{2}$ cup	0.040

Adapted from Orr, M.L.: Pantothenic acid, vitamin B$_6$ and vitamin B$_{12}$ in foods, Home Economics Research Report No. 36, Washington, D.C., 1969, U.S. Department of Agriculture.

Summary

The nutrient needs of individual children vary at any age depending on body size, patterns of activity, and rates of growth. They are greatest per unit of body size in infancy and decline with age.

The recommended dietary intakes during childhood are extrapolated from needs of infants and adult males or are calculated on the basis of presumed energy or protein intake. Intakes of individual children should be evaluated not in relation to the total amounts listed on the RDA chart but on the same basis the RDA was calculated.

Studies indicate that intakes of protein are generally adequate in North America. Nutrients most likely to be consumed in low or deficient amounts are calcium, iron, and vitamins A and C.

Children at risk for nutrient inadequacies are those from deprived families; those who have an excessive appetite, poor eating habits, or anorexia, or those on regimens to manage obesity; pregnant teenagers; and those who consume vegan diets.

SUGGESTED LEARNING ACTIVITIES

1. Calculate the energy intake of two children of the same age and sex whose heights are in

the 10th and 90th percentile. Compare this with the RDA on the basis of total calories, calories per kilogram, and calories per centimeter.

2. Calculate the grams of protein provided by a preschool and a school lunch. What percentage of the RDA does this provide?

3. Discuss the bioavailability of iron and zinc in foods acceptable to preschool children. How can one ensure an adequate intake?

4. Compare the content of a popular children's vitamin-mineral supplement with an adult vitamin-mineral supplement.

5. Compare the cost of the vitamins available in drug stores, health food stores, or sold door-to-door by individuals.

6. Compare the cost of meeting the RDA for vitamins with food or with vitamin-mineral supplementation.

REFERENCES

1. Food and Nutrition Board: Recommended dietary allowances, rev. ed. 10, Washington, D.C., 1989, National Academy of Sciences, National Research Council.

2. Ashworth, A., and Millward, D.J.: Catch-up growth in children, Nutr. Rev. 44:157, 1986.

3. Spady, D.W.: Total daily energy expenditure of healthy, free ranging school children, Am. J. Clin. Nutr. 33:766, 1980.

4. Butte, N.F., and others: Human milk intake and growth in exclusively breast-fed infants. Pediatr 104:187, 1984.

5. Adair, L.I.: The infant's ability to self regulate calorie intake: a case study, J. Amer. Diet. Assoc. 85:543, 1987.

6. Food and nutrient intakes of individuals in 1 day in the United States, Spring, 1977, U.S.D.A. Nationwide Food Consumption Survey, 1977-1978, Preliminary Rep. No. 2, Washington, D.C., 1980, Science and Education Administration.

7. White House Conference on Child Health and Protection: Growth and development of the child. III. Nutrition. Report of the Committee on Growth and Development, New York, 1932, Century House, Inc.

8. Holt, L.E., Jr., and Snyderman, S.E.: The amino acid requirements of infants, J.A.M.A. 175:100, 1961.

9. Fomon, S.J., and others: Requirements for protein and essential amino acids in early infancy, Acta Paediatr. Scand. 62:33, 1973.

10. Fomon, S.J., and Filer, L.J.: Amino acid requirements for normal growth. In Nythan, W.L., editor: Amino acid metabolism and genetic variations, New York, 1967, McGraw-Hill Book Co.

11. Report of a Joint FAO/WHO Ad Hoc Expert Committee: Energy and protein requirements, World Health Organization Technical Series No. 522, FAO Nutr. Meet. Ser. No. 52, Geneva, 1973, World Health Organization.

12. Nakagawa, I., and others: Amino acid requirements of children: nitrogen balance of the minimal level of essential amino acids, J. Nutr. 83:115, 1964.

13. Lozy, M., and Hegsted, D.M.: Calculation of the amino acid requirements of children at different ages by the factorial method, Am. J. Clin. Nutr. 28:1052, 1975.

14. Abernathy, R.P., and Ritchey, S.J.: Position paper on RDA for protein for children, Adv. Med. Biol. 105:1, 1978.

15. Committee on Nutrition, American Academy of Pediatrics: Commentary on breastfeeding and infant formula, Pediatrics 57:278, 1976.

16. John, T.J., and others: Kwashiorkor not associated with poverty, Pediatrics 90:730, 1977.

17. Chase, H.P., and others: Kwashiorkor in the United States, Pediatrics 66:972, 1980.

18. Holman, R.J., Caster, W.O., and Weise, H.F.: The essential fatty acid requirement of infants and the assessment of their dietary intake of linoleate by serum fatty acid analysis, Am. J. Clin. Nutr. 14:70, 1964.

19. Fomon, S.J.: Infant nutrition, ed. 2, Philadelphia, 1974, W.B. Saunders Co.

20. Committee on Nutrition, American Academy of Pediatrics: Plant fiber intake in the pediatric diet, Pediatrics 67:572, 1981.

21. Maller, O., and Desor, J.A.: Effect of taste on ingestion by human newborns. In Bosma, J.F., editor: Oral sensation and perception, Publication No. (NIH) 73-546, Bethesda, Md., 1973, Department of Health, Education and Welfare.

22. Hey, E.N., and Katz, G.: Evaporative water loss in the newborn baby, J. Physiol. 200:605, 1969.

23. Ziegler, E.E., and Fomon, S.J.: Fluid intake, renal solute load, and water balance in infancy, J. Pediatr. 78:561, 1971.

24. Stolley, H., and Schlage, C.: Water balance and water requirement of preschool children, Nutr. Metab. 21 (suppl. 1):15-17, 1977.

25. Arnaud, S.B., and others: Serum parathyroid hormone and blood minerals: interrelationships in normal children, Pediatr. Res. 7:485, 1973.

26. Committee on Nutrition, American Academy of Pediatrics: Calcium requirements in infancy and childhood, Pediatrics 62:826, 1978.

27. Shaw, J.C.L.: Evidence for defective skeletal mineralization in low birth weight infants: the absorption of calcium and fat, Pediatrics 57:16, 1976.

28. Garn, S.M.: The earlier gain and the later loss of cortical bone in nutritional perspective, Springfield, Ill., 1970, Charles C. Thomas, Publisher.

29. Christiansen, C., Rödbro, P., and Neilsen, C.T.: Bone mineral content and estimated total body calcium in normal children and adolescents, Scand. J. Clin. Lab. Invest. 35:507, 1975.

30. Trotter, M., and Hixon, B.B.: Sequential changes in weight, density, and percentage ash weight of human skeleton from the early fetal period through old age, Anat. Rec. 179:1, 1974.

31. Leitch, I., and Aitken, F.C.: The estimation of calcium requirements: a re-examination, Nutr. Abstr. Rev. 29:393, 1959.

32. Kooh, S.W., and others: Rickets due to calcium deficiency, N. Engl. J. Med. 297:1264, 1977.

33. Marie, P.J., and others: Histological osteomalacia due to dietary calcium deficiency in children, New Engl. J. Med. 307:584, 1982.

34. Sheikh, M.S., and others: Gastrointestinal absorption of calcium from milk and calcium salts. New Eng. J. Med. 317:532, 1987.

35. David, L., and Anast, C.S.: Calcium metabolism in newborn infants, the interrelationship of parathyroid function and calcium, magnesium, and phosphorus metabolism in normal, "sick," and hypocalcemic newborns, J. Clin. Invest. 54:287, 1974.

36. Snodgrass, G.J.A.I., and others: Interrelations of plasma calcium, inorganic phosphate, magnesium, and protein over the first week of life, Arch. Dis. Child, 48:279, 1973.

37. Schedewh, H.K., and others: Parathormone and perinatal calcium homeostasis, Pediatr. Res. 13:1, 1979.

38. Salle, B.L.: Prevention of early neonatal hypocalcemia in low birth weight infants with continuous calcium infusion: effect on serum calcium, phosphorus, magnesium, and circulating immunoreactive parathyroid hormone and calcitonin, Pediatr. Res. 11:1180, 1977.

39. Gittleman, I.F., and Pincus, J.B.: Influence of diet on the occurrence of hyperphosphatemia and hypocalcemia in the newborn infant, Pediatrics 8:778, 1951.

40. Gardner, L.: Tetany and parathyroid hyperplasia in the newborn infant: influences of dietary phosphate load, Pediatrics 9:534, 1952.

41. Pierson, J.D., and Crawford, J.D.: Dietary dependent neonatal hypocalcemia, Am. J. Dis. Child. 123:472, 1972.

42. Harris, I., and Wilkinson, A.W.: Magnesium depletion in children, Lancet 2:735, 1971.

43. Barness, L.A.: Nutrition and nutritional disorders. In Behrman, R.E., Vaughan, V.C. and Nelson, W.E., editors: Nelson's textbook of pediatrics, ed. 13. Philadelphia, 1987, W.B. Saunders Co.

44. Fomon, S.J.: Reflections on infant feeding in the 1970s and 1980s, Amer. J. Clin. Nutr. 46:171, 1987.

45. Herbert, V.: Recommended dietary intakes (RDI) of iron in humans, Amer. J. Clin. Nutr. 45:679, 1987.

46. Hallberg, L., and others: Menstrual blood loss— a population study, Acta Obstet. Gynecol. Scand. 45:320, 1966.

47. Monsen, E.R., and others: Estimation of available dietary iron, Am. J. Clin. Nutr. 31:134, 1978.

48. McMillan, J.A.: Iron absorption from human milk, simulated human milk, and proprietary formulas, Pediatrics 60:896, 1977.

49. Cullen, R.W., and Oace, S.M.: Iodine: current status, J. Nutr. Educ. 8:101. 1976.

50. Widdowson, E.M.: Chemical analysis of the body. In Brozek, J., editor: Human body composition, Oxford, 1965, Pergamon Press, Ltd.

51. Krebs, N.F., and Hambidge, K.M.: Zinc requirements and zinc intakes of breast-fed infants, Amer. J. Clin. Nutr. 43:288, 1986.

52. Hambidge, K.M., and others: Low levels of zinc in hair, anorexia, poor growth, and hypogeusia in children, Pediatr. Res. 6:868, 1972.

53. Hambidge, K.M., and others: Zinc nutrition of preschool children in the Denver Headstart Program, Am. J. Clin. Nutr. 29:734, 1976.

54. Vanderkooy, P.D.S. and Gibson, R.S.: Food consumption patterns of Canadian preschool children in relation to zinc and growth status, Amer. J. Clin. Nutr. 45:609, 1987.

55. MacDonald, L.D., Gibson, R.S., and Miles, J.E.: Changes in hair zinc and copper concentrations of breast fed and bottle fed infants during the first six months, Acta Paediatr. Scand. 71:785, 1982.

56. Butrimovitz, G.P., and Purdy, W.C.: Zinc nutrition and growth in children, Am. J. Clin. Nutr. 31:1409, 1978.

57. Cavell, P.A., and Widdowson, E.M.: Intakes and excretions of iron, copper and zinc in the neonatal period, Arch. Dis. Child. 39:496, 1964.

58. Schlage, C., and Wortberg, B.: Zinc in the diet of healthy preschool and school children, Acta Paediatr. Scand. 61:421, 1972.

59. Engel, R.W., Miller, R.F., and Price, N.O.: Metabolic patterns of preadolescent children. XIII. Zinc balance. In Prasad, A.S., editor: Zinc metabolism, Springfield, Ill., 1966, Charles C. Thomas, Publisher.

60. Tribble, H. M., and Scoular, F. I.: Zinc metabolism of young college women on self-selected diets, J. Nutr. 52:209, 1954.

61. Picciano, M.F., and Guthrie, H.A.: Copper, iron, and zinc contents of mature human milk, Am. J. Clin. Nutr. 29:242, 1976.

62. Johnson, P.E., and Evans, G.W.: Relative zinc availability in human milk, infant formulas, and cow's milk, Am. J. Clin. Nutr. 31:416, 1978.

63. Dean, H.T., Arnold, F.A., and Elvove, E.: Domestic water and dental caries. V. Additional studies of the relation of fluoride domestic water to dental experience in 4425 white children, Public Health Rep. 57:1155, 1942.

64. Committee on Nutrition, American Academy of Pediatrics: Flouride supplementation: revised dosage schedule, Pediatrics 63:150, 1979.

65. Dirks, O.B., and others: Total and free ionic fluoride in human and cow's milk as determined by gas-liquid chromatography and the flouride electrode, Caries Res. 8:181, 1974.

66. Singer, L., Ophaug, R.H., and Harland, B.F.: Dietary fluoride intakes of 15 to 19 year old males residing in the United States. J. Dent. Res. 64:1302, 1985.

67. Leverett, D.H.: Fluorides and the changing prevalance of dental caries, Science 217:26, 1982.

68. Galagan, D.J., and Vermillion, J.R.: Determining optimum fluoride concentrations, Public Health Rep. 72:491, 1957.

69. Baker, H., and others: Vitamin profile of 174 mothers and newborns at parturition, Am. J. Clin. Nutr. 28:59, 1975.

70. Olson, J.A.: Recommended dietary intakes of vitamin A in humans, Amer. J. Clin. Nutr. 45:704, 1987.

71. Horwitt, M.K.: Interpretations of requirements for thiamin, riboflavin, niacin, tryptophan, and vitamin E plus comments on balance studies and vitamin B_6, Amer. J. Clin. Nutr. 44:973, 1986.

72. Knott, E.M., Kleiger, S.C., and Schultz, F.W.: Is breast milk adequate in meeting thiamine requirements in infants? J. Pediatr. 22:43, 1943.

73. Boyden, R.F., and Erikson, S.E.: Metabolic patterns of preadolescent children: thiamine utilization in relation to nitrogen intake, Amer. J. Clin. Nutr. 19:398, 1966.

74. Dick, E.C., and others: Thiamine requirement of eight adolescent boys, as estimated from urinary thiamine excretion, J. Nutr. 66:173, 1958.

75. Sebrell, W.H., and others: Human riboflavin requirement estimated by urinary excretion of subjects on controlled intake, U.S. Public Health Rep. 56:510, 1941.

76. Herbert, V.: Recommended dietary intakes (RDI) of folate in humans, Amer. J. Clin. Nutr. 45:661, 1987.

76b. Committee on Nutrition, American Academy of Pediatrics: Commentary on breast-feeding and infant formulas, including proposed standards for formulas, Pediatrics 57:279, 1976.

77. Herbert, V.: Recommended dietary intakes (RDI) of vitamin B_{12} in humans, Amer. J. Clin. Nutr. 45:671, 1987.

78. Olson, J.A., and Hodges, R.E.: Recommended dietary intakes (RDI) of vitamin C in humans, Amer. J. Clin. Nutr. 45:693, 1987.

79. Committee on Nutrition, American Academy of Pediatics: Vitamin and mineral supplement needs in normal children in the United States, Pediatrics 66:1015, 1980.

80. Cook, C.C., and Payne, I.R.: Effect of supplements on the nutrient intake of children, J. Am. Diet. Assoc. 74:130, 1979.

81. Farris, R.P. and others: Dietary studies of children from a biracial population: intakes of vitamins in 10- and 13- year olds. J. Amer. College Nutr. 4:539, 1985.

82. Breskin, M.W., and others: Water soluble vitamins: intakes and indices in children, J. Am. Diet. Assoc. 85:49, 1985.

3

Collecting and Assessing Food Intake Information

Peggy L. Pipes
Judith Bumbalow
Robin Pritkin Glass

OBJECTIVES

After studying this chapter, the student should:

1. Be cognizant of all of the information that needs to be collected for a comprehensive evaluation of infants' and children's food intake.

2. Be able to select the appropriate dietary methodology for any particular case or setting.

3. Recognize the advantages and limitations of the various approaches to evaluating dietary intake.

4. Be able to appropriately screen children who need evaluation of motor and psychosocial parameters that affect food intake.

5. Be aware of the advantages and limitations of computer programs designed to calculate nutrient intake.

Nutrition screening, evaluation, counseling, and education have become integral parts of many health care, public health, and supplemental food programs that provide services to infants and children. In addition, children perceived as having feeding problems, those who must consume therapeutic diets, and those whose parents are concerned about the adequacy of their food intakes are frequently referred to a program for a team management approach. Plans for modifying food intake in childhood should be based on information more comprehensive than that which identifies excesses or deficits in energy and nutrient intakes and cultural food practices. Health care professionals must work jointly to synthesize information and establish programs that can be carried out by children or their parents. Goals for change in food intake should be identified and periodically reassessed. It is imperative therefore that health care professionals recognize the necessity of accurate data collection in relation to the nutrient intake from the food consumed, the developmental level of feeding behavior (oral motor screening), psychosocial issues that affect behavior, and mother-child interactions that affect food and nutrient intake.

It is important to recognize that an assessment of food intake is not an **assessment** of nutritional status. The latter requires anthropometric data and biochemical and clinical evaluations as well as dietary intake data. Adequately collected food intake data can, however, provide information on which judgements of the adequacy of a child's current food intake can be made and plans for resolving concerns of food and nutrient intake can be designed and assessed. It is important for individuals who collect this information to be aware of the variety of methods of collecting food intake information and to develop skills for screening oral motor difficulties of feeding and psychosocial factors that compromise a child's nutrient intake.

TOOLS FOR COLLECTING DIETARY INTAKE DATA

Health care professionals in clinical settings use a variety of tools for collecting dietary data, each tool having limitations and varying degrees of reliability. The choice of tool depends on the purpose of the interview, the time commitment of the professional, and the cooperation of the child or parents. Information sought will vary with the problem. For example, detailed documentation of an early feeding history may be important for counseling parents of young children with feeding problems, whereas this would be inappropriate if the patient were an obese adolescent. Only one tool will be used in some instances, whereas a combination of tools is appropriate at other times. It is important to recognize that valid methods for assessing the dietary intake of groups differ from those designed to collect information on one child for whom plans for nutrition education and counseling

are to be developed. The tools most often used in the clinical setting are the 24-hour recall, the dietary history, and the 3- and 7-day food records. Food frequencies have been considered to be applicable in come circumstances.

The interview is the most important aspect of any of the tools used, the validity of the information obtained being dependent on the client's understanding of the reasons for the interview and the information sought, the client's comfort with the interviewer, and the interviewer's skills at probing for and validating information. Whether the child or parents should be interviewed depends on several developmental and psychosocial factors. Beal found that with few exceptions girls under 12 years of age and boys under 13 to 14 years of age were unlikely to give reliable nutrition histories.[1] However, if there is considerable conflict between a preadolescent and the parents about food intake, it may be important to interview the child both individually and with the parents so that an appropriate counseling relationship can be established.

It must be remembered that assessment data is only as valid as the child's or parents' willingness to share information with the interviewer. It is important that they feel comfortable with the interview and the individual conducting the assessment. The interviewer should give a friendly greeting, a clear definition of the purpose of the interview, and the reasons for the questions asked, which aid in establishing rapport with the client. Providing an adequate diet for children is a very important aspect of parenting. Parents may feel threatened when questioned about a child's food intake. In addition, the interviewer must have reasonable expectations for the respondent. The parent of several children cannot be expected to give information as precisely for one child as does a parent who devotes his or her time to an only child. A number of meals or snacks may be consumed outside the home in a day-care center or at school, and parents may not know what children receive in these settings.

During the interview the interviewer must be careful to avoid suggesting time, meals, food, or amounts consumed. For example, the question "When does your child first have something to eat or to drink?" is appropriate, whereas the question "When does your child first eat breakfast?" is inappropriate. The tone of voice is also important. Neither approval nor disapproval should be expressed verbally or nonverbally by facial expression. Food preferences of the interviewer should never be indicated. Silences must be accepted with comfort, and parents should be permitted time to formulate answers to questions and to ask questions of their own.

24-Hour Recall

The most common method used for collecting dietary data to characterize the nutrient intake of populations is the 24-hour recall, often used in combination with 1-, 3-, or 7-day food records. The 24-hour recall has also been used successfully to screen children at nutritional risk and can give some indication as to compliance with a dietary regimen during clinical follow-up. It cannot be substituted for more intensive methods when judgments regarding the adequacy of an individual child's food intake are to be made.

Parents or the child are asked to relate every food in portion sizes that the child has consumed for the past 24 hours. Errors in the 24-hour recall have been reported to result from inability of the parents or children to remember exactly what was eaten, difficulties in estimating portion sizes, and lack of commitment of the individual who is being interviewed.[2] Often, parents are not aware of the foods consumed between meals. There is no assurance that the recall of the day selected is typical of other days. The accuracy with which portion sizes are reported can be increased by the use of food models and by skillful probing.

Klesges and others found that parental reports of 24-hour intakes of 24- to 48-month-old children correlated highly with weighed food intake.[3] However, Todd, Hudes, and Calloway[2] compared the 24-hour recall and 30-day recorded food intakes by graduate students and found that a single recall did not give an accurate assessment of the intake for that day or for the 30-day mean. There was, however, no consistent bias. Some subjects overestimated their intake, and others underestimated it.

Self-Administered Workbooks

In an effort to find a cost effective approach to collecting nutrient intakes of groups of children, Farris and others compared a self-administered workbook with the 24-hour recalls of 10- to 18-year-old children.[4]

When the workbook was completed by the children after instruction on how to record food intake, it was found that the evening meal accounted for the greatest difference in recorded intake between the two methods. The workbook method yielded higher intakes of energy, protein, carbohydrates and cholesterol than did the 24-hour recall. Omitted foods and inaccurate portion size were the reasons for differences.

The workbook method is considered effective only when studies with a large sample size are made.[4]

3- and 7-Day Food Records

The 3- or 7-day food record or a written diary of all food and beverages consumed is a tool commonly used to characterize current intakes of individual children (see Food Diary for Children, p. 62, and Food Diary for Infants, p. 61). Parents are instructed to measure or weigh portions of food offered and amounts not eaten and record the amounts consumed. Parents report that measuring and weighing pose no problems but that they find the rigidity of recording each time the child eats difficult. Sometimes they forget foods that are added to other foods; for example, catsup,

Food Diary for Infants
(Birth to 1 year)

Instructions

1. Record *all* formula, milk, and food that the baby consumes immediately *after* each feeding.
2. If your baby is breast-fed, record the time of day the baby is fed and how long the baby feeds.
3. If your baby is formula-fed, record the time of day the baby eats, the kind of formula the baby is fed, and the amount actually consumed.

   Infant formula preparation:

   Is the formula iron fortified?

   ☐ Yes   ☐ No

   Formula (brand name): _____

   _____oz liquid *or*

   _____tbsp powder

   Water

   _____oz

   Other (describe): _____

   _____oz

   _____tbsp

   Total prepared formula

   _____oz

4. If the baby spits up or vomits, estimate the amount.
5. Measure the amounts of any other foods carefully in terms of ounces of liquid (e.g., 2 oz apple juice), level tbsp (e.g., 2 tbsp dry rice cereal), or portions of commercially prepared or home prepared foods (e.g., $\frac{1}{2}$ of a 4.7 oz jar or level tablespoon of strained peaches).
6. Does the baby take a vitamin supplement? ☐ Yes   ☐ No

   If yes, what kind? _____

Day 1

Date _____ Day of week _____

Most recent weight _____ on (date) _____

Time	Food or Formula	Amount	Time	Food or Formula	Amount

Adapted from Food Diary for Infants used at the Child Development and Mental Retardation Center, University of Washington, Seattle, Wash.

Food Diary for Children

Instructions
1. Record all foods and beverages immediately after they are consumed.
2. Measure the amounts of each food carefully with standard measuring cups and spoons. Record meat portions in ounces or as fractions of pounds, e.g., 8 oz of milk; 1 medium egg; $\frac{1}{4}$ lb of hamburger; 1 slice of bread, white; $\frac{1}{2}$ of small banana.
3. Indicate method of preparation, e.g., medium egg, fried; $\frac{1}{2}$ cup baked beans with a 2-inch slice of salt pork; 4 oz of steak, broiled.
4. Be sure to record any condiments, gravies, salad dressings, butter, margarine, whipped cream, relishes, e.g., $\frac{3}{4}$ cup of mashed potatoes with 3 tbsp of brown gravy, $\frac{1}{4}$ cup of cottage cheese salad with 2 olives, $\frac{1}{2}$ cup of cornflakes with 1 tsp of sugar and $\frac{1}{3}$ cup of 2% milk.
5. Be sure to record all between-meal foods and drinks, e.g., coffee with 1 oz of cream, 12 oz of cola, 4 sugar cookies, 1 candy bar (indicate brand name).
6. If you eat away from home, please put an asterisk (*) in the food column beside the food listing.

Day 1
Date _____ Day of week _____ Weight _____

Time	Food	Amount	How Prepared

Adapted from Record of Food Intake used at the Child Development and Mental Retardation Center, University of Washington, Seattle, Wash.

butter, or jelly may be unintentionally omitted from the record. Therefore careful instruction as to how to record food intake is important.

McHenry, Ferguson, and Gurland[5] found that records covering less than 20 consecutive meals or 7 days may not provide valid information.

Stuff and others[6] compared 1-, 3-, and 7-day records of food intake with food frequency records and found the 3-day records did not provide good individual estimates of nutrient intake compared with 7-day records but did provide an estimate of the general quality of the diet.

A study comparing calculated nutrient intake of weighed and estimated portion size recorded in food diaries found intraindividual variations smaller for weighed food records than diary estimates. However, weighing food was reported to be tedious for the client and expensive for the investigator, who provided scales.[2] The provision of cassette recorders, which made it possible for individuals to record their intake on tape, seems to have alleviated some of this difficulty in the study with graduate students.[2]

Dietary History

Another method to review dietary intake in retrospect is the research dietary history method developed by Burke[7] and modified and redescribed by Beal.[1] During an interview the investigator obtains an estimate of the frequency and amounts of food and nutrient supplements consumed in a specified period, usually 1 to 6 months. Parents are questioned about the child's food likes and dislikes. If parent-child interaction or early feeding experiences are suspected to be factors in the nutrition concern, information is elicited on the early feeding history. The interview is often cross-checked with a 24-hour recall and/or 3-day record of food consumed.

This method requires a skilled interviewer. The dietitian or nutritionist must gain the confidence of the parent or child, make good estimates, and judge if the answers are reliable. The process is time consuming and cannot be adequately completed in less than 1 hour. The finding that dietary histories administered to 5-, 9- and 13-year-old children could not be replicated is not surprising in view of previous studies, and it emphasizes the need to include parents in obtaining food intake information for young children.[8]

Several researchers have cautioned against using this tool as the sole source of data. Huenemann and Turner[9] compared the research-type dietary history with 10- to 14-day weighed food records for a group of subjects 6 to 16 years of age and found that no history agreed within 20% for all constituents; the greatest deviations were for vitamins A and D, calories, riboflavin, and thiamine. Other investigators compared dietary histories with 7-day food records and 24-hour recalls and found that dietary histories gave distinctly higher values than 7-day food records and 24-hour recalls for groups.[10] Trulson[11] compared 7-day food records, an average of three or more 24-hour recalls, and dietary histories of clinic patients 7 to 12 years of age. She found no proof that one method was more reliable than another, but she preferred the interview method since it might reveal long-range dietary practices. The 7-day food records and detailed dietary histories gave results showing closest similarity, but findings were not consistent.

Food Frequency Questionnaires

Several researchers have developed food frequency questionnaires. Clients are asked to estimate the portion size and frequency with which they currently consume specified foods and mixed dishes. Since the format is computer compatible, it can be keypunched and calculations quickly returned.

Abramson, Slome, and Kosovsky[12] found the food frequency questionnaire was a simple and economical method of detecting differences in the usual diet patterns among groups. Stuff and others[6] found that this method provided estimates of intake higher than the 7-day food record.

When collecting food intake information the interviewer must keep in mind that dietary history and food frequency methods yield higher intakes than 3- or 7-day food intake records. Using both the dietary history and a record of food intake is likely to add credibility to the assessment. The interviewer must, however, recognize the life-style demands of the respondent and negotiate a reasonable approach for both the client and health care professional. It parents are literate, concerned, and motivated, they may be happy to keep the food records. Day-care workers and preschool teachers are generally very agreeable about keeping records. However, it may be necessary to accept a 3-day rather than a 7-day record from a working mother with a large family. If the parents clearly do not want to keep the diet diary, the interviewer must be satisfied with the dietary history but recognize its limitations.

ASSESSING DIETARY INTAKE INFORMATION

When the dietary intake information has been collected, the adequacy of nutrients in the foods consumed is assessed. The decisions of which method of evaluation should be used and which nutrients will be calculated are based on the precision and reliability of the information collected, the foods that appear in the dietary records, the interviewer's knowledge of foods as sources of nutrients, and the problem presented for evaluation.

In some instances intake data may be compared to food groups; other times, knowledge of foods that are present or absent in the dietary history as sources of nutrients may give sufficient indication of the presence or absence of problems of nutrient intake. If precise and complete information has been collected, hand or computer calculations of nutrients in the foods consumed may be compared with a standard.

When parents are unable or unwilling to give information that can be quantitated, such as when they report intake as bites of meat instead of one fourth of a 2 oz hamburger patty or when cross-checks reveal inconsistencies, the analysis of food groups or foods as sources of nutrients seems appropriate. However, if the child is underweight or overweight or if food sources of a particular nutrient appear on the record only occasionally, calculations of nutrient intake are important.

Computer Programs

A number of computer software programs for calculating nutrient intakes are commercially available. Each program has limitations and advantages. Programs vary in the number of foods (from 645 to 16,000) and the number of food constituents (from 1 to 56) listed. Not all values are provided for all foods. Most programs are not updated as frequently as new foods enter the market.[13] Periodic checks should be effected to assess the quality and comparability of the data base with other programs.[14]

Appropriate use of the programs requires coders who are well trained. This is usually not a problem. However, coder reliability should be evaluated periodically.

While these programs need care in selection, maintenance and periodic evaluation, they provide a time efficient way of making calculations once the evaluator learns to use the programs. A much larger number of nutrients can be calculated by computer than is possible by hand.

Evaluating Intake Information

When calculations are complete, the data must be compared with a standard. All formulated standards are intended to be used to interpret data on groups of people and are

Table 3-1 Computer report of one day's food intake*

Quantity	Food	Gram	Calorie (kc)	Calcium (mg)	Total Protein (gm)	Vit C (mg)	Vit B$_1$ (mg)	Niacin (mg)	Vit B$_2$ (mg)	Folic Acid (mg)	Vit A (IU)	Vit D (IU)	Fe (mg)
1 large	Egg, whole, hardboiled	50.0	79.0	28.1	6.1	0.0	0.0	0.0	0.1	0.0	260.0	‡	1.0
1 slice	White bread, enriched	25.0	67.5	21.0	2.2	0.0	0.1	0.8	0.0	0.0	0.0	‡	0.7
12 fl oz	Whole milk, fluid	366.0	224.9	437.0	12.0	3.4	0.1	0.3	0.6	0.0	461.20	150.1	0.2
0.25 cup	Rice, white enriched	51.25	55.9	5.1	1.0	0.0	0.1	0.5	0.0	‡	0.0	‡	0.5
1 NO (8/lb)	Frankfurter Oscar Mayer, cooked	57.0	182.4	4.6	6.3	16.5	0.2	1.4	0.1	0.0	0.0	22.8	0.5
1 cup	Orange juice, fresh	248.0	111.6	27.3	1.7	124.0	0.2	1.0	0.1	0.1	496.0	0.0	0.5
125 gm	Macaroni & cheese Stouffer's	125.0	201.2	175.0	8.4	‡	0.2	0.8	0.2	‡	255.0	‡	0.8
45 gm	Green beans, cut style canned solids drained	45.0	10.8	20.3	0.6	1.8	0.0	0.1	0.0	0.0	211.5	‡	0.7
35 gm	Chicken drumstick fried in veg. fat	35.0	85.8	4.2	9.4	0.0	0.0	2.1	0.1	0.0	29.4	‡	0.5
1	Tortilla, wheat baked/steamed	43.4	123.3	5.6	2.8	0.0	0.1	0.9	0.1	0.0	‡	‡	0.8
	TOTAL		1142.25	728.08	50.58	145.77	1.05	8.04	1.35	0.21	1713.06	172.86	6.03

*Data is for a 2-year-old female child with a height of 82.4 cm and weight of 14.5 kg.
†A dagger beside an amount indicates that the food database record used has no data for that nutrient.
‡A double dagger indicates there is no data on the item specified for that nutrient.

not intended to be used for evaluating the adequacy of nutrient intakes of individuals.

Many of the computer programs compare nutrient intake to the RDA. These allowances for children are generally based on studies of adults from which extrapolations were made for children. A margin of safety above the average requirement is applied to each nutrient. This margin is not standard but varies for each nutrient.

When interpreting the data one must be keenly aware of the **bioavailability** of the nutrients. In addition, changes in nutrient concentration of foods during storage and food preparation must be considered.[15]

Some programs define children at nutritional risk as those who consume less then two thirds or three fourths of the recommended daily dietary allowances of any nutrient and include these children and their families in intensive nutrition follow-up. It may also be important for these children to have a more intensive nutrition evaluation, including biochemical evaluation of their nutritional status.

Anthropometric measurements (height, weight, and fatfold measurements) can give indications of the appropriateness of the child's energy intake. If rates of weight gain are excessive or inadequate, calculations of the child's energy intake provide important data on which plans for adjustments in energy intake can be made.

SCREENING CHILDREN AT NUTRITIONAL RISK

The objective of screening is to identify infants and children who appear to have nutritional problems that require further investigation. The interview is brief and information sought is qualitative. It is often performed by paraprofessionals (e.g., community health workers, nutrition aides), nurses, or other professionals who assume the role of case manager. The 24-hour recall screening questionnaires or questionnaires filled out by parents may be used. (See Screening Questionnaire for Infants, pp. 67-68 and Screening Questionnaire for Young Children, pp. 69-70.)

Screening programs are designed to reach as many individuals as possible at a minimum cost. Adequately nourished individuals may be mistaken as at risk, however, this is acceptable, since many others who are not adequately nourished will be identified.

Anthropometric data plotted on growth grids are also used in screening. In general, when children's growth patterns plot at less than the 10th percentile, when they are underweight or overweight for their lengths (Chapter 1), or when interviews show patterns of intake that indicate a nutrient consumed in short supply, the children are referred for more intensive counseling.

From information on the screening questionnaire, parents of infants and children who need further evaluation or counseling can also be identified. A red flag could be rasied when the infant screening questionnaire indicates that an infant was offered overdiluted or underdiluted formulas, if homogenized milk was offered to infants under 6 months of age, or if nonfat or 2% milk was offered any time in the first year. Other infants who may be identified as at risk include those who receive semisolid foods before 4 months of age and those who are bottle fed as they go to sleep.

As the child ages, the quantity of milk consumed and the frequency with which the listed food groups are eaten can identify older children at risk.

All infants or children who require a modified diet to control chronic disease or whom parents perceive as having a feeding problem need further assessment.

DIETARY ASSESSMENT

Parents and children referred for intensive evaluation of nutrient and energy intake should anticipate a more extensive interview. Even so, the dietitian/nutritionist should carefully explain the purpose of the questions to be asked and reasons for continuing "how much" and

Screening Questionnaire for Infants

Infants (from birth to 1 year of age)	Yes	No
1. Is the baby breast fed?	☐	☐
If yes, does he/she also receive milk or formula?	☐	☐
If yes, what kind? _____		
2. Does the baby receive formula?	☐	☐

If yes ☐ Ready-to-feed
     ☐ Concentrated Liquid
     ☐ Other: _____

How is formula prepared (especially dilution)?

_____

	Yes	No
Is the formula iron fortified?	☐	☐
3. Does the baby drink milk?	☐	☐

If yes ☐ Whole milk
     ☐ 2%milk
     ☐ Skim milk
     ☐ Other: _____

4. How many times does he/she eat each day, including milk or formula? ___

	Yes	No
5. Does the baby usually take a bottle to bed?	☐	☐

If yes, what is usually in the bottle? _____

6. If the baby drinks milk or formula, what is the usual amount in a day?
☐ Less than 16 oz
☐ 16 to 32 oz
☐ More than 32 oz

7. Please indicate which (if any) of these foods the baby eats and how often:

	Never or hardly ever (less than once a week)	Sometimes (not daily but at least once a week)	Every day or nearly every day
Eggs	☐	☐	☐
Dried beans or peas	☐	☐	☐
Meat, fish, poultry	☐	☐	☐
Bread, rice, pasta, grits, cereal, tortillas, potatoes	☐	☐	☐
Fruits or fruit juices	☐	☐	☐
Vegetables	☐	☐	☐

8. If the baby eats fruits or drinks fruit juices every day or nearly every day, which ones does he/she eat or drink most often (not more than three)? _____

9. If the baby eats vegetables every day or nearly every day, which one does he/she eat most often (not more than three)? _____

Continued.

Screening Questionnaire for Infants—*cont'd*

10. Does the person who cares for the baby have use of a
    Stove?   □ □
    Refrigerator?   □ □
    Piped water?   □ □
11. Does the baby take vitamin or iron drops?   □ □
    If yes, how often? _____
    What kind? _____
12. Is the baby on a special diet now?   □ □
    If yes, what is the reason?
    Allergy—specify type of diet: _____
    Weight reduction—specify type of diet: _____
    Other—specify type of diet: _____
    Who recommended the diet? _____
13. Does the baby eat clay, paint chips, dirt, or anything else that is not   □ □
    usually considered food?
    If yes, what? _____
    How often? _____
14. Do you think the child has a feeding problem?   □ □
    If yes, describe: _____

From Fomon, S.J.: Nutritional disorders of children: prevention, screening, and follow-up, Publication No. 76-5612, Rockville, Md., 1976, Department of Health, Education, and Welfare.

"how often" questions. Decisions regarding which tool will be used may be made after the parents and/or children arrive and express their concern or lack of concern.

The dietary history, in combination with a 7-day food record, is the preferred tool currently available for dietary assessment in a clinical setting. These procedures require a skilled nutritionist and are costly in time, and not all parents and/or children can respond with validity even though they may wish to do so.

Some programs use a food frequency questionnaire and 24-hour recall, a method that requires less time and is less taxing on the client but yields less valid and less useful information.

During this interview the nutritionist collects information about family interactions that affect a child's food intake (e.g., family members present at mealtimes, the use of food as rewards), the food budget and money spent for food, the frequency with which family and children eat away from home, and the family's use of community resources that provide food or nutrition education (Figure 3-1).

The case of a 13-month-old girl referred for dietary assessment because of inadequate weight gain may clarify the process. The girl was the unplanned child of the second marriage of a couple who also had teenage children in their home. All medical reasons for failure to thrive had been ruled out. The interview with both father and mother proceeded as follows:

Interviewer: Let's begin with the early feeding history. Was the baby breast- or bottle-fed?
Mother: She was and still is breast-fed. I do not want her to drink formula or cow's milk. I have given her a little's goat's milk from a cup.
Interviewer: Did she have any problems sucking at the breast?
Mother: None at all until she was 6 months. Then she wouldn't take much at a time but wanted

Screening Questionnaire for Young Children

Preschool children and young school-age children   Yes   No

1. Does the child drink milk?   ☐   ☐
   If yes ☐ Whole milk
          ☐ 2% milk
          ☐ Skim milk
          ☐ Other: _____
   If yes, how much?
   ☐ Less than 8 oz
   ☐ 8 to 32 oz
   ☐ More than 32 oz
2. Does the child drink anything from a bottle (for children less than 4 years   ☐   ☐
   of age)?
   If yes ☐ Milk
          ☐ Other: _____
3. Does the child take a bottle to bed?   ☐   ☐
   If yes, what is usually in the bottle? _____
4. How many times a day does the child usually eat (including snacks)? _____
5. Please indicate which (if any) of these foods the child eats and how often:

	Never or hardly ever (less than once a week)	Sometimes (not daily but at least once a week)	Every day or nearly every day
Cheese, yogurt, ice cream	☐	☐	☐
Eggs	☐	☐	☐
Dried beans, peas, peanut butter	☐	☐	☐
Meat, fish, poultry	☐	☐	☐
Bread, rice, pasta, grits cereal, tortillas, potatoes	☐	☐	☐
Fruits or fruit juices	☐	☐	☐
Vegetables	☐	☐	☐

6. If the child eats fruits or drinks fruit juices every day or nearly every day,
   which does he/she eat or drink most often (not more than three)? _____
   _____

7. If the child eats vegetables every day or nearly every day, which one does
   he/she eat most often (not more than three)? _____
8. Does the child usually eat between meals?   ☐   ☐
   If yes, name the 2 or 3 snacks (including bedtime snacks) that the child has
   most often: _____
9. Does the person who cares for the child have use of a
   Stove?   ☐   ☐
   Refrigerator?   ☐   ☐
   Piped water?   ☐   ☐

Continued.

10. Does the child take vitamin or iron drops or tablets?   ☐ ☐
    If yes, how often? _____
    What kind? _____
11. Is the child on a special diet now?   ☐ ☐
    If yes, what is the reason? _____
    ☐ Allergy—specify type of diet: _____
    ☐ Weight reduction—specify type of diet: _____
    ☐ Other—specify reason for diet and type of diet: _____
    Who recommended the diet? _____
12. Does the child eat clay, paint chips, dirt, or anything else that is not   ☐ ☐
    usually considered food?
    If yes, what? _____
    How often? _____
13. How would you describe the child's appetite?
    ☐ Good
    ☐ Fair
    ☐ Poor
    ☐ Other: _____

From Fomon, S.J.: Nutritional disorders of children: prevention, screening, and follow-up, Publication No. 76-5612, Rockville, Md., 1976, Department of Health, Education and Welfare.

to feed often. I want to breast-feed her as long as she wants to.

Interviewer: When was she introduced to foods other than milk?

Mother: I gave her cereal when the doctor told me to, about 5 months, then vegetables and fruits, and I think meat about 9 months. I made them for her from only fresh pure foods. I give her only "natural foods" now.

Interviewer: When did she begin finger-feeding?

Mother: About 6 months, I think. She feeds herself rice crackers.

Interviewer: When did she eat table foods that were not pureed?

Mother: I began mashing up vegetables and grinding meat when she was 8 months old.

Interviewer: Does she drink from a cup?

Mother: She has a little goat's milk from a cup, but I have to help her hold it.

Interviewer: Does she try to feed herself?

Mother: She tries to get the spoon, but I can't stand the mess she makes so I feed her.

Interviewer: Now I would like for you to tell me how she lives her day with food. When does she first have something to eat or drink?

Mother: Well, she wakes about 3:00 or 4:00 in the morning and breast-feeds.

Interviewer: Then when does she have something to eat or drink again?

Mother: Well, she wakes again about 8:00, and I give her rice cereal from the health food store.

Interviewer: How much does she eat?

Mother: She's not too interested. Maybe 1/4 cup.

Interviewer: Do you put anything on the cereal?

Mother: A little goat's milk.

Interviewer: How much?

Mother: An ounce or so.

Interviewer: Do you put anything else on the cereal?

Mother: Nothing else.

Interviewer: How often (out of 7 days) does she have rice cereal?

Mother: Oh, she has it 7 days at breakfast.

Interviewer: When does she have something else to eat or to drink?

Mother: She usually breast-feeds sometime in the morning.

Interviewer: How long does she stay at the breast?

Mother: About 10 minutes. She's learning to bite.

Figure 3-1   Nutritionist evaluates the nutritional adequacy of a preschooler's food intake.

Interviewer: And when does she have something to eat again?

Mother: Between 11:00 and 12:00 I give her lunch. She likes yogurt and sardines. Sometimes I give her a cracker with sunflower seed butter on it, or if I have leftovers from the night before, I may give them to her.

Interviewer: What's next?

Mother: She usually breast-feeds after lunch and again midafternoon, and she has a bottle of pear juice some time in the afternoon.

Interviewer: How much pear juice does she drink?

Mother: Six or seven ounces.

Interviewer: How often does she have the juice?

Mother: Three for four times a week. If she doesn't have juice, she gets half of a small banana.

Interviewer: When does she eat again?

Mother: She eats with us about 7:00.

Interviewer: What does she usually eat?

Mother: I offer her fish, or yogurt, or cottage cheese, but she won't eat much. If we have hamburger or a vegetable she'll eat, I'll give her that.

Interviewer: How much does she eat?

Mother: About a tablespoon of two or three foods.

Interviewer: What do you do when she does eat?

Mother: I offer her more.

Interviewer: What do you do when she refuses to eat?

Mother: I try to find something else for her to eat or try to get her to eat another bite.

It became apparent during the interview that the mother was unable to give information that could be quantitated so a 7-day record of the child's food intake was requested. A sample of the record received is shown in the box on p. 72. Quantitation of the 7-day food record showed an intake of 500 kcal/day or less in addition to the breast milk consumed. On this basis, inadequate energy and nutrient intake was diagnosed to be the cause of the infant's inadequate weight gain. Therapy for this family involved much more than nutrition counseling. Psychosocial and parenting issues had to be dealt with as well.

If children are overweight, activity patterns are explored. Discussions about the consumption of vending machine food and the effects of television on eating patterns may also provide important information.

It may be necessary to discontinue the

Food Intake Record

4:30 AM	Breast-fed
8 AM	Rice bran, 2 tsp
	Rice puffs, 1 tbsp
	Goat's milk, $\frac{1}{2}$ oz
9 AM	Breast-fed
10:15 AM	Banana, $\frac{3}{4}$ small
11:30 AM	Wheat grain crackers, $\frac{1}{3}$
	Goat's milk, 2 oz
	Raw sunflower butter, 1 tsp
	Alfalfa sprouts, 1 tsp
	Mozarella cheese, grated, 1 tsp
	Beets, 1 tsp
	Sardines, 3
	Goat's milk yogurt, 2 tbsp
1 PM	Breast-fed
4:30 PM	Pear juice, 6 oz
5:30 PM	Sardines, 2
	Brown rice cracker, 1
	Sprouts, taste
7:50 PM	Goat's milk yogurt, 2 tbsp
8 PM	Breast-fed

detailed probing necessary for dietary history and use only a cross-check if parental tolerance for the continued questions is limited. It is also important to recognize that it may not be possible to obtain sufficient information during one interview; several follow-up clinic or home visits may be necessary to obtain a true picture of the child's feeding history and food intake.

Preschool teachers and public health nurses often provide information about a child's food intake at school and family food patterns.

When dietary data have been collected, an assessment is made of the following:

1. Parental knowledge of nutrition and appropriate foods for children
2. The adequacy of nutrients provided by the food offered to the child
3. The adequacy of the diet consumed by the child
4. Parental knowledge of and use of community resources to improve the nutritional status of the child
5. Delays in feeding skills that affect food and nutrients consumed
6. Real or potential behavior patterns that can or do compromise a child's nutrient intake
7. The motivation of parents and the child to change the patterns of food intake

If this assessment indicates that adjustments need to be made only in the kinds of food or size of portions offered to and consumed by the child, or if a therapeutic diet is indicated, plans for modifying the child's food intake should be made with the child or parents. The counselor should be aware of community resources that help with the provision of food, such as the Supplemental Food Program for Women, Infants, and Children, the food stamp program, and school lunch programs. Clients may need help in contacting agencies that administer the programs. Plans for modifying food intake should be communicated to teachers, school lunch personnel, and others in the child's food environment.

If it appears that the child has delays in feeding skills or eating patterns or that parent-child interactions are also operative in problems presented, the investigator may need to screen for these specific problems so that appropriate referrals can be made.

ORAL MOTOR EVALUATIONS

Children who are developmentally delayed and those who have abnormal muscle coordination may have difficulty with the various skills needed for the process of eating. These skills are normally learned or are already present so early in life that they are taken for granted. A knowledgeable therapist should be involved in the evaluation and planning for any person with motor feeding problems. Infants and children with these problems, however, are often identified during a dietary intake interview and observation of feeding behavior.

Motor coordination problems may be identified by interviewing parents and by observing children as they eat food and drink liquid. It is important to observe the degree of assistance assumed by parents, as well as the child's abilities. The observer may offer food textures with which the child is not familiar to determine if oral developmental delays are caused by a lack of oral motor skills or a lack of opportunities for a more mature performance. For example, more tongue, jaw, and lip movement may be seen when a piece of cheese is placed between the molars than when pureed spoon food is offered (Figure 3-2).

When making the transition to solid foods, the child initially attempts to use oral patterns that are familiar and habitual, even though they may not be effective. Loss of food from the mouth may be caused by immature tongue movement and should not be interpreted as dislike for the food. Placement of food at the side of the mouth reduces food ejection caused by immature tongue movement. Occasional choking and coughing are not unusual during the transition period from pureed spoon foods to soft table foods. Hiding lumps of solid foods within pureed or strained food will not help in making the transition. For a child with primitive oral patterns it is much more difficult to handle a multitextured food that requires him or her to sort pieces that must be chewed from pieces that can be swallowed without chewing. Gradual introduction of increasingly more textured and drier foods is a better approach to making the transition from pureed foods to table foods. It is most important not to get upset when a child chokes. Ordinarily, the child does not need assistance when choking. However, if there is no coughing or breathing, the evaluator can quickly perform the **Heimlich maneuver** or bend the child forward and tap sharply between the shoulders. Fortunately, few genuine emergencies arise, but it is important to be prepared by knowing how to han-

Figure 3-2 Occupational therapist evaluates oral motor patterns of child with cerebral palsy.

dle emergencies. When asking a parent to try offering new food textures, one needs to assure them that simple choking is not life threatening if one knows how to deal with it.

The Screening of Eating Abilities form (pp. 75 to 79) can be used by the dietitian or nutritionist during the dietary assessment when the child has not yet been seen by a skilled therapist or no therapist is available. This screening tool was developed at the Child Development and Mental Retardation Center of the University of Washington to be used by their comprehensive child evaluation teams. The form can serve as a guideline on which to record information. When completed, the evaluator should be able to determine if the child's eating problems are caused by difficulties in body and oral coordination and if further appropriate resources are necessary. It should be noted that when age guidelines are mentioned they are intended to be lenient in recognition of the normal range of acquisition of skills. Morris[16] provides more detailed description of the age range at which various oral skills are acquired and provides more examples of guiding questions that can be used during a parent interview.

If the oral motor screen identifies delays in feeding behavior in the absence of abnormal movement patterns, changes in the diet can be suggested to support development progress as outlined in Chapter 13. If abnormal oral and movement patterns are identified, however, referral to a specialized therapist is important. When motor control problems and abnormal muscle tone are observed throughout the body and the mouth, an occupational or physical therapist who specializes in pediatrics or neurological disorders should be contacted. If the problem seems to be primarily oral, a speech therapist may be the first contact. Resources for names of treatment centers or private therapists are the United Cerebral Palsy Association in each state, the local Easter Seal Society, or the Neurodevelopmental Treatment Association.[17]

When specialized services are not immediately available, initial steps may be attempted to improve the quality of food intake by using the basic principles of positioning discussed in Chapter 13. It is important to use a problem-solving approach that includes feedback from client and caregiver. The rationale for suggested changes should be thoroughly explained, and expectations for follow-through must be reasonable. It may take more time to feed a child in the desired position, especially at first, so parents can be asked to try the new procedure at the beginning of each meal or at the meal that is the least stressful. Consideration of the client's and caregiver's comfort, feelings, and opinions should be clearly communicated.

When the caregiver does not want to make any changes in the feeding procedure, a compromise suggestion may be to allow a therapist to use the new procedures for a while, until the client is more comfortable and successful. Changes in motor control may be slow to achieve, but changes in the feeding environment are not as difficult to achieve and may have great significance in the long-term social, nutritional, and physical development of the child.

CONSIDERATION OF PSYCHOSOCIAL FACTORS

Whenever and wherever the nutrition of a child is discussed, consideration must also be given to factors that have no direct relationship on the feeding process. Eating behavior serves as a sensitive barometer of the general adjustment of child, parent, and family. For this reason intrapersonal and interpersonal factors that influence food intake should also be taken into consideration when collecting and assessing information.

Since parents are primarily responsible for providing infants and children with both food and the environment in which it is consumed, attention should be given to the parents' psychosocial well-being, adaptation to the parenting role, and general level of parenting skills. Because patterns of food intake, even in young

Text continued on p. 79.

Screening of Eating Abilities

Child's name: _____ ID#: _____ B.D.: _____
Medical diagnosis, if known: _____
Name of evaluator: _____
Name of parent or caregiver: _____ Phone: _____
Other agencies involved: _____

  I. Questions to ask of parent or caregiver
     A. What are your greatest concerns in regard to feeding?
     B. What are the food likes and dislikes of your child in relation to texture, temperature,
         color, and flavor?
     C. Are some foods more difficult for your child to eat than others?
     D. Are there any foods that your child cannot eat?
     E. Does he/she take any medication or food supplements?
     F. When does he/she have meals and snacks?
     G. Does he/she eat with the family?
     H. Who assists at mealtimes (home, school, other)?
      I. How much assistance is given?
     J. What textures are usually eaten (thin liquid, thick liquid, soft spoon food, soft chewy
         food, ground food, chopped food, crunchy food—see list below)?
 II. Tactile sensitivity
         These stimuli are applied toward the beginning of the evaluation before offering food
     but after the child has had some opportunity to adjust to you as a stranger. Tell the child
     what you are going to do before applying the stimuli. Be cautious in overinterpreting
     inappropriate responses that may be social or behavioral and not necessarily tactile.
         First, lightly stroke the front and back of each of the child's hands. Then stroke the
     front aspect of the skin on each arm. Finally, stroke the face, lips, and gums with firm
     pressure of your fingertips.

APPROPRIATE	QUESTIONABLE APPROPRIATENESS
Neutral or positive response to touch	Muscle tension, moving away from
☐ Hand, arm	stimulus or vocal protest
☐ Face	☐ Hand, arm
☐ Gums, outside teeth, when stroked	☐ Face
with a fingertip	☐ Gums, outside teeth, when stroked
	with a fingertip

     Questionable appropriate responses may be caused by situational variables, but if the
     caregiver reports consistent negative responses, a therapy referral is indicated.
III. Food offered
         These foods are listed in sequence according to difficulty and are grouped into three
     levels of corresponding normal developmental skills. Ask the caregiver to first offer foods
     commonly eaten at home, then try some of the other textures at more difficult levels.

Adapted from Carman, P.: Screening of eating abilities. Occupational Therapy Department, Child Development and Mental
Retardation Center, WJ-10, Seattle, 1980, University of Washington.

Continued.

Screening of Eating Abilities—*cont'd*

Watch carefully for amount of chewing, movement of food within the mouth; and tendency to choke. Small amounts of food are offered from each category appropriate to the child's developmental level so that satiation does not occur too quickly. Thin liquid is offered to every child, but soft spoon foods or soft chewy foods should be omitted when the child has demonstrated higher level skills. Thick liquid is offered only when thin liquids are difficult (evidenced by choking, liquid running out of mouth).

A. *Child less than 5 months of age developmentally* (needs head and trunk support while eating, i.e., needs to be held in adult's arms, infant seat, special support chairs).
- ☐ Thick liquid (optional, offered when thin liquid is taken with difficulty): milkshake, thinned applesauce, thinned yogurt
- ☐ Thin liquid: milk, water, fruit juice
- ☐ Soft spoon food: applesauce, pudding, yogurt
- ☐ Soft chewy food: cheese, fish, vienna sausage

B. *Child 5 to 12 months of age developmentally* (good head control, needs some trunk support while eating, sits upright in chair).
- ☐ Ground solid food: "junior foods," ground table foods (dry consistency)
- ☐ Crunchy food that dissolves readily: cracker, potato stick
- ☐ Oblong finger food (easier to grasp): potato stick, green bean
- ☐ Small finger food (harder to grasp): Cheerio, puffed cereal
- ☐ Hard crunchy food: melba toast, bread stick

C. *Child more than 12 months of age developmentally* (with good head and trunk control and tongue mobility, lateralization).
- ☐ Chopped table foods
- ☐ Bite-sized table foods: raisins
- ☐ Multitexture foods (solid plus liquid): apple, celery, soup
- ☐ Chewy food: chicken, hamburger, small pieces of well-cooked meat
- ☐ Hard foods that break into diffuse pieces: carrots, nuts (if older than 2 years of age)

IV. Observations of child eating

Caregiver is asked to feed the child in the usual way. Ask whether any particular equipment or furniture is used that may not be present for this observation.

Mark NA (not applicable) if child is younger than stated age. Asterisks indicate posture or movement that is always abnormal; other activity of questionable appropriateness may be caused by neurological immaturity or other factors.

A. *Positioning*

APPROPRIATE	QUESTIONABLE APPROPRIATENESS
☐ Held by caregiver (if younger than 1 year of age) within 30° of upright	☐ Held by caregiver (lying back, asymmetrical, or otherwise unusual)
☐ Within 30° of upright, propped, or special seat (hips flexed 90° in usual sitting angle)	☐ Held by caregiver (older than 1 year of age)
☐ High chair	☐ Lying on flat surface
☐ Other: _____	☐ Other: _____

The health professional may wish to discuss alternative means of positioning if the usual method is questionably appropriate. If the child has abnormal muscle tone, appropriate positioning is much more difficult to achieve. Consultation with a physical therapist or occupational therapist should be obtained. Any of the following behaviors under the "questionable" column indicate need for a consultation or a therapy program.

B. *Posture and movement*

APPROPRIATE

- ☐ Head in alignment with body
- ☐ Head control stable (expected by 4 or 5 months of age)
- ☐ Arms forward, hands midline (frequent by 4 to 6 months of age)
- ☐ Hands, legs, and feet move freely, without stiffness
- ☐ Hips flex easily for sitting, knees spread apart spontaneously for wide sitting base
- ☐ Trunk straight when sitting (expected by 5 to 6 months of age)

QUESTIONABLE APPROPRIATENESS

- ☐ Head frequently back or to one side, rotated to one side
- ☐ Lack of head stability, excess motions, floppy, pushes back, falls forward (older than 5 months of age)
- ☐ Arms frequently retracted at shoulders, hands do not come together (older than 4 to 5 months of age)
- ☐ Legs and feet seem stiff, seldom move, or move in stereotyped patterns
- ☐ Hips resist bending or intermittently extend; narrow sitting base, knees pull together
- ☐ Trunk tilted, slumped, rotated, or arched backwards (older than 5 months of age)

C. *Oral motor coordination*

APPROPRIATE

JAW

- ☐ Jaw opens and closes easily, controlled to receive food
- ☐ Jaw stabilized with little movement
- ☐ Jaw moves up and down with slight lateral movements when chewing ("rotary")

QUESTIONABLE APPROPRIATENESS

- ☐ Jaw opens too wide or with tension
- ☐ Delayed jaw opening response to receive food
- ☐ Jaw moves up and down while drinking from a cup so liquid is lost (older than 12 months of age)
- ☐ Jaw clamps down intermittently (older than 2 years of age)
- ☐ Lack of up and down movement with solid food

APPROPRIATE

TONGUE

- ☐ Tongue stays within mouth while drinking
- ☐ Tongue stays within mouth with foods
- ☐ Tongue lateralized, food placed at side (6 months of age); food placed midline (9 months of age)

QUESTIONABLE APPROPRIATENESS

- ☐ Tongue protrudes past border of lips while drinking
- ☐ Tongue protrudes with spoon foods
- ☐ Tongue moves forward and backward when solid foods are placed at side of mouth or presented midline, no lateral movement

Continued.

Screening of Eating Abilities—*cont'd*

APPROPRIATE	QUESTIONABLE APPROPRIATENESS
LIPS	
☐ Lips seal on nipple or cup rim	☐ Liquids not retained well by lips with nipple, with cup (older than 24 months of age)
☐ Lips close on and clean spoon	
☐ Lips move actively while chewing	☐ Spoon foods not retained well by lips (older than 8 months of age)
	☐ Passive lips while chewing
SWALLOW	
☐ Swallows readily	☐ Delayed swallow, slows eating
☐ Swallows liquids, no choking	☐ Chokes two or more times when drinking liquid from a cup
☐ Swallows solids, seldom chokes	☐ Chokes two or more times when drinking liquids other than from a cup (bottle, etc.)
	☐ Chokes two or more times when solids are fed
GAG REFLEX	
☐ Normal gag reflex (readiness to vomit when pressure applied to pharyngeal wall, soft palate, posterior tongue)	☐ Gag reflex hyposensitive (slow or absent)
	☐ Gag reflex hypersensitive (occurs to pressure on middle or front of tongue or at sight of certain food)
SALIVA CONTROL	
☐ Swallows saliva (doesn't drool)	☐ Drools when not eating (older than 24 months of age) and when not teething

D. *Prehension*

Grasping of objects starts with a reflexive closing when the palmar surface of the hand is stimulated; the grasp becomes voluntary with maturity and is gradually refined to use of opposed fingertips. Any observations of questionable quality or prolonged primitive skill level should be cause for further evaluation.

APPROPRIATE	QUESTIONABLE APPROPRIATENESS
☐ Reflexive grasp (fading by 3 months of age	☐ Wrist flexed, hand often in awkward position
☐ Raking grasp, whole hand (by 6 months of age)	☐ Hand usually fisted (older than 3 months of age)
☐ Thumb to side of fingers (8 months of age and older)	☐ Hand usually limp or grasp weak
	☐ Grasps food too tightly
☐ Thumb to fingertips of index and/or middle fingers	☐ Raking, use of whole hand (older than 12 months of age)
	☐ Difficulty releasing grasp (older than 12 months of age)

Continued.

E. *Hand and arm movement*

A child must have head and upper trunk control before the hand can be used for purposeful reaching. At first the hand and arm movements appear to be random. Purposeful movements are first seen as a child brings the hands to the mouth and the hands together at midline. Reaching for toys and bringing them to the mouth precedes finger-feeding. As control of the trunk improves, arm and hand use matures. A child will usually grap the spoon and help bring it to the mouth long before he or she is able to control it independently. The effort of holding a cup is seen initially as the cup is pushed tightly against the mouth to stabilize it; it is difficult at this stage to stop drinking and put a partially full cup back to the table without spilling. Abnormal muscle tone or lack of head and trunk stability interferes with the quality and effectiveness of hand use.

APPROPRIATE
- ☐ Hand to mouth
- ☐ Hands to midline, hands together
- ☐ Hand touches object purposefully
- ☐ Toy to mouth
- ☐ Holds bottle or drinks from cup (hands may be on cup, adult controls)
- ☐ Self-feeds finger foods
- ☐ Helps with spoon
- ☐ Independent with spoon, spills
- ☐ Independent with spoon, no spills
- ☐ Holds cup with some assistance
- ☐ Independent with cup

QUESTIONABLE APPROPRIATENESS
- ☐ Arms tight, limited movement
- ☐ Hands usually fisted (older than 2 to 3 months of age)
- ☐ Hand frequently misses object, over-shoots (older than 6 months of age)
- ☐ No attempt to reach for food or spoon, even when hungry and food is within reach (older than 6 months of age)
- ☐ Uses spoon with much extraneous movement and spilling
- ☐ Other: _____

F. *Cooperation*

APPROPRIATE
- ☐ Motivated to eat
- ☐ Accepts food passively
- ☐ Participates to best of ability
- ☐ Socially appropriate behavior

QUESTIONABLE APPROPRIATENESS
- ☐ Does not seem to care about eating
- ☐ Actively resists eating (turns mouth away or slow to open mouth)
- ☐ Physical skills not used to potential for self-assistance
- ☐ Socially disruptive, attention seeking

Any observations of questionable cooperation tend to reduces the validity of other observations. A more thorough evaluation of parent-child interaction during mealtime may be indicated and may be the primary area requiring assistance.

children, can be altered by emotional status, screening should also consider the socioemotional development of the child. When appropriate food is available and there no evidence of biological or organic problems in the child, it is not unusual to find that the cause of a disturbance in food intake is within the psychosocial/emotional category. Such problems can manifest themselves in a variety of ways, for instance parent or child dissatisfaction with the feeding or mealtime situation, parental neglect or overconcern with food or feeding, anorexia or vomiting, and food aversions or food gorging.

Level of Stress and Family Coping

Infants and children are sensitive to the feelings and attitudes of parents, particularly at feeding time or bedtime. Research by Brandon[18] on the epidemiological factors of childhood eating disturbances found that the parents of the maladjusted group, as compared with control group, were younger, were more dependent on relatives, were regarded as unstable or suffering from mental problems, reported unhappy childhoods, experienced marital conflict, or were regarded as showing disturbed relationships with their children. It is reasonable to hypothesize that parents who are anxious or distressed somehow communicate these states to their babies and young children, which in turn affects feeding behavior. Older children are also quick to identify tension or conflict between adults at the dinner table and to respond accordingly. Reality stressors like a job or financial worries, recent change of domicile, and illness or injury of child or parent are additional factors that can disrupt routines and can be associated with temporary symptoms related to food or feeding behavior. Personal problems of adult family members, for instance, marital discord, unresolved grief, depression, drug use, or lack of self-esteem, may also influence the feeding situation involving children. When the feeding problem appears to be nonorganic, it is appropriate to ask parents a few simple questions to determine the emotional climate in the home. This can be done selectively in an interview or by using a questionnaire as a routine part of the assessment process (see Screening Questionnaire for Family Stress on p. 81).

Parental Feelings of Competence and Satisfaction

Clinical observations indicate that parental *feelings* of competence and satisfaction or dissatisfaction with the parental role are psy-

chological factors that also have an influence on the food intakes and feeding behaviors of children. When an individual, for whatever reason, experiences minimal feelings of success in carrying out the activities associated with parenting, the opportunity for experiencing satisfaction decreases proportionately and the stage is set for problems in parent-child interaction. If the parent does not feel adequate in handling child-care activities outside the feeding sphere, lack of confidence or feelings of incompetence can eventually be manifested in a dysfunctional feeding situation. The mother who reported the following impressions was trying to deal with a 3-year-old boy whose diet consisted only of olives, avocados, and salmon:

> I'll never forget what I felt like when he was 2 weeks old and I had to care for him completely on my own. It wasn't at all what I expected. I was scared to death and sure that every time he cried I must have done something wrong. There were half-filled bottles all over the house because I worried that the milk might spoil if Gary didn't drink it in 10 or 15 minutes. My mother-in-law didn't help. She is still always giving me suggestions for a better way to do something.

In early infancy the close relationship to and dependence on the mother, in particular, often become linked with the feeding process. For this reason many individuals equate successful mothering with a well-nourished infant or child and a nonproblematic feeding situation. The comments of the mother of a developmentally delayed toddler with congenital heart disease (still on a diet of pureed foods) are illustrative:

> I couldn't do anything about his heart, but I did pretty well at feeding him by that nasogastric tube. Nobody else could do it as well as I did. Now when he doesn't eat I fix a special high-calorie pudding for him so that he doesn't lose weight. He really gobbles it down!

Factors like past experience, age, knowledge of child growth and development, and the input of significant family members or professionals are important determinants of parental feelings

---

Screening Questionnaire for Family Stress

	Yes	No
1. During the past year have any of the following occurred in your immediate family?		
Family moved?	☐	☐
Death, divorce, separation, loss of family member?	☐	☐
Marriage, reconciliation, pregnancy, new family member?	☐	☐
Serious injury or illness, problem with aging relative?	☐	☐
Loss of work, change of job, retirement?	☐	☐
Frequent or serious arguments or fights?	☐	☐
Money problems?	☐	☐
Drug or drinking problems?	☐	☐
Trouble with the law?	☐	☐
Some other serious problem?	☐	☐
If yes, what? _____		
2. During the past year:		
Has anyone in your family been seriously upset, depressed, or moody?	☐	☐
Have you been generally happy with your family's way of life?	☐	☐
Have you often felt lonely or cut off from other people?	☐	☐
Have you or your mate had serious differences that you feel may be related to differences in religion, race, nationality, family background?	☐	☐
3. Have you and your children been separated for more than 1 day in the past year?	☐	☐
Do you have someone reliable to take care of your children when you need it?	☐	☐
Are your children cared for daily by someone outside the family?	☐	☐
If yes, has it been the same person for the past year?	☐	☐

Adapted from Metz, J.R., and others: Pediatrics 58:4, 1976. Copyright American Academy of Pediatrics, 1976.

---

of competence.[19] The standards of performance or values that parents hold for themselves, along with their more general feelings of self-esteem, are also related to perceptions of competence. But probably the most significant influence on parental feelings of success or satisfaction is the responsiveness of the child; that is, does the child show developmental and social evidence of a positive response to parenting? With these determinants in mind the following questions can serve as guidelines for eliciting data on the adjustment to parenting and its associated emotional responses:

1. As you were growing up, did you observe or assist with the upbringing of younger children such as brothers or sisters, relatives, friends, or neighbors?
2. How would you rate your maternal feelings on a scale of 1 to 5, with 1 being very maternal and 5 being nonmaternal?
3. What has been the biggest surprise or thing you least expected about being a parent?
4. How satisfied are you with your child's physical growth and development?
5. How satisfied are you with your child's social adjustment?

6. How much influence does your spouse have on your ideas about child rearing? Do you usually agree or disagree on child-rearing concerns?
7. Who or what has had the most influence on your ideas about child rearing? Books, magazines, or the media? Religion? Friends, neighbors, or relatives? Professionals? Formal education or parenting classes?
8. When you and your child are getting along as you usually do, how does your relationship with your child make you feel as a parent?
9. How competent do you feel about how you handle your life in general?
10. How competent do you feel as a parent?
11. How competent a parent do you think you are *from the viewpoint of others* who know you well?
12. Before you had your own family, how did you feel about children?

Parent-Child Interaction

An integral component of assessment and data collection related to food intake is consideration of the interaction between child and parent. To have an indication of the effects of food and the feeding situation on the parent-child dyad, such data should be based on observation of both mealtime and non-mealtime situations. It is important to determine if food-related parent-child problems are situation specific or part of a more basic discord. Ideally, the assessment should be done in the home setting during mealtime *and* free-play situations. If this is not possible, every attempt should be made to simulate natural conditions in the clinic, office, or hospital environment.

Several research methods and standardized tools have been developed to evaluate parent-child interaction, for instance, Verbal Interaction Record,[20] Mutual Problem-Solving Task,[21] Nursing Child Assessment Feeding Scales,[22] and Nursing Child Assessment Teaching Scales.[23] Some practitioners may want to obtain training in the use of standardized assessment techniques; however, less formalized methods can also be helpful in collecting data. Using the concepts of affectional ties, propensity to interact, and feedback and reciprocity as organizers, it is possible to identify the essential elements of most interacction between parents and children.

I. **Affectional ties** (refers to the emotional attachment and degree of psychological involvement between parent and child)
   A. Appropriate interview questions
      1. Do you believe in such a thing as unconditional mother love? Would you ever use such a term to describe your feelings about _____ ?
      2. How old was _____ when you really felt that he/she was *your* child?
      3. How does _____ know that you love and care abouthim/her?
      4. How do you know that _____ loves you?
      5. Who or what is _____ most attached to?
      6. Have you ever regretted the decision to become a parent? Occasionally? Frequently?
   B. Direct observation
      1. Attentiveness of parent to child's distress; physical comforting
      2. Use of expressions of love or special designations to refer to child *or* use of negative terms to refer to child; no reference to child by name
      3. Evidence of parental pleasure when child is complimented or comments are made regarding parent-child physical resemblances
      4. Evidence of strong mutual need for togetherness and a maximum avoid-

ance of separation *or* parent or child tendency/preference for isolated activity
5. Willingness to relinquish child to care of a stranger

II. **Propensity to interact** (refers to the ability and desire of parent or child to give and receive communication)
A. Appropriate interview questions
1. When ＿＿ is not around, do you ever find yourself thinking of something you want to do with him/her or something you want to tell him/her?
2. Have you been (or are you ever) so preoccupied with adult worries or concerns that you don't have any energy left to interact with ＿＿ ?
3. Can you identify any person, thing, or situation that interferes with your relationship or communication with ＿＿ ?
4. How would you describe your relationship with ＿＿ ?
B. Direct observation
1. Evidence of physical intactness (especially sensory and perceptual) of parent and child
2. Evidence of emotional intactness of parent and child
3. Presence or absence of reality stressors (as per Family Stress Questionnaire)

III. **Feedback and reciprocity** (refers to chains of response between parent and child; activity of one that occurs as a direct result of stimuli from the other)
A. Appropriate interview questions
1. How does ＿＿ let you know that he/she needs something or wants your attention? What is you usual response to this?
2. Who or what usually initiates the interaction between you and your child?

3. What do you do for ＿＿ ? What does ＿＿ do for you?
B. Direct observation
1. Efforts on the part of either parent or child to remain in touch (physically or verbally) that are successful
2. Conversation, singing, laughing, or smiling that maintains an extended interaction (one partner answers the other, the latter responds in turn, and so on)
3. Presence or absence of eye contact between parent and child
4. Presence or absence of caregiving activity on the part of the parent in response to behavior (e.g, cry, yawn, request)
5. Manner in which infant or young child is held
6. Attention of parent to cues in the feeding situation (e.g., satiation, hunger, pacing)

When data indicate that the cause of a child's feeding or food intake problem is most likely psychosocial, intervention must be planned accordingly. The primary focus of treatment most likely is on strategies to alleviate stress and support family coping abilities, on increasing parental knowledge and skill regarding child rearing, or on facilitating the parent-child relationship. In some situations these goals may be accomplished within the context of the feeding situation; however, in the majority of instances more specific treatment is indicated. Reality-based family needs demand rapid provisions of concrete services to relieve situational demands. For this reason, referral to a public or private family service or social welfare agency may be appropriate. Those situations that require supportive counseling or education and anticipatory guidance may be handled in a variety of ways, for instance, with family therapy, enrollment in parenting classes, referral to a parent group, or one-to-one work with a qualified professional.

The variety of concerns presented about infants' and children's food intake clearly indicates that information sought must be based on problems presented and the health care professional's judgment. In some instances dietary intake data may profide sufficient information to design plans with parents and children to modify energy and nutrient intakes. In many cases, if plans are to be effective, the behavioral and psychosocial influences on a compromised food intake must be investigated. Parents of children with oral motor and self-feeding delays may need help in identifying specific foods to support developmental progress. Those with abnormal motor patterns need therapy.

Screening procedures may identify children with feeding problems of multiple etiological factors for whom an interdisciplinary assessment is appropriate. Factors that must be considered are adequacy of nutrient intake, structural abnormalities of the oral cavity, oral tissue health, medical status, speech development, living environment, social environment, and neurological integrity (including sensation). The collective data provide a base on which the cause of the problem may be determined, effective treatment plans may be designed, and progress may be assessed.

The team approach facilitates identification of priorities for treatment and use of logical step-by-step approach. Periodic reevaluations of identified concerns indicate the effectiveness of programs designed.

Summary

Several studies have attempted to assess dietary methods. Most of these studies have found that children who provide information are not as reliable as adults. Even so, all methods have inherent limitations that should be recognized. The results of diet histories have not agreed with those of weighed food records when applied to individual children. Most studies have indicated that diet histories of children overestimate intake by individuals compared with 3- and 7-day food records. Children who have delays in feeding skills should be screened to determine whether the delays are because of abnormal motor patterns or because of an overall delay, which should determine the need for an occupational or physical therapy evaluation. Because many feeding difficulties in childhood are caused by parent-child interactions, it may be necessary to evaluate the family level of stress and coping and the interaction between parent and child.

SUGGESTED LEARNING ACTIVITIES

1. Interview parents of a preschool child to collect a diet history. Assess the validity of the information collected.
2. Measure (in standard household measures) portions appropriate for children for 1 day; compare these with adult size portions.
3. Keep a 7-day record of all food and beverages consumed. Assess the difficulty in keeping such a record.
4. Assess stress in the family of a preschool child whose parents consider him or her to have a feeding problem.
5. Observe a comprehensive nutrition/feeding evaluation of a child who has oral motor feeding delays. Using appropriate tools, record dietary intake information, eating abilities, and level of family stress.

REFERENCES

1. Beal, V. A.: The nutrition history in longitudinal research, J. Am. Diet. Assoc. 51:426, 1967.
2. Todd, K. S., Hudes, M., and Calloway, H.: Food intake measurements; problems and approaches, Am. J. Clin. Nutr. 37:139, 1983.
3. Klesges, R. C., and others: Validation of the 24-hour dietary recall in preschool children, J. Am. Diet. Assoc. 86:1383, 1986.
4. Farris, R. P., and others: A group method for obtaining dietary recalls of children, J. Am. Diet. Assoc. 85:1315, 1985.

5. McHenry, E. W., Ferguson, H. P., and Gurland, J.: Souces of error in dietary surveys, Can. J. Public Health, 36:355, 1945.

6. Stuff, J. E. and others: A comparision of dietary methods, Am. J. Clin. Nutr. 37:300, 1983.

7. Burke, B. S.: The dietary history as a tool in research, J. Am. Diet Assoc. 23:1031, 1947.

8. Rasanen, L.: Nutrition survey of Finnish rural children. VI. Methodological study comparing the 24-hour record and dietary history. Am. J. Clin. Nutr. 32:2560, 1979.

9. Huenemann, R. I., and Turner, D.: Methods of dietary investigation, J. Am. Diet. Assoc. 18:562, 1942.

10. Young C. M. and others: A comparison of dietary study methods. I. Dietary history vs. 7 day record, J. Am. Diet. Assoc. 28:124, 1952.

11. Trulson, M. F.: Assessment of dietary study methods. I. Comparison of methods for obtaining data for clinical work, J. Am. Diet. Assoc. 30:991, 1954.

12. Abramson, J. N., Slome, C., and Kosovsky, C.: Food frequency tool as an epidemiological tool, Am. J. Public Health 53:2093, 1963.

13. Hoover, L. W. and Pelican, S.: Nutrient data bases - considerations for educators, J. Nutr. Ed. 16:58, 1984.

14. Adelman, M. O., and others: Computerized dietary analysis systems, J. Amer. Diet. Assoc. 83:421, 1983.

15. Rogan, A., and Stella, Y.: Some problems with nutritional analysis software, J. Nutr. Ed. 16:58, 1984.

16. Morris, S. E.: The normal acquisition of oral feeding skills: implications for assessment and treatment, New York, 1982, Therapeutic Media, Inc.

17. Neurodevelopmental Treatment Association Inc., Executive Secretary, P. O. Box 14613, Chicago, IL 60614.

18. Brandon, S.: An epidemiological study of eating disturbances, J. Psychosom. Res. 14:253, 1970.

19. Sutherland, S.: An exploratory study of the factors which contribute to a material sense of competence among mothers of children in preschools, parenting classes and a day care center, Unpublished masters thesis, Seattle, 1980, University of Washington.

20. Lambie, D. L., Bond J. T., and Weikart, D. P.: Verbal interaction record, monograph 2, High Scope Monograph Series, Home teaching with mothers and infants. The Ypsilanti-Carnegie infant education project: an experiment, Ypsilanti, Mich., 1974, High Scope Press.

21. Epstein, A., and Weikart, D. P.: Mutual problem-solving task, monograph 6, High Scope Monograph Series. The Ypsilanti-Carnegie infant education project: longitudinal follow-up, Ypsilanti, Mich., 1980, High Scope Press.

22. Nursing child assessment feeding scales. In Barnard, K. E. and Eyres, S. J. editors: Child health assessment, part 2: the first year of life, Publication No. HRA 79-25, Washington, D. C., June 1979, U. S. Department of Health, Education and Welfare.

23. Nursing child assessment teaching scales. In Barnard, K. E. and Eyres, S. J. editors: Child health assessment, part 2: the first year of life, Publication No. HRA 79-25, Washington, D. C., June 1979, U. S. Department of Health, Education and Welfare.

4

Infant Feeding and Nutrition

Peggy L. Pipes

OBJECTIVES

After studying this chapter, the student should:

1. Recognize differences in human and other milks available for infants.

2. Define the appropriate use of the various formulas and whole milk for infants.

3. Recognize developmental landmarks during infancy that indicate a readiness for the infant to progress in feeding behaviors and in the varieties and textures of food that should be offered.

4. Be aware of infant foods as sources of nutrients and appropriate use of foods to optimize the baby's nutritional status.

5. Be aware of the variability among the personalities, growth patterns, and nutrient needs of infants at any age and the need to individualize what, when, how often, and how much each baby should be fed.

At no time in the life cycle are as many changes in food and nutrient intake observed as during the first year of life. Influenced by a rapid but declining rate of physical growth, maturation of the oral, fine, and gross motor skills, and relationships established with their parents, infants prepared at birth to suck liquids from a nipple are at 1 year of age making attempts to feed themselves table food with cul-turally defined utensils. The need for nutrients and energy depends on the infant's requirement for maintenance, physical growth, and energy expenditure, while the foods offered to infants reflect culturally accepted practices. Infants' acceptance of food is further influenced both by neuromotor maturation and their interactions with their parents. Because of the variability of the above parameters among infants, a variety of combinations of foods and milks are consumed by well-nourished children at any month during the first year.

MATURATION OF DIGESTION AND ABSORPTION

The newborn is a functionally immature organism. Although the normal neonate is well prepared to digest and absorb human milk, cow's milk, or soy formulas at birth, maturation of many of the enzyme systems occurs during and after the first year.

The stomach capacity of infants increases from 10 to 20 ml at birth to 200 ml by 12 months of age. The rate of stomach emptying depends on the size and composition of the meal. During the first weeks after birth, gastric acidity decreases, and for the first few months it remains lower than in the adult.

Protein

Proteolytic activity of duodenal juice is as great in infancy as in adulthood. However, the total quantity of protein that can be digested per hour is less during infancy and childhood and increases with age.[1]

Fat

A greater percentage of fat is absorbed in later life than in infancy. Adults absorb about 95% of ingested fats, whereas newborns absorb about 85% to 90% of the fat provided by human milk. Many infants absorb less than 70% of the fat in cow's milk.[2] Mixtures of vegetable oils in commercially prepared infant formulas are well absorbed, although the reason for the degree of absorption of those containing oleo oil remains unclear.[2] Absorption of fat begins to reach adult levels between 6 and 9 months of age.

Pancreatic lipase activity is low in the newborn, especially the premature infant. The bile acid pool, although present, is reduced. When compared with an adult on the basis of body surface, the newborn, although able to synthe-size bile, has a bile acid pool one half that of the adult.[3]

During infancy the position the saturated fatty acid occupies on the glycerol molecule influences absorption. Stearic acid is poorly absorbed in any position. Free palmitic acid hydrolyzed from positions 1 and 3 is poorly absorbed, whereas palmitic acid, which occupies position 2 on the glycerol molecule, remains as a monoglyceride and appears to be well absorbed.[4]

Carbohydrates

Maltase, isomaltase, and sucrase activity reach adult levels by 28 to 32 weeks' gestation. Lactase, present at low levels at 28 weeks' gestation, increases near term and reaches adult levels at birth.[5] Salivary and pancreatic **amylase** are low during the first months after birth. Concentrations of salivary amylase rise to adult values between 6 months and 1 year of age.[6] Concentrations of salivary amylase increase to two thirds of adult values by 3 months of age. However, large variations in enzyme activity have been noted among groups of infants. There appears to be no relationship between salivary amylase activity, the size of the infant, and intakes of starch-containing food before 3 months of age.[8] Concentrations of pancreatic amylase increase from birth through the preschool years. Hadorn and others[7] found that output of amylase per kilogram in children less than 6 months of age was two to four times less than in children 1 year of age. There also appears to be an increase in output of amylase from the preschool to the school-age years.

Most health care professionals believe the introduction of infant cereal before 3 to 4 months of age is inappropriate.

RENAL FUNCTION

The newborn has a functionally immature kidney. The ratio of glomerular surface area to tubular volume in an infant's kidney is high, compared with the kidney of an adult.[10] The glomerular filtration rate is low. The concentrating capacity of some neonates has been reported to be as limited as 700 mOsm/L, and for others it is as great as that of older children and adults, 1200 to 1400 mOsm/L. Infants therefore are vulnerable to water imbalance.[11]

MILK IN THE INFANT'S DIET

That human milk from adequately nourished lactating mothers offers nutritional, immunological, and psychosocial benefits to infants has never been questioned. Even so, the incidence of breast-feeding of the newborn infant fell to 18% in 1966. Renewed interest in promoting breast-feeding and supporting the lactating mother caused the incidence of breast-feeding during hospitalization to increase to 56.9% in 1986. However, many infants are breast-fed for only a few months. At 3 to 4 months of age, 28.7% were breast-fed; by 5 to 6 months of age, only 21.6% of infants continued to be breast-fed in 1986.[12] The incidence of breast-feeding in the hospital is highest among mothers who have some college education, are not employed outside the home, and who have just delivered their first infant. It is higher in upper-income families than among those with lower incomes.[5,13]

Instruction and support in breast-feeding has been found to influence its continuation. Of mothers who received instruction both before and after birth, 40% continued to breast-feed at 6 months, whereas 37.2% of mothers who received instruction only before birth and 31.3% of mothers who received instruction only after birth were breast-feeding at 6 months.

Most normal full-term infants who are not breast-fed receive a cow's milk-base formula; very few receive fresh cow's milk. Milk-free formulas, including soy and hydrolyzed casein formulas, are fed to infants who do not tolerate milk.

Colostrum and Transitional Milk

For the first few days after birth, the breast-fed infant ingests a yellowish, transparent fluid called **colostrum**. Human colostrum contains more protein but less fat, carbohydrate, and energy than does mature human milk. Concentrations of sodium, potassium, and chloride are greater in colostrum than in later milk. Between the third and sixth day colostrum changes to a milk that, compared with mature milk, has a high protein content. By the tenth day the breast-fed infant receives mature milk.

Comparison of Nutrient Compositions of Human Milk and Cow's Milk

Nutrients secreted in human milk vary and reflect individual biochemical variability among women, and diet consumed, the stage of lactation, and the length of time the mother has breast-fed.[14] When milk is analyzed for nutrient content, the time of day the milk was expressed, and whether foremilk or hindmilk is analyzed influenced its nutrient composition. Wide ranges of many vitamins and minerals have been reported. Table 4-1 lists average nutrients contained in pooled human milk and minimum federal standards for homogenized milk.

Both human and cow's milk are complex liquids containing more than 200 components in the fat-soluble and water-soluble fractions. There are, however, considerable differences in the quantity and availability of the nutrients in the two milks. Differences are thought to reflect species specific nutrient needs to support individual maintenance and growth needs of the offspring. This hypothesis is further supported by the fact that there are changes in the nutrient composition of human milk during lactation. For example, the concentration of iron, copper, and zinc decline between 2 weeks and 5 to 9 months of lactation.[14,15] Protein concentration decreases from the first week through 6 to 9

Table 4-1   Nutrient content of human milk and cow's milk

Constituent (Per Liter)	Human Milk	Cow's Milk	Constituent (Per Liter)	Human Milk	Cow's Milk
Energy (kcal)	690	660	Minerals		
Protein (gm)	9	35	Calcium (mg)	241-340	1200
Fat (gm)	40	38	Phosphorus (mg)	150	920
Lactose (gm)	68	49	Sodium (mg)	160	506
Vitamins			Potassium (mg)	530	1570
Vitamin A (IU)	1898	1025	Chlorine (mg)	400	1028
Vitamin D (activity)	40	14	Magnesium (mg)	38-41	120
Vitamin E (IU)	3.2	0.4	Sulfur (mg)	140	300
Vitamin K (μg)	34	170	Iron (mg)*	0.56-0.3	0.5
Thiamine (μg)	150	370	Iodine (mg)	200	80
Riboflavin (μg)	380	1700	Manganese (μg)[+]	5.9-4.0	20-40
Niacin (mg)	1.7	0.9	Copper (μg)	60	110
Pyridoxine (μg)	130	460	Zinc (mg)[‡]	4-.5	3-5
Folic acid (μg)	41-84.6	2.9-68	Selenium (μg)	20	5-50
Cobalamine (μg)	.5	4	Fluoride (mg)	0.05	0.03-0.1
Ascorbic acid (μg)	44	17	Chromium (μg)	4	2

Data from Hambreaus, L.: Pediatr. Clin. North Am. **24**:17, 1977; Blanc, B.: World Rev. Nutr. Diet. **36**:I, 1981; Jensen, R.G., Haggerty, M.M., and McMahon, K.E.: Am. J. Clin. Nutr. **31**:990, 1978; Jansson, L., Akesson, B., and Holmberg, L.: Am. J. Clin. Nutr. **34**:8, 1981; Reeve, L.E., Chesney, R.W., and DeLuca, H.F.: Am. J. Clin. Nutr. **36**:122, 1982; Cooperman, J.M., and others: Am. J. Clin. Nutr. **36**:576, 1982; Keimpulainen, J., and Vuori, E.: Am. J. Clin. Nutr. **33**:2299, 1980; Siimes, M.A., Vuori, E., and Kuitunen, P.: Acta Paediatr. Scand. **68**:29, 1979; Vuori, E.: Acta Paediatr. Scand. **68**:571, 1979; Vuori, E., and Kuitunen, P.: Acta Paediatr. Scand. **68**:33, 1978; and Nayman, R., and others: Am. J. Clin. Nutr. **32**:1279, 1979.

*Median values at 2 weeks and 5 months of lactation.

+ Median values at 2 weeks and 5 months of lactation, after which time the manganese content of human milk tends to increase.

‡Median values at 2 weeks and 37 weeks of lactation.

months of age and then rises slightly, reflecting the infant's declining needs during declining rates of growth.

Human milk and cow's milk provide similar amounts of water and approximately the same quantity of energy. The nutrient sources of the energy are, however, different. Protein supplies approximately 7% of the calories in human milk and 20% of the calories in cow's milk; the carbohydrate lactose supplies approximately 42% of the calories in human milk and 20% of the calories in cow's milk. The percentage of calories supplied by fat is similar in both milks.

The protein content of human milk approximates 0.9 gm/100 ml, compared with 3.5 gm/100 ml in cow's milk. Nonprotein nitrogen accounts for 25% of total nitrogen in human milk, 5% of total nitrogen in cow's milk. During lactation protein levels decrease. Anderson, Atkinson, and Bryan[16] noted a linear decrease in protein nitrogen content of milk during the first 4 weeks of lactation. Chavalittamrong and others[17] found a decrease from 1.56 gm/100 ml at 1 to 7 days to 0.60 gm/100 ml at 180 to 270 days, then a gradual increase at 270 days in milk of the mothers.

Casein and **whey** constitute the protein in both milks. Amounts of whey protein are similar in each. Cow's milk contains six to seven times as much casein as does human milk, and differences in the casein/whey ratios of the two milks are great. The casein/whey ratio of human milk is 40:60, whereas the casein/whey ratio of cow's milk is 82:18. β-Lactoglobulin, the dominant whey protein in cow's milk, is absent in human milk, in which α-Lactoglobulin and lactoferrin are the predominant whey proteins.

During digestion in the stomach, the protein of milk mixes with hydrochloric acid. The result of this process is the formation of curds from the casein and calcium and of a liquid that contains the whey. Because of its lower casein content, human milk forms a soft, flocculent, easy-to-digest curd in the infant's stomach. The increased casein content of fresh cow's milk causes it to form a tough, cheesy, hard-to-digest curd. Homogenization, boiling, and dilution of cow's milk modify the curd and prevent the formation of the hard curd in the stomach so that it is easily digested by the infant.

The amino acid composition of human milk meets the needs of the neonate with an immature enzyme system, whereas that of cow's milk may be inappropriate. The newborn has a limited ability to metabolize phenylalanine to tyrosine. Human milk has a low content of tyrosine and phenylalanine compared with cow's milk. Cystathionase, an enzyme that catalyzes the transulfuration of methionine to cystine, is low in the neonate. Taurine and cystine are present in much higher concentrations in human milk than in cow's milk.

The total fat content of human milk and cow's milk is similar. Saturated fatty acids predominate in cow's milk. The fatty acid pattern of human milk resembles that of the maternal diet. About 98% of the fat in human milk is triglycerides in which palmitic acid is in position 2, enhancing its absorbability. The average content of linoleic acid is 10% of fat, but ranges of 1% to 43% have been reported. Linoleic acid provides an average of 4% of the calories in human milk but only 1% of the calories in cow's milk. The cholesterol content of human milk averages 20 mg/100 ml, but there is considerable variability. Values up to 47 mg/100 ml have been reported. Cow's milk contains 7 to 25 mg/100 ml of cholesterol.[18] Diurnal variations occur in human milk, the fat content being higher in early mornings. The content of short-chain fatty acids is greater in cow's milk. Human hindmilk has a higher percentage of fat than foremilk.

Both cow's milk and human milk contain lipoprotein lipase in the cream fraction that is stimulated by serum and inhibited by bile salts. Human milk contains an additional lipase that is stimulated by bile salts and contributes significantly to the hydrolysis of milk triglycerides. These enzymes contribute significantly to a higher percentage absorption of human milk fat as compared with butter fat.

The concentration of lactose is greater in human milk than in cow's milk. This nutrient is incorporated into galactolipids in the brain and spinal cord. Trace amounts of glucose, galactose, glucosamines, and other nitrogen-containing carbohydrates are also present in both milks. Human milk contains L-bifidus factor, a nitrogen-containing carbohydrate, in concentrations 40 times greater than in cow's milk. This carbohydrate is required by the bacteria *Lactobacillus* for growth.

Human milk from adequately nourished mothers is a reliable source of fat-soluble vitamins A and E and the water-soluble vitamins. The concentration of vitamin D in human milk has been shown to be influenced by maternal intake of vitamin D. The effect of sunlight on the infant is difficult to quantitate. However, when vitamin D deficient rickets has been identified in breast-fed infants, it has occurred most often in infants with dark skin and who have had little exposure to sunlight. Most breast-fed infants have exhibited normal growth and development without symptoms of vitamin D deficiency. A vitamin D supplement continues to be recommended for breast-fed infants, but evidence that supplements are necessary for infants with light skin is not convincing.[9]

Cow's milk is a reliable source of vitamin A and the B vitamins. It contains less vitamin E and more vitamin K than human milk. Most dairies fortify homogenized, 2%, and nonfat milk with vitamin D. Evaporated milk that is reconstituted with equal amounts of water is fortified with 400 IU/quart. The milk is low in vitamin C.

Cow's milk contains four times as much vitamin K as human milk. In breast-fed infants the prothrombin level is 20% to 50% of that of the adult in the first few days. Hemorrhagic disease of the newborn may occur if vitamin K is not given. A prophylactic dose of 0.5 to 1 mg is usually given to breast-fed infants at birth.

The increase in home deliveries with subsequent breast-feeding has caused concern. O'Connor and others[19] describe two infants delivered at home who were not given vitamin K and required hospitalization at 4 to 5 weeks of age because of vitamin K deficiency. Women who plan to have home deliveries should be counseled about the infant's need for vitamin K before delivery.

Inadequate amounts of water-soluble nutrients in the maternal diet are reflected in milk produced for the infant. Infantile beriberi is well known in East Asians when maternal intakes of thiamine are inadequate. Vitamin B_{12} deficiency has been reported in a breast-fed infant whose mother had been a vegan for 8 years before her pregnancy and in the infant of a mother who had pernicious anemia.[20] Supplementation of a folate-deficient woman resulted in a prompt increase in her milk folate.[21]

Because vitamin B_6 is critical to the development of the central nervous system, researchers have investigated the need for maternal supplementation to support optimal levels in their milk. They have found that only when mothers are supplemented with 10 to 20 mg pyrodoxidal hydrochloride does their milk meet American Academy of Pediatrics standards.[22]

The mineral content of cow's milk is several times greater than that of human milk. Cow's milk contains more than three times as much calcium and six times as much phosphorus as does human milk. The high phosphate load and calcium/phosphate ratio have been implicated as causes of late hypocalcemic tetany of the neonate.

The iron content of human milk declines from 0.5 to 0.3 mg/100 ml between 2 weeks and 5 months of age; that of cow's milk remains at 0.5 mg/100 ml. It has been reported that 5- to 7-month-old infants absorbed 49% of the iron in human milk but only 10% of the iron in cow's milk.[23]

Studies of the iron status of solely breast-fed infants indicate that a substantial number will become iron deficient by 9 months of age as evidenced by low total body iron. Iron supplements are desirable for breast-fed infants.[9]

Human milk contains less zinc than does cow's milk. In cow's milk zinc binds strongly to casein, but very little is bound to the whey. The zinc-binding capacity of human milk protein is assumed to be minimal. As the stomach acid secretion is low in early infancy, ingested zinc may not be released from casein or its curd, making zinc from cow's milk inaccessible to infants.[24] Studies suggest that the bioavailability of zinc in human milk is 59%, in cow's milk, 43% to 51%.[25]

Plasma fluoride is poorly transferred to breast milk, and breast-fed infants receive almost no fluoride.

The high protein and mineral content of cow's milk places a much greater osmolar load on the kidney of the infant and obligates a greater amount of water for excretion. The margin of safety is smaller. Cow's milk may not supply sufficient amounts of water when the environmental temperature is high. Neither milk may provide adequate amounts of water when requirements are increased by fever, vomiting, or diarrhea.

Anti-infective Characteristics of Human Milk

In addition to nutrients, human colostrum and milk contain antibodies, enzymes, and other factors absent or present in only minute amounts in cow's milk—factors that provide infants with protection against enteric infections.[26] Table 4-2 gives the antibacterial and antiviral factors that are present in breast milk.

Lactobacillus microorganisms in the gastrointestinal tract, whose growth is dependent on L-bifidus factor, produce acetic and lactic acids. The resulting acidic environment interferes with the growth of certain pathogenic organisms such as *Escherichia coli* and *Shigella* organisms and provides a medium in which lysozymes are stable. Lysozymes exert their effect by destroying bacterial cell membranes after the organisms have been inactivated by peroxides and ascorbic acid also present in human colostrum and milk.

Immunoglobulins (antibodies) to many different types of organisms, including pertussis, staphylococci, *E. coli,* and *Salmonella,* have been identified in colostrum and, in smaller amounts, in mature human milk. Since these immunoglobulins are not absorbed, they exert an effect only through the gastrointestinal tract. Infants who are breast-fed by mothers with high titers of antibodies to poliomyelitis are resistant to infection with orally administered polio vaccine. It is, however, believed that

Table 4-2   Antibacterial and antiviral factors in breast milk

Factor	Shown in Vitro to Be Active Against
Antibacterial factors	
L. bifidus growth factor	Enterobacteriaceae, enteric pathogens
Secretory IgA	E. coli, E. coli enterotoxin, C. tetani, C. diphtheriae, D. pneumoniae, Salmonella, Shigella
C1-C9	Effect not known
Lactoferrin	E. coli, C. albicans
Lactoperoxidase	Streptococcus, Pseudomonas, E. coli, S. typhimurium
Lysozyme	E. coli, Salmonella, M. lysodeikticus
Lipid (unsaturated fatty acid)	S. aureus
Milk cells	By phagocytosis: E. coli, C. albicans
	By sensitized lymphocytes: E. coli
Antiviral factors	
Secretory IgA	Polio types 1, 2, 3; Coxsackie types A9, B3, B5; ECHO types 6, 9; Semliki Forest virus, Ross River virus, rotavirus
Lipid (unsaturated fatty acids and monoglycerides)	Herpes simplex; Semliki Forest virus, influenza, dengue, Ross River virus, Murine leukemia virus, Japanese B encephalitis virus
Nonimmunoglobulin macromolecules	Herpes simplex; vesicular stomatitis virus
Milk cells	Rotavirus; induced interferon active against Sendai virus; sensitized lymphocytes; phagocytosis

Modified from Welsh, J. K., and May, J. T.: J. Pediatr. **94:**1, 1979.

human milk does not completely inhibit the effectiveness of the vaccine. Lactoperoxidase, an enzyme present in human milk and saliva, aids in killing streptococci and may act on other organisms.

Large amounts of lactoferrin and small amounts of transferrin (iron-binding proteins) in human milk exert a bacterial effect. Lactoferrin is less than 50% saturated with iron. In fact, Fransson and Lönnerdal[27] found the iron saturation of lactoferrin to be only 1% to 4%. It is bacteriostatic because it deprives bacteria of the iron-containing environment necessary for their normal cell growth.

Because of the presence of these and other antiinfective factors, infants who receive human milk have a lesser incidence of gastrointestinal and other infections than those fed other milks. This is true of those who live in well-sanitized environments as well as those who live under constant risk of environmental contamination.

Antiallergenic Characteristics of Human Milk

The intestine of the newborn infant is permeable to macromolecules. Secretory IgA in human milk promotes closure of the gut and therefore decreases the permeability of **allergens**. Cow's milk protein β-lactoglobulin and serum bovine albumin are the most common allergens in infancy. Breast-feeding is the best prophylaxis for food allergy during infancy.

Modified Cow's Milk Formula for Infants

Modified, commercially manufactured formulas prepared from nonfat cow's milk are readily available and are generously used for feeding in early infancy. In fact, the increase in the incidence of breast-feeding since 1966 has been accompanied by an increase in the use of formula products for older infants. There has been a decrease in the use of whole cow's milk in the first year.[9]

Cow's milk formulas are prepared by modifying whole cow's milk to reduce the solute load by reducing the protein and mineral content. The curd tension is reduced through homogenization and heat treatment to produce an easily digested protein.

Two manufacturers (Wyeth and Mead Johnson) combine demineralized whey with nonfat milk to produce a product with a whey/casein ratio similar to that of human milk. Minerals removed from the whey by electrodialysis are added in concentrations similar to that of human milk, resulting in simulated human milk. One manufacturer (Ross Laboratory) markets a modified casein predominant formula.

Combinations of vegetable oils, a high percentage of which are absorbed in infancy, are included, and carbohydrate is added to increase the caloric concentration to approximately that of human milk and cow's milk. Vitamins and minerals are added. Formulas are marketed both with and without ferrous sulfate in amounts that provide 12 mg of iron/quart.

Formulas for Infants

The Committee on Nutrition of the American Academy of Pediatrics, concerned about the composition of proprietary infant formulas, issued a policy statement on standards for these products. These standards are based on the composition of milk from a healthy mother and are given in Table 4-3. The minimum amount for each nutrient is close to that of human milk and thus is the preferable quantity. The maximum amount is given for formulas intended for low birth weight or sick infants who take less formula and therefore need the higher nutrient content.

Nutrients provided by commonly used formula preparations are given in Table 4-4.

Hypoallergenic Formulas

The most commonly used products for infants who have conditions that contraindi-

Table 4-3 Nutrient levels of infant formulas (per 100 kcal)

Nutrient	CON 1976 Recommendations			
	Minimum		Maximum	
Protein (gm)	1.8		4.5	
Fat				
(gm)	3.3		6.0	
(%cal)	30.0		54.0	
Essential fatty acids (linoleate)				
(%cal)	3.0		—	
(mg)	300.0		—	
Vitamins				
A (IU)	250.0	(75 μg)*	750.0	(225 μg)*
D (IU)	40.0		100.0	
K (μg)	4.0		—	
E (IU)	0.3	(with 0.7 IU/gm linoleic acid)	—	
C (ascorbic acid) (mg)	8.0		—	
B$_1$ (thiamine) (μg)	40.0		—	
B$_2$ (riboflavin) (μg)	60.0		—	
B$_6$ (pyridoxine) (μg)	35.0	(with 15 μg/gm of protein in formula)	—	
B$_{12}$ (μg)	0.15		—	
Niacin				
(μg)	250.0		—	
(μg equiv)	—		—	
Folic acid (μg)	4.0		—	
Pantothenic acid (μg)	300.0		—	
Biotin (μg)	1.5		—	
Choline (mg)	7.0		—	
Inositol (mg)	4.0		—	
Minerals				
Calcium (mg)	50.0+		—	
Phosphorus (mg)	25.0+		—	
Magnesium (mg)	6.0		—	
Iron (mg)	0.15		—	
Iodine (μg)	5.0		—	
Zinc (mg)	0.5		—	
Copper (μg)	60.0		—	
Manganese (μg)	5.0		—	
Sodium (mg)	20.0	(6 mEq)‡	60.0	(17 mEq)‡
Potassium (mg)	80.0	(14 mEq)‡	200.0	(34 mEq)‡
Chloride (mg)	55.0	(11 mEq)‡	150.0	(29 mEq)‡

From Committee on Nutrition, American Academy of Pediatrics: Pediatrics 57(2):278, 1976. Copyright American Academy of Pediatrics, 1976.

*Retinol equivalents.

+Calcium to phosphorus ratio must be no less than 1.1 nor more than 2.0.

‡Milliequivalent for 670 kcal/L of formula.

Table 4-4   Nutrient content of commercially available cow's milk–base formula

	Similac	Enfamil	S.M.A.
Nutrient source			
Protein	Casein	Reduced mineral whey, casein	Demineralized whey, casein
Fat	Soy oil, coconut oil	Soy oil, coconut oil	Oleo; soybean, oleic, and coconut oils
Carbohydrate	Lactose	Lactose	Lactose
Nutrients per 100/ml— normal dilution			
Energy (kcal)	68.0	67.0	67.0
Protein (gm)	1.5	1.5	1.5
Fat (gm)	3.6	3.8	3.6
Carbohydrate (gm)	7.2	6.9	7.2
Vitamin A (IU)	250.0	210.0	200.0
Vitamin D (IU)	41.0	42.0	40.0
Vitamin E (IU)	2.0	2.0	1.0
Vitamin C (mg)	6.0	5.4	5.5
Thiamine (μg)	68.0	52.0	67.0
Riboflavin (μg)	10.0	11.0	10.0
Niacin (μg)	710.0	840.0	500.0
Pyridoxine (μg)	41.0	42.0	41.0
Vitamin B_{12}(μg)	0.17	0.15	0.13
Folic acid (μg)	10.0	10.5	5.0
Calcium (mg)	51.0	46.0	42.0
Phosphorus (mg)	39.0	32.0	28.0
Magnesium (mg)	4.0	4.1	5.2
Iron (mg)	tr.	tr.	tr.
Zinc (mg)	0.5	0.5	0.5
Copper (μg)	60.0	63.4	48.0
Iodine (μg)	10.0	6.8	6.0

cate the use of cow's milk are the soy milks. The most frequently used formulas are constructed of protein isolated from soy meal fortified with methionine, corn syrup and/or sucrose, and soy or vegetable oils to which vitamins and minerals have been added. The trypsin inhibitor in raw soybean meal is inactivated during heat processing. The *goitrogenic effect* of soy is diminished by heating and the addition of iodine.

The American Academy of Pediatrics has stated that the soy formulas are useful for potentially allergic infants but should not be used for infants with a documented allergy to cow's milk.[29] Soy formulas are commonly used for infants who are recovering from diarrhea, and for children with galactosemia and lactase deficiency because they contain no lactase.

Other formulas are marketed for infants who do not tolerate either soy or cow's milk. Nutramigen, prepared from a casein hydrolysate and corn oil, and Progestimil, which contains a casein hydrolysate and medium-chain triglycerides, are commonly used when infants do not tolerate soy or cow's milk. They have an unpleasant odor and taste and are rarely accepted by infants if not introduced before 8 or 9 months of age. A whey-based predigested product for infants allergic to soy and cows milk has recently been marketed by another manufacturer. The composition of non-cow's milk-base formulas is given in Table 4-5.

Table 4-5　Nutrient content of soy formulas and other milk substitutes for infants

	Prosobee	Isomil	Nutramigen	Progestimil
Nutrient source				
Protein	Soy protein	Soy protein	Casein hydrolysate	Casein hydrolysate
Fat	Soy and coconut oil	Coconut and soy oil	Corn oil	Corn oil, medium-chain triglycerides
Carbohydrate	Corn syrup solids	Sucrose, corn syrup solids	Modified tapioca, sucrose	Corn syrup solids, modified tapioca starch
Nutrient per 100/ml— normal dilution				
Energy (kcal)	67.0	68.0	67.0	68.0
Protein (gm)	2.0	1.8	1.9	1.9
Fat (gm)	3.6	3.7	2.6	2.7
Carbohydrate (gm)	6.7	6.8	9.1	9.1
Vitamin A (IU)	21.0	20.3	17.0	21.0
Vitamin D (IU)	42.0	41.0	42.0	42.0
Vitamin E (IU)	2.1	2.0	1.0	2.0
Vitamin C (mg)	5.4	5.4	5.5	5.5
Thiamine (μg)	53.0	41.0	53.0	53.0
Riboflavin (μg)	63.0	61.0	63.4	63.4
Niacin (mg)	0.8	0.9	0.8	0.8
Pyridoxine (μg)	42.0	41.0	42.0	42.0
Vitamin B_{12} (μg)	0.2	0.3	0.2	0.2
Folic acid (μg)	10.5	10.0	10.5	10.5
Calcium (mg)	63.0	71.0	63.0	63.0
Phosphorus (mg)	50.0	51.0	42.0	42.0
Magnesium (mg)	7.3	5.1	7.4	7.4
Iron (mg)	1.3	1.2	1.3	1.3
Zinc (mg)	0.5	0.5	0.5	0.4
Copper (μg)	63.0	51.0	63.0	63.0
Iodine (μg)	6.8	10.0	4.8	4.8

Goat's milk should be used with care during infancy. It is low in iron, folate, and vitamins B, C, and D. It has a high solute load relative to cow's milk and may cause metabolic **acidosis** if fed in the first month of life.[30] If goat's milk is to be used before 6 months, it should be diluted with water and carbohydrate should be added.

Feeding infants formulas made from recipes that have not been proved to support adequate nutrition should be strongly discouraged. Malnutrition has been observed in infants fed a barley water, corn syrup, and whole milk formula.[31] Kwashiorkor has been reported in infants fed a non-diary creamer as a substitute for milk.[32] Beriberi has been diagnosed in a 6-week-old infant whose intake was limited to a non-dairy creamer.[33]

Formula Preparation

Manufacturers market formulas as liquid concentrates to be prepared for feeding by mixing equal amounts of the liquid and water. Ready-to-feed formulas that require no preparation are available in an assortment of sizes (4-, 6-, 8-, and 32-oz bottles and cans). Powdered formula that is prepared by mixing 1 level tbsp of powder in 2 oz of water is also available. One recommended evaporated milk formula is prepared by mixing 13 oz (one can) of evaporated milk with 2 tbsp of corn syrup and 18 oz of water. All of the formulas, when properly prepared and adequately supplemented, provide the nutrients important for the infant in an appropriate caloric concentration and present a solute load reasonable for the normal full-term infant. Errors in dilution caused by misunderstanding the proper method of preparation, improper measurements, or the belief of the parents that their child should have greater amounts of nutritious food can lead to problems.

Result of errors in formula preparation

Failure to gain appropriately in height and weight has been observed as a result of dilu-

tion of ready-to-feed formulas in the manner concentrates are prepared. Mothers have been known to add extra water to formula in the belief that a more dilute formula might reduce spitting up by their infants.

Feeding undiluted concentrated formula increases calories, protein, and solutes presented to the kidneys for excretion and may predispose the young infant to **hypernatremia**, tetany, and obesity. Problems of improper formula preparation have most frequently been reported with the use of powdered formula and occur most often when an increased need for water caused by fever or infection is superimposed on consumption of an already high-solute formula. Infants fed concentrated formula during such illnesses may become thirsty, demand more to drink, or refuse to consume more liquid because of anorexia secondary to illness. When presented with more milk concentrated in the protein and solutes, the osmolality of the blood increases and hypernatremic dehydration may result. Cases of cerebral damage and gangrene of the extremities have been reported to be the result of hypernatremic dehydration and metabolic acidosis.[34,35] The feeding of undiluted evaporated milk for 5 days after an illness during infancy has been reported to be the cause of gangrene resulting in the loss of limbs in a $6\frac{1}{2}$-week-old infant.[34] Infants who have been fed improperly prepared concentrated and ready-to-feed formulas with less dramatic long-term effects have been noted by many who counsel parents of very young infants.

Overdiluting formula or offering water as a substitute for milk or as a pacifier can lead to serious consequences. Water intoxication resulting in hyponatremia, irritability, and coma has been reported in several infants fed 8 oz of water after each feeding or fed water as a substitute for milk because of financial inability of parents to buy more formula.[36,37]

Anticipatory guidance of parents of young infants should include information on the variety of formulas available with which to feed their infants, differences in methods of preparation of each product, and the dangers of overdiluted formula and excessive water intake.

Sterilization of formulas

Although terminal sterilization is recommended for infant formulas, many parents do not follow this practice but prepare formulas by the clean technique, one bottle at each feeding time, and immediately feed the infant. Several researchers have found no differences in incidence of illness or infection of infants fed formulas prepared by the clean technique or by terminal sterilization regardless of socioeconomic background or housekeeping practices.[38,39] Formulas prepared by both methods result in milk that produces aerobic bacteria.

If formulas are to be prepared by the clean technique, it is important that the hands of the person preparing the formula are first carefully washed. All equipment to be used during preparation, including the cans that contain the milk, the bottles, and the nipples, must be thoroughly washed and rinsed. Once opened, cans of formula must be covered and refrigerated. The formula is prepared immediately before each feeding. After the formula has been heated and the infant has been fed, any remaining milk should be discarded. Warm milk is an excellent medium for bacterial growth.

The age at which it is appropriate to offer whole cow's milk to infants is controversial. Reasons for discouraging the use of whole cow's milk in infancy includes its relation to anemia caused by occult blood loss from the gastrointestinal tract, its high renal solute load compared to both human milk and commercially prepared infant formulas, and a potential allergy to milk.[40]

That occult blood loss occurs in infancy and is associated with whole milk is known. It has usually been noted in younger infants and those who have consumed large volumes of milk.

However, Fomon and associates have shown that after 140 days of life there is no difference in the number of guaiac positive stools of infants fed whole cow's milk compared to those fed commercially prepared formula.[41]

Cow's milk does have a higher renal solute load than human milk and infant formula. However, by 6 months of age the kidneys of the normal infant have matured sufficiently that the use of whole milk should cause no problem in the absence of diarrhea or hot weather.

The problem of food **allergy** is the difficulty in achieving a definitive diagnosis since many of the symptoms of food allergy mimic those of other conditions. A properly controlled elimination/challenge test under controlled conditions can confirm or negate the suspected allergy.

The Committee on Nutrition of the Academy of Pediatrics has stated that if infants receive at least one third of their calories from supplemental foods and consume no more than 1 L of milk per day, they see no disadvantage to the use of whole milk after 6 months of age.[40]

Nonfat and 2% milk are not recommended in the first year. Infants fed nonfat milk increase their intake and continue to gain weight but at a slower rate. They lose body fat, as evidenced by decreases in skinfold thickness, and lose energy reserves. Because milk solids are often added to 2% milk it may increase the renal solute load. Even though one researcher suggested infants over 6 months of age can achieve adequate growth and nurture consuming this milk in combination with infant food, it is not recommended.[42]

Substitute or imitation milks should not be offered to infants. These milks, defined by the Food and Drug Administration as nutritionally equivalent to whole or skim milk based on the content of only 14 or 15 nutrients, omitting many nutrients recommended as components for infant formulas, are not appropriate for infants.[43]

One manufacturer (Ross Laboratories) markets a formula for the older infant that consists of nonfat milk, corn oil, and sucrose, the caloric concentration of which is reduced to 16.5 kcal/oz as compared with 20 kcal/oz in standard formulas. The formula is fortified with both iron and vitamins. Infants fed this milk and pureed foods have been noted to increase their volume of intake, so that when compared with infants consuming a standard formula supplying 20 kcal/oz energy intakes are similar.

Economics of Infant Feeding

Several attempts have been made to compare the economic impact of the provision of energy and nutrients to support human lactation with the use of prepared infant formula. Investigators have reported disadvantages both to breast-feeding and to formula-feeding.

It must be remembered that the numbers of foods that supply important nutrients for lactation are large. Therefore the economic impact can range from a minimal increase to a sizeable increase over basic food costs.

Young infants who consume a whole milk or evaporated milk formula prepared with added carbohydrate are hypothesized to be receiving the least expensive feeding. However, many infants malabsorb as much as 34% of butterfat ingested. Any savings may be lost in the feces. The cost of commercially prepared formula varies with packaging. Concentrated formulas are the least expensive; ready-to-feed formulas are the most costly. The nutrient support for breast-feeding cost about 50% to 60% as much as the ready-to-feed formula.

Feeding the infant human milk can be less expensive or more expensive than commercially prepared formula, depending on the parents' food purchasing practices and selection of foods. The many advantages of human milk far exceed any small monetary advantage to the use of prepared formula. Money saved can be obligated by additional medical care when the resistance factors are not present in the young infant's diet. Parents may need help in the selection of appropriate low-cost foods, but breast-feeding should never be discouraged on an economic basis.

Bonding

Klaus and Kennell[44] have shown that the first few minutes and hours of life are important to maternal-infant **bonding**. This leads to attachment, the unique relationship between two people that is special and lasts forever. Mothers who have immediate skin contact with their infants shortly after birth have significantly more attachment behaviors. Breast-feeding facilitates this attachment.

FOODS IN THE INFANT'S DIET

In spite of the fact that no nutritional advantage can be expected from the early introduction of semisolid foods, many families feed them in the first month of life. Semisolid foods are introduced by parents on the advice of physicians, neighbors, and friends and because parents think that it is time for their infants to eat foods other than milk. Some parents add semisolid foods in the hope that they will encourage their infants to sleep through the night, a commonly held belief that has been proved untrue. Other parents feed semisolid foods because they think that their infants are hungry or because they consider the acceptance of these foods a developmental landmark.

Many infants receive table food by the time they can sustain a sitting posture. After infants begin to finger feed, increasing amounts of table food are included in their diets.

Semisolid Foods

The age of introduction of semisolid foods to infants in the United States declined from 1920, when these foods were seldom offered before 1 year of age, to 1960 to 1970, when they were frequently offered in the first weeks and months of life. Concern that this early introduction of semisolid foods predisposed infants to obesity and allergic reactions caused many health care professionals in the pediatric community to reexamine the appropriate age for the introduction of these foods. It is currently recommended that the feeding of semisolid foods be delayed until the infant's consumption of food is no longer a reflexive process, and the infant has the fine, gross, and oral motor skills to appropriately consume them (i.e., at approximately 4 to 6 months of age). Even so, many parents are reported to offer semisolid foods in the first month of life. Table 4-6 gives suggested guidelines for the introduction of semisolid foods to normal infants.

It appears to make little difference whether fruits or vegetables are introduced first. New foods should be added singly at intervals of no more than every 3 days. The introduction

of nitrate-containing vegetables (e.g., carrots, beets, and spinach) is usually delayed until the infant is at least 4 months of age, because the nitrate can be converted to nitrite in the stomach of the young infant. This can result in **methemoglobinemia.**

Infant's acceptance of semisolid foods

Parents report both immediate acceptance and rejection of semisolid foods, a fact that may relate to the mother's skill in feeding and her attitudes and feelings about these foods. Some parents who believe that the use of semisolid foods is important add them to the formula, cut a larger hole in the nipple, and feed the semisolid foods in this manner. One manufacturer markets a syringe with a plunger and a nipple with which mothers can force feed their babies by pushing the strained food through the nipple. These practices increase the

Table 4-6 Suggested ages for the introduction of semisolid foods and table foods

Food	Age (Months)		
	4 to 6	6 to 8	9 to 12
Iron-fortified cereals for infants	Add		
Vegetables		Add strained	Gradually delete strained foods, introduce table foods
Fruits		Add strained	Gradually delete strained foods, introduce chopped well-cooked or canned foods
Meats		Add strained or finely chopped table meats	Decrease the use of strained meats, increase the varieties of table meats
Finger foods such as arrowroot biscuits, oven-dried toast		Add those that can be secured with a palmar grasp	Increase the use of small-sized finger foods as the pincer grasp develops
Well-cooked mashed or chopped table foods, prepared without added salt or sugar			Add
Juice by cup			Add

energy and nutrient composition of the formula and may deprive the infant of experiences that are important in the development of feeding behavior.

Commercially prepared strained and junior foods are offered to many infants. They are available in jars and as dried flakes. Some mothers prefer to make their own with a blender or strainer. Ready-to-serve single-grain dry cereals such as rice cereal are commonly the first food offered to infants because rice is considered the least allergenic of the cereal grains and because most cereals are fortified with electrolic iron. Parents are reported to mix milk with cereal until it is almost liquid. Fruits are commonly reported as favorites. Vegetables appear to be accepted without problems. Preferences have been suggested for yellow vegetables, green beans, and peas; spinach and beets are often reported to be rejected. Strained meats, especially liver, are frequently rejected by infants. Parents state that the infants reject the sticky, granular texture rather than the taste of meats. Older infants are, as a result, often fed strained and junior vegetable and meat mixtures and high-meat dinners.

Food additives and fortification in semisolid foods

Concern that intakes of sodium in the first year might predispose infants to later **hypertension** has resulted in the deletion of salt from commercially prepared infant foods. Sugar is added only to desserts. All cereals are fortified with niacin, thiamine, riboflavin, calcium, and phosphorus. All dry infant cereals are fortified with electrolytically reduced iron. Strained, jarred cereals with fruit are fortified with ferrous sulfate. High-meat and mixed dinners are prepared with rice or wheat flour or tapioca to increase shelf life. Modified corn or tapioca starch is included in some desserts. Fruits and fruit juices are enriched with vitamin C.

Home preparation of semisolid foods

It is both possible and economical for parents to prepare semisolid foods for their infants with a food grinder, blender, or strainer. The foods should be carefully selected from high-quality fresh, frozen, or canned fruits, vegetables, and meats and should be prepared so that nutrients are retained. The area in which the foods are prepared and the utensils used in preparation should be meticulously cleaned. Salt and sugar should be used sparingly, if at all. When the food has been cooked, pureed, and strained, it should be packaged in individual portions and refrigerated or frozen so that a single portion can be heated and fed without compromising the quality and bacterial content of the entire batch. Directions for preparation of infant foods are given in the box on p. 102.

Home-prepared infant foods have a greater energy content than commercially prepared foods and many have a higher salt content. One study found that home-prepared infant foods had 1005% more salt than commercially prepared food.[45] Mothers who feed higher sodium intakes to infants are reported to salt their food more vigorously and have less education than mothers who offer lower sodium intakes.[46]

Fruit juice

When a high percentage of infants were fed evaporated milk formulas, vitamin C–containing fruit juices were commonly introduced in the first month of life; the widespread use of vitamin-fortified formula and vitamin supplements made this practice unnecessary. Because a sucrose-containing liquid consumed as infants go to sleep sometimes results in extensive dental caries (see Chapter 11), it is generally recommended that the introduction of fruit juice be delayed until it can be consumed from a cup.

Nutrients in semisolids

Ranges of nutrients found in any group of foods for infants are sizeable (Table 4-7).

Directions for Home Preparation of Infant Foods

1. Select fresh, high-quality fruits, vegetables, or meats.
2. Be sure all utensils, including cutting boards, grinders, and knives are thoroughly clean.
3. Wash your hands before preparing the food.
4. Clean, wash, and trim the foods in as little water as possible.
5. Cook the foods until tender in as little water as possible. Avoid overcooking, which may destroy heat-sensitive nutrients.
6. Do not add salt. Add sugar sparingly. Do not add honey to foods for infants less than 1 year of age.*
7. Add enough water so that the food has a consistency that is easily pureed.
8. Strain or puree the food using an electric blender, a food mill, a baby food grinder, or a kitchen strainer.
9. Pour puree into ice cube tray and freeze.
10. When food is frozen hard, remove the cubes and store in freezer bags.
11. Unfreeze and heat in serving container the amount of food that will be consumed at a single feeding (in water bath or microwave oven).

From Pipes, P.L.: Nutrition in infancy. In Krause, M.V., and Mahan, L.K.: Food, nutrition, and diet therapy, ed. 7, Philadelphia, 1984, W.B. Saunders Co.

*Botulism spores have been reported in honey, and young infants do not have the immune capacity to resist this infection.

Table 4-7 Ranges of selected nutrients per ounce in commercially prepared infant foods

Food	Energy (kcal)	Protein (gm)	Iron (mg)	Vitamin A (IU)	Vitamin C (mg)
Dry cereal	102-114	2.0-10.2	17.0-21.0	0-20	0-1.4
Strained and junior fruits	11-23	0.0-0.2	0.0-2.0	3-206	0.2-35.3
Strained and junior vegetables	7-18	0.2-1.0	0.1-0.4	9-3348	0.6-3.6
Strained and junior meats	27-42	3.6-4.4	0.3-1.5	8-10811	0.3-0.7
Strained egg yolks	58	2.8	0.8	355	0.4
Strained and junior meat and vegetable dinners	20-33	1.6-2.6	0.0-0.3	22-237	0.1-0.5
Strained and junior vegetable and meat dinners	9-70	0.1-1.5	0.1-0.3	4-1114	0.2-1.2
Strained and junior desserts	17-25	0.0-0.8	0.0-0.1	4-71	0.2-8.9

From Gebhardt, S.E., Cutrufelli, R., and Matthews, R.H.: Composition of foods, baby foods, raw, processed, prepared, Agriculture Handbook No. 8-3, Washington, D.C., 1978, U.S. Department of Agriculture.

Jarred cereals are fortified with ferrous sulfate, dry infant cereals are fortified with electrolytically reduced iron. Absorption of electrolytically reduced iron is approximately 5% of that of ferrous sulfate.

Strained and junior fruits contribute one third more calories, only a fraction of the vitamin A, but twice as much vitamin C as do vegetables when fed in equal amounts. Vegetables contribute small but important amounts of iron. Fruit juice is fortified with abundant amounts of vitamin C.

Strained and junior meats contribute significant amounts of protein and iron. High-meat dinners contribute less than half as much protein as pure meat; vegetables and meat contribute less than one fifth as much protein as pure meat. Strained and junior meats and high-meat dinners contribute similar amounts of iron; strained vegetables and meat contribute much less iron. Strained vegetables and meat provide slightly less than half as many calories as meat; high-meat dinners provide 75% as many calories as pure meat. Strained egg yolks have the highest calorie concentration of the prepared infant foods.

Strained and junior desserts are rich in carbohydrate and calories. A few are fortified with vitamin C. All have a sweet taste, and indiscriminate use of these items should be discouraged.

Infants receive table food soon after the introduction of supplemental foods. Most often the foods offered the infants are the same foods prepared for the remainder of the family. Data from the HANES II study indicate that 7 to 12 months of age the energy intake from table food increases dramatically and that from commercially prepared foods declines. At 1 year of age over 50% of the energy intake of infants is provided by table food.[47] Little guidance has been provided parents in appropriate table foods for infants, and cases of choking and aspiration have occurred. Hot dogs, nuts, grapes, carrots, and round candies should be

---

Appropriate Introductory Table Food for Infants

Mashed potatoes
Well-cooked mashed vegetables (carrots, stringless green beans)
Soft, mashed fruits (bananas, peaches, pears)
Peeled, mashed vienna sausage
Well-cooked, *finely ground*, ground meats
Yogurt
Canned, drained tuna or salmon (no bones)
Egg yolk, mashed with milk or water
Mashed or refried beans

---

avoided. Appropriate table foods for infants are shown in the box above.

Honey, sometimes used as a sweetener for home-prepared infant foods and formulas and recommended for use on pacifiers to promote sucking in hypotonic infants, has been implicated as the only food source of spores of *Clostridium botulinum* during infancy. These spores are extremely resistant to heat and are not destroyed by present methods of processing honey. **Botulism** in infancy is caused by ingestion of the spores, which germinate into the toxin in the lumen of the bowel. Honey should not be fed to infants less than 1 year of age.[48]

Stages of development of feeding behavior indicate readiness to progress in textures of food and are discussed in the section on development of feeding behavior. The energy and nutrient composition of foods offered must also be considered. Examples of table foods often offered and their contribution to an infant's dietary intake are given in Table 4-8.

INTAKES OF INFANTS

Volume of intake and energy consumption is influenced not only by the infant's requirements for maintenance, growth, and activity

Table 4-8   Nutrient content of selected table foods commonly fed to infants

Food	Portion size	Energy (kcal)	Protein (gm)	Iron (mg)	Vitamin A (IU)	Vitamin C (mg)
Cooked cereal (farina)	$\frac{1}{4}$ cup	26	0.8	Dependent on level of fortification		
Mashed potato	$\frac{1}{3}$ cup	34	1.1	0.2	10	5
French fried potato	3, 1" to 2"	29	0.4	0.2		
Spaghetti	2 tbsp	19	0.6	0.2		
Macaroni and cheese	2 tbsp	54	2.1	0.2	107	
Liverwurst	$\frac{1}{2}$ oz	45	2.1	0.8	925	
Hamburger	$\frac{1}{2}$ oz	41	3.4	0.5	5	
Eggs	1 medium	72	5.7	1.0	520	
Cottage cheese	1 tbsp	5	1.9		23.7	
Green beans	1 tbsp	3	0.15	0.2	43	1
Cooked carrots	1 tbsp	2.81			952	
Banana	$\frac{1}{2}$ small	40	0.5	0.35	90	5
Pudding	$\frac{1}{4}$ cup	70	2.2	Trace	102	
Lollipop	1 oz hard candy	109				
Saltine crackers	1	12	0.2			
Vanilla wafer	$\frac{1}{4}$" thick, $1\frac{3}{4}$" diameter	18	0.2			
Cheese strips	$\frac{1}{4}$ oz	28	1.78		92	

From Adams, C.F.: Nutritive value of American foods in common units, Agriculture Handbook No. 456, Washington, D.C., 1975, U.S. Department of Agriculture.

but also by the parents' sensitivity to and willingness to accept cues of hunger and satiety, parental eagerness for the infant to feed, and the parents' skill at feeding. The caloric concentration of the formula is also a determinant of the volume of intake, calorie intake, and growth in early infancy.[41, 49]

Infants feed differently, and mothers vary in their sensitivity to their child's cues. Thoman[50] found that primiparous mothers spent more time stimulating their infants during feeding than did multiparous mothers, yet their infants spent less time sucking during breast-feeding and consumed less from bottles at feeding than did infants of multiparous mothers in the newborn period. Primiparous mothers stimulated their infants during pauses between sucking. The stimulation prolonged the pause and reduced the total consumption of food.

Growth Response to Feeding

Normal breast-fed infants regulate their intakes of milk to meet their needs for normal growth and development. Formula-fed infants have been reported to regain their birth weights more rapidly than breast-fed infants.[51]

Exclusively breast-fed infants grow in length more slowly then infants fed formula and semisolid foods; they are heavier for their length. These infants experience catch-up growth when their diet is expanded.[52] Weight gains of formula-fed infants have been found to be equal to or slightly greater than those of breast-fed infants in the first 4 months of life.[53]

Energy Intakes

Per unit of size, infants consume the greatest number of calories between 14 and 28 days of age, a time known to many pediatricians as the hungry period.[49] Mothers who are breast-feeding often find it necessary to provide supplemental bottles at the end of a breast-feeding (when the breasts are emptied) for several days during this hungry period, after which lactation adjusts to increased intakes and breast-feeding alone can be resumed. After this time, although total quantity and energy intakes increase, intakes per unit of size decrease. Infants consume greater amounts of food and nutrients as they grow older but less and less per unit of body size.

Wide ranges of volume of intake and energy consumption throughout the first year of life have been noted in formula-fed infants by several researchers.[54,56] Table 4-9 gives ranges reported in Boston and Denver studies.[54,55]

Table 4-10 shows ranges of breast-fed and bottle-fed infants in an Australian study.

Studies by Fomon and others[49] have shown that the caloric concentration of the formula influences calorie intake during the first 41 days of life. Female infants who were fed formulas calorically concentrated to 100 kcal/100 ml (30 kcal/oz) reduced their volume of intake but consumed greater numbers of calories, whereas those who were fed for-

Table 4-9 Ranges of volume of intake and energy consumption of normal infants

Age (Months)	Denver Studies (Calories/kg/Day)	Boston Studies (Calories/kg/Day)
2-3	89-141	90-159
5-6	75-139	82-163
9-12	74-152	75-152

From Rueda-Willamson, R., and Rose, H.E.: Pediatrics 30:639, 1962.

Table 4-10 Consumption in kcal/kg body weight (mean and range of breast milk substitutes [BMS] and breast milk [BM] by 150 infants aged 1-3 months and fed ad libitum)

Age (Months)	BMS (kcal/kg)	BM (kcal/kg)
1	120 (78-201)	112 (74-146)
2	107 (75-168)	108 (74-145)
3	101 (76-130)	96 (70-120)

From Hofvander, Y., and others: The amount of milk consumed by 1-3 month old breast or bottle fed infants, Acta Paediatr. Scand. 71:953, 1982.

mulas calorically diluted to 54 kcal/100 ml (16.5 kcal/oz) increased their volume of intake but consumed fewer calories, as compared with infants who were fed formulas of normal caloric concentration. After this period, adjustments in volume of intake were sufficient so that calorie intakes were similar for the entire 111-day study period. Infants who were fed the calorically concentrated formula were, however, heavier for their lengths at 111 days of age than were infants who had been fed the calorically dilute formulas.[56] Male infants who were fed formulas concentrated to 133 kcal/100 ml (40 kcal/oz) reduced their volume of intake but consumed greater numbers of calories during the first 84 days of life and experienced supernormal rates of growth in both length and weight during the first 42 days of life, as compared with infants who were fed formulas providing 67 kcal/100 ml (20 kcal/oz).[49]

FEEDING BEHAVIORS

Defining developmental readiness for changes in textures of food and the acquisition of self-feeding skills is important in establishing realistic goals for normal and handicapped infants and children. Illingworth and Lister[57] have defined a critical or sensitive period of development in relation to eating, a time at which a specific stimulus, solid food, must be applied for the organism to learn a particular action, that of accepting and eating table food, which is more difficult to masticate. They point out that an infant learns to chew at about 6 or 7 months of age, thus he or she is, at this point, developmentally ready to consume food. If solid foods are withheld until a later age, the child will have considerably more difficulty in accepting them.

In 1937 Gesell and Ilg[58] published observations of their extensive studies of the feeding behavior of infants. Their observations are as valid today as they were then. Cineradiographic techniques developed since then have permitted more detailed descriptions of sucking, suckling, and swallowing.[59,60]

Development of feeding behavior depends on the maturation of the central nervous system, which controls the acquisition of fine, gross, and oral motor skills, each of which influences the child's ability to consume food and the manner in which he or she suckles, sucks, chews, and swallows. Normal development proceeds in an orderly and predictable **cephalocaudal** sequence. Likewise, the sequence of acquisition of feeding skills occurs in a predictable order influenced by the acquisition of function and behavior.

It is important to recognize that even though the normal neonate is well prepared to suck and swallow at birth, the physical and neuromotor maturation during the first year alter both the form of the oral structure and the methods by which the infant extracts liquids from a nipple. Each of the parameters of change influences the infant's eating skills. At birth the tongue is disproportionately large in comparison with the lower jaw and essentially fills the oral cavity. The mandible is retruded relative to the maxilla, the maxilla protruding over the mandible by approximately 2 mm. When the mouth is closed, the jaws do not rest on top of each other, but the tip of the tongue lies between the upper and lower jaws. There is a fat pad in each of the cheeks. It is thought that these pads serve as a prop for the buccinator muscle, maintaining rigidity of the cheeks during suckling. The lips of the neonate are also instrumental in sucking and suckling and have characteristics appropriate for their function at this age. A mucosal fold on the free edge of the gums in the region of the eyetooth buds of both jaws is instrumental in sealing off the oral cavity as the lips close around a nipple. The mucosal fold disappears by the third or fourth month, when the lips have developed muscular control to seal the oral cavity.

The sucking, swallowing, and respiratory centers are located in close proximity within the brain stem. The rhythmic functions must be coordinated to allow for the crossing of the alimentary and respiratory pathways in the **pharynx**. The newborn infant coordinates sucking, breathing, and swallowing.

The newborn infant sucks reflexively; the young infant (beginning at 2 to 3 weeks of age) suckles, and, as the infant grows older, he or she learns mature sucking. Some description of the two processes therefore seems important.

Suckling

Cineradiographic studies by Ardan, Kemp, and Lind[59,60] have shown that the processes of breast suckling and bottle suckling are similar. The nipple of the breast becomes rigid and elongated during breast feeding so that it closely resembles a rubber nipple in shape, and both assume a similar position in the infant's mouth. The infant grasps the nipple in his or her mouth. The oral cavity is sealed off by pressure from the median portions of the lips assisted by the mucosal folds in the jaws. The nipple is held in the infant's mouth with the tip located close to the junction of the hard and soft palates.

During the first stage of suckling, the mandible and tongue are lowered while the mouth is closed, thus creating a negative pressure. The tip of the tongue moves forward. The mandible and tongue are next raised, compressing the anterior end of the nipple. The compression is moved anteroposteriorly as the tip of the tongue withdraws, thus stroking or milking the liquid from the nipple. The retruded position of the mandible maximizes the efficiency of the stroking action. As the tongue moves back, it comes in contact with the tensed soft palate, thus causing liquid to squirt into the lateral food channels. The location of the larynx is much higher during infancy that it is in adulthood, and the larynx is further elevated by muscular contractions during swallowing. The **epiglottis** functions as a breakwater during swallowing. As the liquid is squirted back in the mouth, the epiglottis is positioned so that it parts the stream of liquid, thus passing it to the sides of the larynx instead of over it. Thus liquid does not pass over the **laryngeal** entrance during early infancy because of the relatively higher position of the larynx and parting of the stream of liquid by the epiglottis.

Sucking

Mature sucking is an acquired feature of the orofacial muscles. It is not a continuous process. Upon accumulation of sufficient fluid in the mouth, sucking and breathing are interrupted by a swallowing movement. The closure of the nasopharyngeal and laryngeal sphincters in response to the presence of food in the pharynx is responsible for the interruption of nasal breathing.

During swallowing the food lies in a swallow preparatory position on the groove of the tongue. The distal portion of the soft palate is raised toward the adenoidal pad in the roof of the epipharynx. The tongue is pressed upward against the nipple so that the bolus of milk follows gravity down the sloping tongue reaching the pharynx. As the bolus moves downward, the posterior wall of the pharynx comes forward to displace the soft palate toward the dorsal surface of the tongue, and the larynx is elevated and arched backward. The bolus is expressed from the pharynx by peristaltic movements of the pharyngeal wall toward the back of the tongue and the larynx. The bolus spills over the pharyngoepiglottic folds into the lateral food channels and then into the esophagus.[60]

The tonsils and lymphoid tissue play an important role as infants swallow; they assist in keeping the airway open and in keeping food away from the posterior pharyngeal wall as the infant is fed in a reclining position, thus delaying nasopharyngeal closure until food has reached the lower pharynx.

As the infant grows older the oral cavity enlarges so that the tongue no longer fills the mouth. The tongue grows differentially at the tip and attains motility in the larger oral cavity. The elongated tongue can be protruded to receive and pass solids between the gum pads and erupting teeth for mastication. Mature feeding is characterized by separate movements of the lip, tongue, and gum pads or teeth.

Sequence of Development of Feeding Behavior

The sequence of development of feeding behavior is given in Table 4-11 and Figure 4-1.

Newborn infants can neither focus their eyes nor direct their hands, yet they find nourishment. The rooting reflex caused by stroking of the perioral skin including the cheeks and lips causes an infant to turn toward the stimulus, so that the mouth comes in contact with it. Stimulus placed on the lips causes involuntary movements toward it, closure, and pouting in preparation for sucking. These reflexes thus enable the infant to suck and receive nourishment. Both rooting and suckling can be elicited when the infant is hungry but are absent when the infant is satiated. During feeding the neonate assumes a tonic neck position, the head rotated to one side and the arm on that side extended while the other is

Table 4-11   Sequence of development of feeding behavior

Age	Reflexes	Oral, Fine, Gross Motor Development
1-3 months	Rooting, suck, and swallow reflexes are present at birth Tonic neck reflex present	Head control is poor Secures milk with a suckling pattern, the tongue projecting during a swallow By the end of the third month, head control is developed
4-6 months	Rooting and bite reflexes fade Tonic neck reflex fades by 16 weeks	Changes from a sucking pattern to a mature suck with liquids Sucking strength increases Munching pattern begins Grasps with a palmar grasp Grasps, brings objects to mouth, and bites them
7-9 months	Gag reflex is less strong as chewing of solids begins and normal gag is developing Choking reflex can be inhibited	Munching movements begin when solid foods are eaten Rotary chewing begins Sits alone Has power of voluntary release and resecural Holds bottle alone Develops an inferior pincer grasp
10-12 months		Reaches for a spoon Bites nipples, spoons, and crunchy foods Grasps bottle and foods and brings them to the mouth Can drink from a cup that is held Tongue is used to lick food morsels off the lower lip Finger feeds with a refined pincer grasp

Modified from Gessell, A., and Ilg, F.L.: Feeding behavior of infants, Philadelphia, 1937, J.B. Lippincott Co.

fisted. The infant seeks the nipple by touch and obtains milk from the nipple with a rhythmic suckle. Semisolid foods, introduced at an early age into diets of many infants fed by spoon, are secured in the same manner as is the milk, by stroking movements of the tongue with the tongue projecting as the spoon is withdrawn. Frequently, food is expelled from the mouth.

By 5 weeks of age the infant can focus the eyes on faces, and by 12 weeks of age the gaze can be shifted. At 10 weeks of age the infant is able to recognize the breast or bottle as the source of food.

4 to 6 months

By 16 weeks of age the more mature sucking pattern has become evident, with the tongue moving back and forth as opposed to the earlier up-and-down motions. Spoon feeding is easier because the infant can draw in the lower lip as the spoon is removed. The tonic neck position has faded, and the infant assumes a more symmetrical position with the head at midline. The hands close on the bottle. By 20 weeks of age the infant can grasp on **tactile** contact with a palmar squeeze. By 24 weeks of age he or she can reach for and grasp an object on sight. In

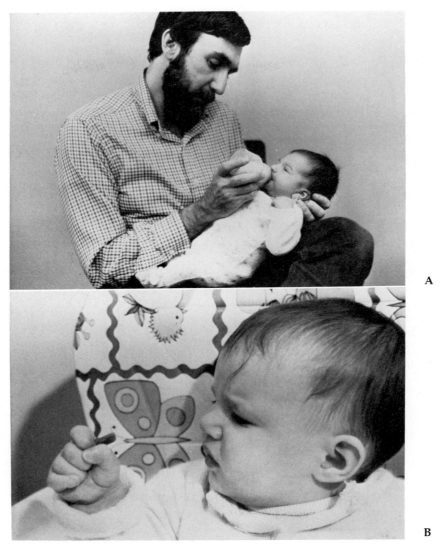

Figure 4-1   Sequence of development of feeding behaviors. **A,** Infant sucks liquids. **B,** Five-month-old infant begins to finger feed.

almost every instance the object goes into the mouth.

7 to 9 months

Between 24 and 28 weeks of age the beginning of chewing movements, an up-and-down movement of the jaws, occurs. This, combined with the ability to grasp, the hand-to-mouth route of grasped objects, and sitting posture, indicates a readiness of the infant to finger-feed. Infants at this age grasp with a **palmar grasp**. Therefore the shape of the food presented for the child to finger-feed is important. Cookies, melba toast, crackers, and teeth-

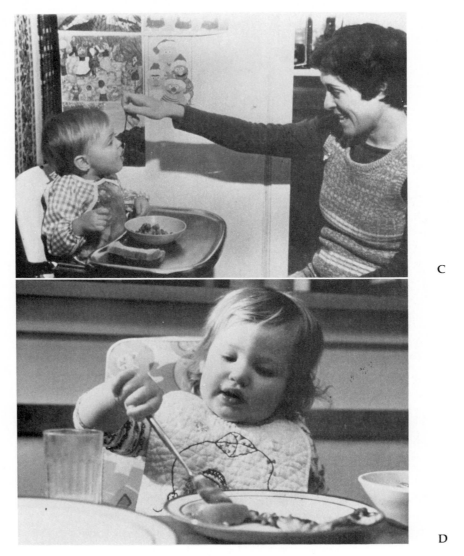

C

D

Figure 4-1 cont'd.   Sequence of development of feeding behaviors. C, Eight-month-old infant is fed table food. D, Eleven-month-old infant begins to feed herself.

ing biscuits are frequently introduced at this stage.

Between 28 and 32 weeks of age the infant gains control of the trunk and can sit alone without support. The sitting infant has greater mobility of the shoulders and arms and is freer to reach and grasp. The grasp is more digital than the earlier palmar grasp. The infant is able to transfer items from one hand to another and learns to voluntarily release and resecure objects. The beginning of chewing patterns (up-and-down movements of the jaws) is

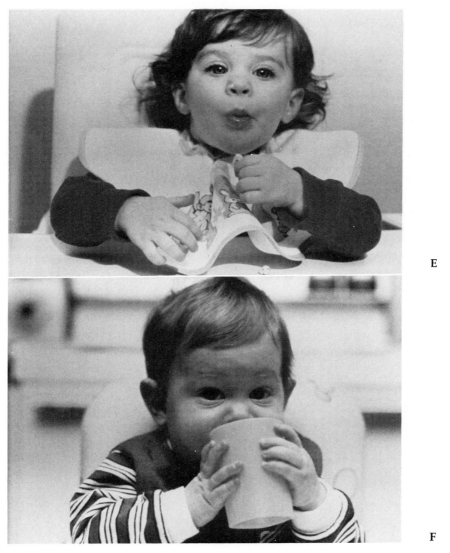

E

F

Figure 4-1 cont'd. Sequence of development of feeding behaviors. E, Ten-month-old infant purses her lips. F, Twelve-month-old infant drinks from a cup.

demonstrated. The tongue shows more maturity in regard to spood feeding than to drinking. Food is received from the spoon by pressing the lips against the spoon, drawing the head away, and drawing in the lower lip. The infant is aware of a cup and can suck from it. Milk frequently leaks from corners of the mouth as the tongue is projected before swallowing.

Critical stage of development

The introduction of soft, mashed (but not strained) foods is appropriate at this stage of development. In fact, it is at this stage of development that Illingworth and Lister[57] believe it is critical to introduce the infant to harder-to-masticate foods.

Between 6 and 12 months of age the infant gradually receives greater amounts of food from the family menu and less and less of the pureed and strained items. Foods should be carefully selected and modified so that they are presented in a form that can be manipulated in the mouth without the potential of choking and **aspiration**, as may occur with small grains of rice or corn. Many parents mash well-cooked vegetables and canned fruits and successfully offer them to their infants. Well-cooked ground meat dishes, such as ground meat in gravies or sauces, appear to be easily accepted, as are liverwurst, minced chicken livers, and drained tuna fish. Custards, puddings, and ice cream soon becomes favorites.

Self-feeding

By 28 weeks of age infants are able to help themselves to their bottle in sitting postures, although they will not be able to tip the bottle adaptively as it empties until about 32 weeks of age. By the end of the first year they can completely manage bottle feeding alone.

By 32 weeks of age infants bring their heads forward to receive the spoon as it is presented to them. The tongue shows increased motility and allows for considerably increased manipulation of food in the mouth before swallowing. At the end of the first year, infants are able to manipulate food in the mouth with definite chewing movements.

9 to 12 months

During the fourth quarter of the first year, the child develops an increasingly precise **pincer grasp**. The bottle can be managed alone and can be resecured if it is lost. Infants at this age are increasingly conscious of what others do and often imitate the models set for them. By 1 year of age the patterns of eating have changed from sucking to beginning rotary chewing movements. Children understand the concept of the container and the contained, have voluntary hand-to-mouth movements and a precise pincer grasp, and can voluntarily release and resecure objects. They are thus prepared to learn to feed themselves, a behavior they learn and refine in the second year.

Feeding the Infant

Presented with the breast of an adequately fed, lactating mother or the nipple on a bottle of properly prepared formula, the hungry infant receives both biochemical and psychosocial nurturance. Most mothers warm the milk to body temperature. The infant held in a semireclining position who is offered the nipple sucks and receives the major portion of nourishment in 20 minutes. Most physicians recommend a flexible self-demand schedule. Newborn infants initially feed six to eight times a day at intervals of 2 to 4 hours and will consume 2 to 3 oz at a feeding (Figure 4-2).

Parents should recognize that infants are quite variable in their eating patterns. Not uncommonly they may want to eat at an interval of 2 hours, then wait 5 hours for the next feeding.

By 2 weeks of age most infants have increased the amount of milk consumed at a feeding and reduced the number of feedings to six. By 2 months of age, most infants are fed five times a day and sleep through the night. By 6 months of age, most consume three meals and four milk feedings a day.

Infants swallow air as well as formula during feeding. Holding the child in an upright position and gently patting the back encourages expulsion of swallowed air and prevents distention and discomfort.

Difficulties in Infant Feeding

During feeding both the parents and the infant receive satisfaction and pleasure. The infant is pleased because hunger is satiated; the parents are pleased because they have fulfilled the needs of their newborn infant. Infants

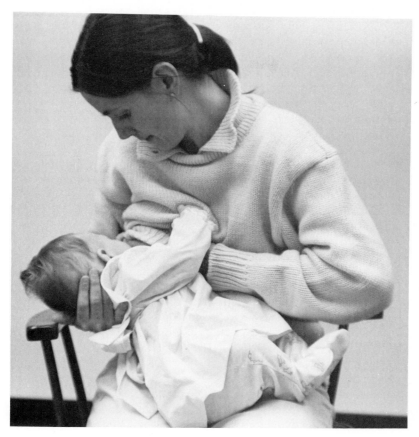

Figure 4-2   Mother breast-feeds her 4-month-old infant.

learn that they can trust their parents to feed them and that they please their parents by eating. Successful feeding provides the basis for the warm, trusting relationship that develops between infants and their parents.

Difficulties in feeding resulting from a weak suck, maternal difficulty in establishing adequate lactation, improper equipment such as firm nipples with small holes, or other causes are frustrating to both infants and their mothers. Hungry infants cry more frequently, demand to be fed more often, and may create anxiety in conscientious and concerned mothers.

Since infants have not yet learned to separate themselves from others in the environment, they perceive the feelings of others as their own immediate feelings in any particular situation. Thus they are easily susceptible to parental anxieties and may reflect these by crying and not eating well. When the infant does not eat well, parental anxieties may increase. Thus the cycle can begin. It is possible that such bottle-fed infants will feed more easily when presented the bottle by a less intense person. However, when the infant is successfully fed by another, the parent's feelings of inadequacy and anxiety may be increased.

To achieve successful parent-child feeding experiences, it is important to work directly with the parents. It may be necessary for the professional to determine any problems with equipment used and positioning, then to model a calm, relaxed feeding situation for the parents. Care should be taken not to usurp the parent's role, thus increasing their feelings of inadequacy. An approach that seems to be beneficial to all concerned is to (1) model a feeding, (2) sit beside the parents and talk them through a feeding while showing them how to use a relaxed position, (3) reinforce parenting behaviors, and (4) help them to become aware of cues from the infant that he or she is relaxed.

This method may need to be used for several feedings until the parent and infant can achieve a successful, relaxed experience. Even then, parents may need further support in their continuing efforts to create a relaxed and warm relationship with their infants during feeding.

Inadequate human milk

Several cases of malnutrition and failure to thrive have been reported in breast-fed infants secondary to an inadequate milk intake, and thus an energy and nutrient intake.[61] Most of the mothers were primiparous women who seemed intelligent and mature. They appeared to not be aware that their babies were not gaining or were losing weight or that their milk production was inadequate.

Feeding the baby at both breasts more frequently may help to increase the mother's milk supply. However, if weight gain continues to be less than adequate, the temporary use of supplemental feedings is appropriate.

It is important for parents to recognize that newborn infants demonstrate a pattern of crying in early life and that a crying infant is not a symptom of inadequate mothering. The amount of time an infant cries increases from 2 weeks of age to approximately 6 weeks of age, when it peaks. After this time crying decreases. The major concentration period is from 6 to 11

PM. Other periods of crying occur in the morning from 4 to 7 AM and 9 to 11 AM. By 10 weeks of age most infants become more quiet.[62] Seldom is this crying a symptom of allergy, and it is no indication for formula change.

Colic

Parents of colicky babies—those who are otherwise healthy and well fed but who cry constantly for several hours, draw their legs onto the abdomens, and pass large amounts of gas—often request changes in the infants' formulas. This rarely resolves colic, and frequent change in formulas should be discouraged. It has been suggested that colic in some breast-fed infants be resolved by eliminating milk from the mothers' diets.[63, 64] A casein hydrolysate formula may alleviate symptoms in some, but not all, bottle-fed infants.

Spitting

Both spitting and regurgitation can occur in infants and usually cause concern for parents. During the early months of life some otherwise healthy infants spit a small amount of any milk or food ingested at each feeding. Although the infants do not fail to thrive, parents may seek help in resolving this situation. There is no therapy. The problem usually resolves itself by the time the infants can sustain sitting. Regurgitation, the effortless expulsion of gastric contents, is a symptom that demands medical evaluation. The most common cause of persistent regurgitation is gastrointestinal reflux, the result of decreased pressure in the lower esophageal sphincter. Positioning the infant in an infant seat at a 45 to 60 degree angle may help, but it will not decrease the amount of contact of gastric acid on the esophageal mucosa. Surgery may be indicated.[65]

Distractions

Some infants are easily distracted by noise or by other influences in the environment. Such infants feed more easily at the night feeding.

Presentation of the bottle in a quiet, partially darkened room by a rested parent may promote successful feeding for both the parent and the infant.

Parental perception of feeding problems

Many parents perceive their infants as having feeding problems. Problems include refusal of a particular food because of taste or texture, dissatisfaction with amount consumed, spitting up, developmentally related problems such as refusing the bottle or refusing to be fed, and only finger-feeding. Such difficulties are usually of short duration and rarely compromise an infant's nutrient intake or physical growth. Parents, however, may need reassurance that their infant's development is normal and that their food-related behaviors are not of nutritional concern.

Recognizing Cues of Satiation and Readiness to Progress

Successful infant feeding is generally regarded in our society as a measure of competent parenthood. As such, it is a reinforcing experience to parents. They must learn to recognize and to accept their infant's cues, as the infant uses a variety of cries and vocalizations to express needs. Frequently parents, for one reason or another, cannot always discriminate their infant's cries. Consequently, they give food to satisfy all types of infant discomforts. The infant, in turn, may not learn to discriminate hunger from other discomforts and may learn to rely on eating to satisfy a wide variety of needs. Parents must learn to recognize satiation of hunger in infants and be willing to accept their infant's expressions of satisfaction, to set limits on amounts of food offered to eager eaters, and to decline the natural inclination to overfeed infants who please others by accepting more food. Satiety behaviors of infants are given in Table 4-12.

Parents who are eager for their infant to empty the bottle encourage excessive intakes of

Table 4-12   Satiety behaviors in infants

Age	Behavior
4-12 weeks	Draws head away from nipple
	Falls asleep
	When nipple is reinserted, closes lips tightly
	Bites nipple, purses lips, or smiles and lets go
16-24 weeks	Releases nipple and withdraws head
	Fusses or cries
	Obstructs mouth with hands
	Increases attention to surroundings
	Bites nipple
28-36 weeks	Changes posture
	Keeps mouth tightly closed
	Shakes head as if to say "no"
	Plays with utensils
	Hands become more active
	Throws utensils
40-52 weeks	Behaviors of above period typical
	Sputters with tongue and lips
	Hands bottle or cup to parent

From Pipes P.L.: Health care professionals. In Garwood, G., and Fewell, R.: Educating handicapped infants, Rockville, Md., 1982, Aspen Systems. With permission by Aspen Systems Corp.; modified from Gessell, A., and Ilg, F.L.: Feeding behavior of infants, Philadelphia, 1937, J.B. Lippincott Co.

food and can reinforce eating to the extent that obesity may result. Infants may be offered food and formula by many people: parents, baby-sitters, aunts, siblings, and others.

Parents who are dissatisfied with their infant's food intake may find that the infant has reduced the intake to compensate for food offered by others. Additional cues that parents must recognize are those that indicate the infant's readiness for increasingly independent feeding experiences. The infant's ability to put objects to his or her mouth and to chew on them indicates a readiness to use increasingly solid foods and to begin finger-feeding. Anticipatory guidance to parents during this period about developmental changes is an important factor in their acceptance of and adaptation to their infant's behavior.

Recognizing Needs for Nutrients and Energy in the Infant's Diet

Most infants consume foods that provide nutrients in excess of recommended amounts, with the exception of iron. Human milk, cow's milk, and formula provide the major source of protein and calcium and important sources of vitamin A and the B vitamins in early life. Breast-fed infants should receive supplements of iron, vitamin D, and fluoride. Iron-fortified formulas contribute appreciable amounts of iron in early infancy.

Most lactating mothers need to be away occasionally when it is time to feed their infant. It is therefore advantageous for the infant to have an occasional bottle with a rubber nipple after lactation is well established. Ready-to-feed formulas can be used, but many mothers prefer to express their milk for such occasions. Manual expression is the choice of most mothers. However, manual and electric pumps are on the market and may be preferred by mothers who work and express for a day or more.

Once expressed, the milk must be stored so that it will be microbiologically safe with a minimal loss of nutrients. Freezing protects it from contamination with minimal change in milk composition. Immunoglobulin levels and nutritional properties are essentially unchanged. Milk should be refrigerated or frozen at once. It can be safely held in a refrigerator for 24 hours and in a freezer for up to 3 months.

Often breast-fed infants refuse a rubber nipple from their mother. They usually accept such a feeding from their father or a friend or baby sitter.

Because of the great variability in calories and nutrients provided by foods offered to infants, selection of foods and the amounts offered should be based on the infant's rate of gain in height and weight as well as on nutrient needs. The introduction and acceptance of heme iron-containing foods before the time homogenized milk replaces iron-fortified formula or before iron supplements are discontinued is important, because the infant must continue to consume foods that provide this nutrient as it is deleted from milk or supplements. Fruit juice offers sources of vitamin C when vitamin-containing formulas are no longer consumed. It seems reasonable to encourage parents of infants whose gains in weight are more rapid than gains in length to feed them lower-calorie infant foods such as vegetables and dinners. Parents of infants whose increments of weight gains are small should be encouraged to feed greater amounts of the higher-calorie strained meats and fruits. Amounts of semisolid foods offered to infants should be adjusted to their appetites and rates of weight gain. Experiences with a variety of flavors and textures are thought to be conducive to acceptance of a variety of foods in later life.

Programs to Help Parents Optimize the Nutritional Status of Infants

A variety of federal and state programs include a component to improve the nutritional status of infants. State and local health departments have always considered nutrition services during pregnancy, lactation, and infancy an essential component of preventive health care. Nutritionists in these programs provide information about nutrition in infancy by preparing materials for public distribution, serving as a resource for other health workers, and participating in mother-infant and other classes.

Nutritionists provide nutrition education and individual counseling to parents in a number of federally funded programs designed to meet the needs of children at risk. These services may be found in Crippled Children, Migrant Health, Appalachian Health, and Indian Health programs. Diagnostic clinics for infants and children also provide nutrition services, including nutrition screening, counseling, education, referral, and follow-up. Such clinics are included in programs funded to serve children and youth and the developmentally delayed.

One program, the Special Supplemental Food Program for Women, Infants, and Children (WIC), provides specific food supplements to pregnant and lactating women and to infants and children to age 5 years who are at nutritional risk because of nutritional needs and inadequate income.

The program provides the following food for formula-fed infants:

Iron-fortified infant formula
Infant cereal containing 45 mg iron/100 gm
Single-strength, frozen concentrated, or infant juices that contain a minimum of 30 mg vitamin C/dl

Mothers of breast-fed infants may be certified to receive the supplemental food themselves. Some breast-fed infants may be certified to receive partial food packages that include iron-fortified cereal and fruit juice. Also, the infants who are both breast-fed and formula-fed may receive a partial package of iron-fortified formula. Nutrition education is a required component of this program.

Summary

A variety of combinations of milks, supplements, and semisolid foods can provide an adequately nourishing diet for infants. Maturation of the oral and fine motor skills indicate appropriate stages for the introduction of semisolid and solid foods. Current recommendations include breast-feeding by an adequately nour-

ished mother, the introduction of semisolid foods at 4 to 6 months of age, and the introduction of finger foods when the infant reaches out, grasps, and brings items to his or her mouth.

If the mother is unable or unwilling to breast-feed, a variety of properly constructed infant formulas are marketed that have been proved to support normal growth and development in infants. It is to the formula-fed baby's advantage to receive a formula with iron.

Infants should be permitted to establish their own feeding schedule and fed to satiety. When they develop a voluntary mature sucking pattern, the introduction of semisolid foods is appropriate. When munching and rotary chewing begin, the introduction of soft-cooked table food is appropriate. Infants can begin to drink from a cup with help between 9 and 12 months of age.

Difficulties in infant feedings that indicate a need for intervention include inadequate milk production by the mother, poor suck, improper formula preparation, and parental anxiety about feeding their infants.

SUGGESTED LEARNING ACTIVITIES

1. Investigate the incidence of breast-feeding in the maternity unit of your local hospital.
2. Investigate local agencies in your community that provide support for the lactating mother.
3. Describe formula products available for feeding infants in your community.
4. Compare the cost of homemade and commercially available foods for infants.
5. Describe how useful mothers find the nutrition information found on commercially prepared baby food container labels.
6. Observe infants feeding at 2, 4, 7, and 9 months of age and describe changes in the way babies secure their food.
7. Describe appropriate therapy for breast-fed babies who are thought to be gaining weight too fast.

REFERENCES

1. Lindberg, T.: Proteolytic activity in duodenal juice in infants, children, and adults, Acta Paediatr. Scand. 63:805, 1974.
2. Fomon, S. J.: Infant nutrition, ed. 2, Philadelphia, 1974, W. B. Saunders Co.
3. Watkins, J. B.: Bile acid metabolism and fat absorption in newborn infants, Pediatr. Clin. North Am. 2:501, 1974.
4. Filer, L. J., Mattson, F. H., and Fomon, S. J.: Triglyceride configuration and fat absorption by the human infant, J. Nutr. 99:293, 1969.
5. Bayless, T. M., and Christopher N. L.: Disaccharidase deficiency, Am. J. Clin. Nutr. 22: 181, 1969.
6. Rossiter, M. A. and others: Amylase content of mixed saliva in children, Acta Paediatr. Scand. 63:389, 1974.
7. Sevenhusen, G. P., and others: Development of salivary a-amylase in infants from birth to 5 months, Amer. J. Clin. Nutr. 39:584, 1984.
8. Hadorn, B., and others: Quantitative assessment of exocrine pancreatic function in infants and children, J. Pediatr. 73:39, 1968.
9. Fomon, S. J.: Reflections in infant feeding in the 1970s and 1980s, Amer. J. Clin. Nutr. 46:71, 1987.
10. Nash, M. A., and Edelmann, C. M.: The developing kidney, Nephron, 11:71, 1973.
11. Polacek, E., and others: The osmotic concentrating ability in healthy infants and children, Arch. Dis. Child. 40:291, 1965.
12. Nagata, M., Ross Laboratory Representative, personal communication.
13. Martinez, G. A., and Krieger, K. W.: 1984 milk-feeding patterns in the United States, Pediatrics 76:1004, 1985.
14. Blanc, B.: Biochemical aspects of human milk, World Rev. Nutr. Diet 36:1, 1981.
15. Siimes, M. A., Vuori, E., And Kuitunen, P.: Breast milk iron—a declining concentration during the course of lactation, Acta Paediatr. Scand. 68:29, 1979.
16. Anderson, G. N., Atkinson, S. A., and Bryan, M. H.: Energy and macronutrient content of human milk during early lactation from mothers giving birth prematurely and at term, Am. J. Clin. Nutr. 34:258, 1981.
17. Chavalittamrong, B., and others: Protein and amino acids of breast milk from Thai mothers, Am. J. Clin. Nutr. 24:1126, 1981.
18. Jensen, R. G., Hagerty, M. M., and McMahon, K. E.: Lipids of human milk and infant formulas: a review, Am. J. Clin. Nutr. 31:990, 1978.
19. O'Connor, M. E., and others: Vitamin K deficiency and breast feeding, Am. J. Dis. Child. 137:601, 1983.
20. Higginbottom, L., Sweetman L., and Nylan, W. L.: A syndrome of methylmalonic aciduria, homocystinuria, megaloblastic anemia, and neurological abnormalities of a B_{12} deficiency in an infant strictly breast-fed by a mother with latent pernicious anemia, J. Pediatr. 100:917, 1982.
21. Cooperman, J. M., and others: The folate in human milk, Am. J. Clin. Nutr. 36:576, 1982.
22. Borschel, M. W., Kirksey, A., and Hannemann, R. E.: Effects of Vitamin B_6 intake on nutriture and growth of young infants, Amer. J. Clin. Nutr. 43:7, 1986.
23. Saarinen, U. M., Siimes, M. A., and Dallman, P. R.: Iron absorption in infants; high bioavailability of breast milk iron as indicated by the extrinsic tag method of iron absorption and by the concentration of serum ferritin, J. Pediatr. 91:36, 1977.
24. Harzer, G., and Kauer, H.: Binding of zinc to casein, Am. J. Clin. Nutr. 35:981, 1982.
25. Johnson, P. E., and Evans, G. W.: Relative zinc availability in human breast milk, infant formulas, and cow's milk, Am. J. Clin. Nutr. 31:416, 1978.
26. Welsh, J. K., and May, J. T.: Anti-infective properties of breast milk, J. Pediatr. 94:1, 1979.
27. Fransson, G. B., and Lönnerdal, B.: Iron in human milk, Pediatr. 96:380, 1980.
28. Committee on Nutrition, American Academy of Pediatrics: Commentary on breast-feeding and infant formulas, including proposed standards for formulas, Pediatrics 57:279, 1976.
29. American Academy of Pediatrics, Committee on Nutrition. Soy-protein formulas: Recommendations for use in infant feeding, Pediatrics 72:359, 1983.
30. Harrison, H. L. and others: Goat milk acidosis, J. Pediatr. 94:927, 1979.
31. Fabius, R. J. and others: Malnutrition associated with a formula of barley water, corn syrups, and whole milk, Am. J. Dis. Child. 135:615, 1981.
32. Sinatra, F. R., and Merritt, R. J.: Iatrongenic kwashiorkor in infants, Am. J. Dis. Child. 135:21, 1981.
33. Wyatt, D. T., Noetzel, M. J., and Hillman, R. E.: Infantile beriberi presenting as subacute necrotizing encephalomyelopathy, J. Pediatr. 110:888, 1987.
34. Comay, S. C. and Karabus, C. D.: Peripheral gangrene in hypernatremic dehydration of infancy, Arch. Dis. Child. 50:616, 1975.
35. Abrams, C. A. L., and others: Hazards of overconcentrated milk formula, J. A. M. A. 232:1136, 1975.
36. Partridge, J. C., and others: Water intoxication secondary to feeding mismanagement, Am. J. Dis. Child. 135:38. 1981.
37. Schulman, J.: Infantile water intoxication at home, Pediatrics 66:119, 1980.
38. Hargrove, C. B., Temple A. R., and Chinn P.: Formula preparation and infant illness, Clin. Pediatr. 13:1057, 1974.

39. Kendall, N., Vaughn, V. C., and Kusakeroglu, A.: A study of preparation of infant formulas, Am. J. Dis. Child. 122:215, 1971.

40. Committee on Nutrition, American Academy of Pediatrics: The use of whole milk in infancy, Pediatrics 72:253, 1983.

41. Fomon, S. J. and others: Cow milk feeding in infancy: gastronintestinal blood loss and iron nutritional status, J. Pediatr. 98:540, 1981.

42. American Academy of Pediatrics, Committee on Nutrition: Pediatric nutrition handbook, Elk Grove Village, IL, 1985, American Academy of Pediatrics.

43. American Academy of Pediatrics, Committee on Nutrition: Imitation and substitute milks, Pediatrics 73:876, 1984.

44. Klaus, M. H., and Kennell, J. H.: Maternal-infant bonding: the impact of early separation or loss on family development, St. Louis, 1976, The C. V. Mosby Co.

45. Kerr, C. M., Reisinger, K. S., and Plankey, F. W.: Sodium concentration of homemade baby food, Pediatrics 62:331, 1978.

46. Schaefer, L. J., and Kumanyika, K.: Maternal variables related to potentially high-sodium infant-feeding practices, J. Amer. Diet. Assoc. 85:434, 1985.

47. Arnon, S. S., and others: Honey and other environmental risk factors for infant botulism, Pediatrics 94:331, 1979.

48. Montalto, M. S., Benson, J. D., and Martinez, G. A.: Nutrient intakes of formula fed infants and infants fed cow's milk, Pediatrics 75:343, 1985.

49. Fomon, S. J., and others: Influence of formula concentration on calorie intake and growth of normal infants, Acta Paediatr. Scand. 64:172, 1975.

50. Thoman, E. B.: Development of synchrony in mother-infant interaction in feeding and other situations, Fed. Proc. 34:1587, 1975.

51. Fomon, S. J., and others: Food consumption and growth of normal infants fed milk-based formulas, Acta Paediatr. Scand. Suppl. 223, 1971.

52. Salmenpera, L., Perheentupa, J., and Siimes, M. A.: Exclusively breast-fed healthy infants grow slower than reference infants, Acta Paediatr. Scand. 19:307, 1985.

53. Fomon, S. J., and others: Growth and serum chemical values of normal breast fed infants, Acta Paediatr. Scand. Suppl. 202, 1970.

54. Beal, V. A.: Nutritional intake of children, I. Calories, carbohydrate, fat and protein; J. Nutr. 50:223, 1953.

55. Rueda-Williamson, R., and Rose, H. E.: Growth and nutrition of infants: the influence of diet and other factors on growth, Pediatrics 30:639, 1962.

56. Fomon, S. J., Owen, G. M., and Thomas L. N.: Milk or formula volume ingested by infants fed ad libitum, Am. J. Dis. Child. 108:601, 1964.

57. Illingworth, R. S., and Lister, J.: The critical or sensitive period with special reference to certain feeding problems in infants and children, J. Pediatr. 65:839, 1964.

58. Gesell, A., and Ilg, F. L.: Feeding behavior of infants, Philadelphia, 1937, J. B. Lippincott Co.

59. Ardran, G. M., Kemp, F. H., and Lind, J.: A cineradiographic study of breast feeding, Br. J. Radiol. 31:156, 1958.

60. Ardran, G. M.: Kemp, F. H., and Lind, J.: A cineradiographic study of bottle feeding, Br. J. Radio. 31:11 1958.

61. Roddey, O. F., Martin, E. S., and Swetenburg, R. L.: Critical weight loss and malnutrition in breast-fed infants, Am. J. Dis. Child. 135:597, 1981.

62. Brazelton, T. B.: Crying in infancy, Pediatrics 29:579, 1962.

63. Jakobsson, I., and Lindberg, T.: Cow's milk proteins cause infantile colic in breast-fed infants: a double blind crossover study, Pediatrics 71:268, 1983.

64. Lothe, L., Lindberg, T., and Jakobsson, I.: Cow's milk formula as a cause of infantile colic, Pediatrics 70:7, 1982.

65. Cohen, S.: Developmental characteristics of lower esophageal sphincter dysfunction: a possible mechanism for infantile chalasia, Gastroenterology 67:252, 1974.

5

Between Infancy and Adolescence

Peggy L. Pipes

OBJECTIVES

After studying this chapter, the student should:

1. Be aware of nutrition concerns of preschool and school-age children.

2. Recognize factors that influence parents' provision of food for children.

3. Recognize factors that must be considered to prevent choking in children.

4. Be aware of the value of snacks to a child's daily total nutrient intake.

5. Be aware of common concerns about food intake encountered by parents of preschool and school-age children.

6. Have knowledge of feeding programs designed to improve the nutritional status of children.

Between infancy and adolescence, changes in children's rates of growth, continuing maturation of fine and gross motor skills, and personality development influence not only the amounts of food children consume but also those foods that are acceptable to them. Food habits, likes, and dislikes are established, some of which are transient and many of which form the base for a lifetime of food and nutrition intake. Environmental influences and parental behavior reinforce or extinguish food-related behavior.

There are common patterns of food and nutrient intake among preschool and school-age children. Feeding programs at day care and school contribute significantly to children's total nutrient intake. Although evidence of malnutrition has been reduced in the past ten years, populations of children who exhibit significant biochemical evidence of inadequate nutrient intake continue to be found in the United States.

NUTRITION OF PRESCHOOL AND SCHOOL-AGE CHILDREN

Although clinical signs of malnutrition are rarely found in children in North America, there is evidence that there are children who receive diets that are inadequate in quantity or quality. Iron and vitamin B_6 are the nutrients most frequently of concern.[1,2] The Nationwide Food Consumption Study identified that in addition to these nutrients, calcium and vitamin C are frequently consumed in less than recommended amounts.[2]

Children from low-income families frequently are shorter than those from families with greater economic resources. However, differences in linear height are not consistently associated with energy intakes.[3] Several studies have indicated that when nutrient intakes are calculated on the basis of nutrients per 1000 kcal consumed, they are similar at all economic levels.[4,5]

The employment status of the male family-head has been found to have an impact on average daily energy intake. Windham and others[4] found, by analyzing data from the Nationwide Food Consumption Survey, that family members in which the male head was employed averaged intakes of 165 kcal/day more than those in which the male head was unemployed. Female family-head employment status was not found to affect energy intake.

Differences in the nutrient density of diets consumed were noted in specific racial and geographical groups. A lower calcium density was noted in the diets of Spanish and black groups than in other populations. The vitamin A density was lowest in the Spanish groups compared with other groups studied. The place of residence also influenced the nutrient density of the diets consumed. Intakes of niacin, vitamin B_6, and C per 1000 kcal were lower in nonmetropolitan areas than in the central city and nonsuburban areas studied.[4]

The National Nutrition Status Study of preschool children conducted by Owen and others[5] found that black children consumed an average of 1 mg of iron/day more than white preschoolers at all ages. Cereal grains were the major contributors of iron. Vitamin C intakes were unrelated to energy intakes, and children of parents who had more money to spend for

food consumed greater amounts of ascorbic acid.

A high percentage of children in all studies have been found to be receiving multiple vitamin and mineral supplements. The use of supplements decreases until about age 13 years.[6,7] At that age the percentage of boys using supplements plateaus, whereas the percentage of girls who take vitamins increases. In general, supplements are more often used by children from families with a head who is white and better educated. Fewer children have been noted to take iron supplements than vitamin supplements. Most often supplemental iron is consumed as part of a multiple vitamin supplement. Analysis of data from the HANES II study found children who received supplements had higher serum levels of vitamins A and C.[7]

Nutrition Concerns of Children

Ethnic and geographical variations in nutrient deficiency concerns have been found in various populations. For example, Navajo Indian children in Montana were found to have low-dietary intakes of calcium and vitamins A and C. Biochemical evidence of inadequate intakes of iron, vitamin A, and riboflavin was also noted.[8] White Mountain Apache children in Arizona were noted to have biochemical evidence of inadequate intakes of vitamins A and C.[9]

A nutritional status study of low-income preschool children in Memphis, Tennessee, indicated that, although improvement in the nutritional status of the children had been affected in the past 10 years, 9% to 18% of the children studied had low or deficient serum levels of vitamins A, C, B_1, B_2, and/or hemoglobin. Also, the income level had dropped and a greater number of the children were categorized as thin than 10 years previously.[10]

Biochemical evidence of vitamin B_6 deficiency has been reported in 9% of children studied in Virginia.[11]

Mothers of 10% of the preschool children in a nutritional status study in the North

Central Region of the United States reported that their children had conditions that required modification of the kinds or amounts of food consumed.[12] Compliance with dietary modifications necessary to control chronic diseases, such as diabetes, celiac disease, and allergies, is difficult in childhood. Children want to eat the same food as their peers and family. Teachers and friends are not always sympathetic with the need to restrict or modify food intake. Restriction of several groups of foods such as may be necessary for children who have multiple allergies makes adequate energy intakes difficult. Thus children who must modify their intakes of food are at risk for nutritional deficits.

In some poverty-level populations, groups of children have been identified that have shown both clinical and biochemical evidence of malnutrition. All preschool children are at risk for iron-deficiency anemia, which appears to be a greater problem in children of low-income families than in children of other groups. Dental caries as a result of excessive intakes of sweet foods, poor dental hygiene, and lack of dental care are common among all groups of children.

FAMILY RESPONSIBILITY AND CHILDREN'S FOOD INTAKES

Children from infancy to adolescence depend on their parents for the selection of food they consume at home. As they grow older, have money to spend, attend school, and interact with larger numbers of individuals, the decisions as to their selection of food become increasingly their own. Since the preschool and the preadolescent periods are important in the formation of attitudes toward food, it is important that foods that supply a variety of nutrients be available to children. Parents also need to understand and support children in their food-related behaviors so that food habits are formed that are conducive to an adequate nutrient intake. Children need some experience

selecting food, yet parents need to set limits so that children eat foods that provide adequate amounts of nutrients.

The educational level and nutrition knowledge of the mother influence the nutritional quality of the diet. Eppright and others[13] noted that as the nutrition knowledge of the mother increased, preschool children's intakes of calcium, iron, riboflavin, and ascorbic acid increased. They also found that nutrition knowledge was significantly related to positive attitudes toward meal planning and food preparation. Caliendo and others[14] found that the more positive mothers felt about meal planning, the importance of good nutrition for their children, and their roles as homemakers, the more likely were the children to receive good quality meals; the more discontent, nervous, and unhappy the mothers were with their roles as homemakers, the lower was the dietary quality of the children's food intakes.

Parents often need both help in interpreting the nutrition information to which they have been exposed and direction to valid sources of information. Sources of nutrition information vary among groups of parents. Low-income families reportedly receive their nutrition information from relatives and friends. Other families rely heavily on lay sources such as magazines, newspapers, books, radio, and television. Some of the information presented in these sources lacks validity, and conflicting information is often presented in any two sources. In addition, advertising and merchandising play on parents' emotional responses to suggestion, and imply a false need for certain foods or supplements.

Also, preschool children often accompany their mothers to the grocery store and request specific foods. In this situation, 68% of mothers have reported that they sometimes buy foods that are requested and 18% stated they always purchase the items. Sugar-coated cereal is the food most frequently requested.[15]

Convenience is another factor many mothers consider when they select food for their families. Working mothers may rely heavily on convenience food and fast-food establishments and have been known to leave the decision to the child as to which one he or she would like for dinner. Parents may need help selecting convenience foods and combinations of other foods that, when served together, provide a balanced nutrient intake. Parents may also need to learn how to plan other meals so that the daily intake is adequate when fast foods are consumed frequently.

Low-income families have less money for food than more affluent families. If the purchasing power is reduced significantly, foods that provide essential nutrients may be partially or wholly eliminated from the diet. However, not all children from low-income families are at risk for undernutrition. One study in Philadelphia found undernourished low-income children had parents who prepared fewer regular meals and who were less likely to eat vegetables and milk than parents of adequately nourished children from homes with similar incomes. More convenience foods and fewer foods requiring preparation were available to undernourished children than to well-nourished children.[16]

FACTORS AFFECTING FOOD INTAKE

Provision of appropriate amounts and kinds of food does not ensure that children will consume foods that support an appropriate nutrient intake. Children imitate the models of food acceptance set for them. They learn to control concerned parents by the food they accept or reject. Emotional factors influence food acceptance and intake.

Parents and siblings provide a model of food acceptance and feeding behavior that children imitate. In a study of parents and 6- to 19-year-old children, Laskarzewski and others[17] found a significant positive correlation between parent and child intakes of calories, carbohydrate, saturated fats, and polyunsaturated fats. The

correlation was greater for black than for white children.

Attitudes of parents toward child rearing influence nutrient intake. Eppright[18] found permissiveness of parents in relation to eating to be negatively related to the nutritive value of food consumed by the children, adversely affecting all dietary components except fat. Less permissive mothers regulated to some degree the child's food intakes, and as a result children consumed greater amounts of protein, vitamins, and minerals. Sims and Morris[19] found that children of more affluent, nonauthoritarian mothers had higher intakes of calcium and ascorbic acid, whereas children of parents with authoritarian attitudes toward child rearing had higher intakes of calories, carbohydrates, iron, and thiamine.

The emotional environment at mealtime may influence food and nutrient intake. The dinner table is not the place for family battles or punitive action toward children. For eating to be successful, it should occur at a time and in a setting that is comfortable and free from stress and unreasonable demands. Lund and Burk[20] found that mealtime criticism about nonfood-related activities reduced the levels of food consumption and adversely affected intakes of vitamins A and C in 9- to 11-year-old children.

THE PRESCHOOL CHILD

During the preschool years rates of growth decrease and as a result appetites decrease. Children learn to understand language and to talk and ask for food. Development of gross motor skills permits them to learn to walk and seek food for themselves. Development of fine motor skills allows them to learn to feed themselves and to prepare simple foods such as cereal with milk and sandwiches. They learn about food and the way it feels, tastes, and smells. Preschool children learn to eat a wider variety of textures and kinds of food, give up the bottle, and drink from a cup. They

Figure 5-1 Children consume food successfully in a comfortable setting free from stress.

demand independence and refuse help in many tasks in which they are not skillful, such as self-feeding. As they grow older they become less interested in food and more interested in their environment. They test and learn limits of behavior that are acceptable.

Self-feeding

Children learn to feed themselves independently during the second year of life. Spilling and messiness are marked during the first half of the year, but by their second birthday most children spill very little. Handedness is not established at 1 year of age. Children may grasp the spoon with either hand and may find when they try to fill the spoon that the bowl is upside down. The 15-month-old child will have difficulty scooping food into his or her spoon and bringing food to the mouth without turning the spoon upside down and spilling its contents because of lack of wrist control. By 16 to 17 months of age a well-defined ulnar deviation of the wrist occurs and the contents of a spoon may be transferred more steadily to the mouth. By 18 months of age the child lifts the elbow as the spoon is raised and flexes the wrist as the

spoon reaches the mouth so that only moderate spilling occurs at this age, in contrast to earlier stages of self-feeding. By 2 years of age spilling seldom occurs.

Children are interested in how food feels and often prefer finger-feeding to spoon-feeding. Foods that provide opportunities for finger-feeding should be provided at every meal. Children not infrequently will place food in the spoon with their fingers and may finger-feed foods commonly spoon-fed, such as vegetables and pudding.

By 15 months of age children can manage the cup, although not expertly. They have difficulty in lifting and tilting a cup and in lowering it to a tray after drinking. The cup is tilted, using the palm, and often is tilted too rapidly. By 18 to 24 months of age the cup is tilted by manipulation of the fingers.

Rotary chewing movements are refined in the second year and are well established by $2\frac{1}{2}$ years of age.

Risk of Choking

Young children, especially preschoolers, are at risk choking on food. Death from food

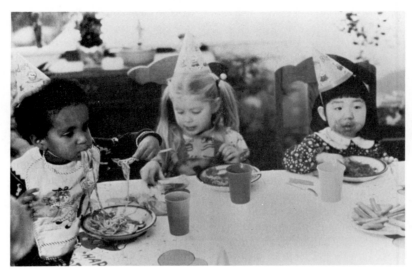

Figure 5-2   Preschool children enjoy learning to self-feed.

asphyxiation has been described in 102 children over a two-year period, mostly in children less than 2 years of age. Foods most often responsible for the deaths include hot dogs, candy, nuts, and grapes.[21]

Actually, children can choke on almost any food but are most likely to have trouble with foods that are hard, slippery, or just the right size to plug up the throat (e.g., hard candy, popcorn). If the food becomes stuck, the plug prevents the child from coughing and bringing it back up. Other foods that may cause problems are thick, sticky foods such as peanut butter. These foods can line the back of the throat and build up so the children cannot clear their throats.

Prevention is the most reasonable approach to childhood choking. Educating parents about developmentally appropriate foods is important. Guidelines for preventing choking are given in the box on p. 126.

Patterns of Food Intake

Few children pass through the preschool years without creating concern about their food intakes. Between 9 and 18 months of age a disinterest in food becomes apparent; this lasts from a few months to a few years.[22] Food jags are common. Likes and dislikes may change from day to day and week to week. For example, a child may demand only boiled eggs for snacks for a week and completely reject them for the next 6 months. Rituals become a part of food preparation and service. Some children, for example, accept sandwiches only when they are cut in half, and when parents quarter the sandwiches the children may throw tantrums. Others demand that foods have a particular arrangement on the plate or that their dishes be placed only in certain locations on the table.

Appetites are usually erratic and unpredictable during this period. The child may eat hungrily at one meal and completely refuse the next. The evening meal is generally the least well received and is of the most concern to the majority of parents. It is possible that a child who has consumed two meals and several snacks has met his or her need for energy and nutrients before dinnertime; in this instance

---

Guidelines for Feeding Safety
—Preschool Children

1. Insist that children eat sitting down. It lets them concentrate on chewing and swallowing.
2. An adult should supervise children while they eat.
3. Food on which preschoolers often choke, such as hot dogs, peanut butter, hard pieces of fruit, and vegetables, should be avoided for children under 3 years of age.
4. Well-cooked foods, modified so that the child can chew and swallow without difficulty, should be offered.
5. Eating in the car should be avoided. If the child starts choking it is hard to get to the side of the road safely.
6. Rub-on teething medications can cause problems with chewing and swallowing because the muscles in the throat may also become numb. Children who receive such medications should be carefully observed during feeding.

---

consumption of limited amounts of food may be appropriate. It is also important to recognize that much social interaction occurs during the evening meal. This may be overwhelming for the preschooler who is learning not only to eat and interact at the same time but also to master the use of utensils and to eat harder-to-masticate foods.

Beal[22] and Eppright and others[18] report a high percentage of parental dissatisfaction with children's appetites and interest in food between 2 and 4 years of age. Concerns most frequently expressed are selection of a limited variety of foods, dawdling, limited consumption of fruits and vegetables, and consumption of too many sweets and too little meat.

More recently, Pelchat and Pliner found that mothers describe feeding problems among 2- to 7-year-old children that are very similar to the concerns previously described (see box p. 127).[23] It is apparent that such problems are those of the parents' lack of insight into normal child development and, if properly managed, need not compromise a child's nutrient intake. Anticipatory guidance about children's food behavior is important for all parents, and intervention is imperative when battles are waged between parents and children about what is to be eaten.

Frequency of eating

Huenemann[24] has pointed out that we are raising a generation of nibblers. Nearly 60% of 3- to 5-year-old children eat more than three times a day.[25] They consume food an average of five to seven times per day, although ranges of three to fourteen times per day have been noted.[24] Crawford, Hankin, and Huenemann found that by 6 years of age 50% of children ate five times per day. Eppright and others[26] noted that the frequency of food intakes was unrelated to nutrient intakes except when children consumed food less than four or more than six times a day. Children in this study who consumed food less than four times a day consumed fewer calories and less calcium, protein, ascorbic acid, and iron than average intakes of other children their age. Those who consumed food more than six times a day consumed more energy, calcium, and ascorbic acid than average intakes of children their age. Snacks have been noted to provide one fourth to one third of the total calories, over one third of the total sucrose, one fifth of the total calcium

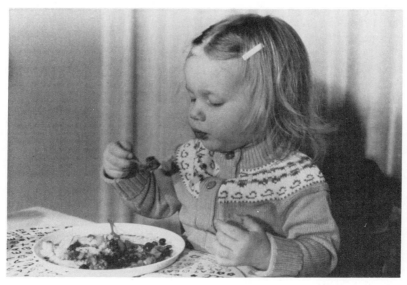

Figure 5-3   Preschool children refine their self-feeding skills as they grow older.

and ascorbic acid, and one fifth of the protein ingested by school-age children.[27,28]

Food preferences

Parents report that preschool children enjoy meat, cereal grains, baked products, fruit, and

---

Food Behaviors of Children 2 to 7 years of Age Viewed as Problems by Mother (in Order of Frequency Cited)

Child consumes a restricted range of foods.
Child's eating habits are poor.
Child eats insufficient quantity of food.
Child is not interested in eating.
Child dislikes new foods.
Child likes "junk foods."
Other.

From Pelchat, M.L. and Pliner, D.: Antecedents and correlates of feeding problems in young children, J. Nutr. Ed. 18:23, 1986.

sweets. They frequently ask for dairy products, cereal, and snack items such as cookies, crackers, fruit juice, and dry beverage mixes.[41] Preschoolers seem to prefer the carbohydrate-rich foods that are easier to masticate. Cereals, breads, and crackers are often selected in preference to meat and other protein-rich foods. The use of dry fortified cereals as a primary source of many nutrients is increasing.[15] Yogurt and cheese appear to be increasing in popularity among young children.

Concerns of Parents

A concern of parents of many children between 1 and 3 years of age is that their children do not like and will not eat meat. In the description of their dissatisfaction, it may become apparent that the children do eat and enjoy chicken, frankfurters, and hamburger but refuse the more fibrous and harder-to-chew steaks and roasts. Foods have not yet been classified in relation to the pressure that must be applied to chew them well. Empirical obser-

Figure 5-4   Snacks are an important part of children's nutrient intake.

vations, however, indicate that fibrous meats require the greatest pressure of any food consumed and may be difficult for the preschooler to eat. It may be important to focus parents' attention on the many softer, easier-to-chew meats and protein-rich foods that their children are consuming.

Food dislikes in childhood consistently include cooked vegetables, mixed dishes, and liver. Children accept raw vegetables more readily than they do cooked ones but often accept only a limited number. Acceptance of new foods appears to be age related. Owen and others[5] found that only 6% of the youngest but 18% of the oldest preschoolers in their study

would flatly refuse a new food. Since familiarity with food is believed to influence its acceptance, new foods should be offered frequently, even though they have been previously refused.

Milk intakes are erratic and change with age. Beal[22] noted that a reduction in milk intake begins at approximately 6 months of age. Milk may be completely refused at times. Intakes of milk between ages 1 and 4 years approximate 1 to $2\frac{1}{2}$ cups per day. After this age, the total volume of milk consumed increases.

Patterns of Nutrient Intake

Both longitudinal and cross-sectional studies of nutrient and energy intakes of children have shown large differences in intakes between individual children of the same age and sex; some children consume two to three times as much energy as others.[15,29] After a rapid rise in intake of all nutrients during the first 9 months of life, reductions can be expected in the intakes of some nutrients as increases occur in intakes of others.

Sex differences in intakes of energy and nutrients have been noted by several researchers. In all studies males consumed greater quantities of food and thus greater amounts of nutrients and energy.

During the preschool years there is a decrease in intakes of calcium, phosphorus, riboflavin, iron, and vitamin A because of the omission of iron-fortified infant cereals in the diets of children, the reduction in milk intake, and the disinterest in vegetables. During this period children increase their intakes of carbohydrate and fat. Protein intakes may plateau or increase only slightly.[29] Between 3 and 8 years of age there is a slow, steady, and relatively consistent increase in intake of all nutrients. Since intakes of vitamins A and C are unrelated to energy intakes, greater ranges of intakes of these nutrients have been noted. Black preschoolers in California have been noted to have higher intakes of sodium than whites because of their frequent use of undiluted commercially prepared soups. They were found also to have greater energy intakes than whites between 2 and 4 years of age.[15]

Selection of a Nutritionally Appropriate Diet

Some clinicians mistakenly believe that, if children are given a wide variety of food choices, they will instinctively select an adequate diet. These opinions are the result of studies designed to prove that infants and young children could tolerate and should receive a variety of foods in the first years of life. The studies, conducted in the 1920s and early 1930s, involved 6-month-old to $4\frac{1}{2}$-year-old foundlings in a Chicago hospital.[30] The children under investigation were presented with 10 different fresh, unprocessed foods selected from those listed in the box below. They could eat as much or as many of the foods presented as they wished. At the completion of this study, the children were described as in good health, judged by physical growth, appearance, and vigor. It is important to note that the foods offered included only nutrient-dense, unsweetened items. There were no environmental factors which influenced food selection during the studies.

These studies do indicate the kinds of food from which young children can select nutritionally adequate diets. They show that when natural, unmixed, unprocessed foods are presented in a neutral environment, children are likely to

---

Foods Used in Experiment

1. *Meats, Muscle Cuts*
   Beef
   Lamb
   Chicken
2. *Meats, Glandular Organs*
   Liver
   Kidney
   Brains
   Sweetbreads (thymus)
3. *Sea Food*
   Sea fish (haddock)
4. *Cereals*
   Whole wheat (unprocessed)
   Oatmeal (Scotch)
   Barley (whole grains)
   Corn meal (yellow)
   Rye (Ry-Krisp)
5. *Bone Products*
   Bone marrow (beef and veal)
   Bone jelly (soluble bone substances)
6. *Eggs*

7. *Milk*
   Grade A raw milk
   Grade A raw whole lactic milk
8. *Fruits*
   Apples
   Oranges
   Bananas
   Tomatoes
   Peaches or Pineapple
9. *Vegetables*
   Lettuce
   Cabbage
   Spinach
   Cauliflower
   Peas
   Beets
   Carrots
   Turnips
   Potatoes
10. Incidentals: Sea salt (Seisal)

From: Davis, C. M.: The Self-Selection of Diet Experiment: It's Significance for feeding in the Home, Ohio State Med. J. 34: 862, 1938.

consume quantities to support normal growth and development. They do not prove that children in the free-living population and exposed to the number of combined and convenience foods available today will innately consume an appropriate nutrient and energy intake.[31]

Feeding Preschool Children

In spite of the reduction in appetite and erratic consumption of food, preschool children do enjoy food and gradually increase their average daily energy intakes. If simply prepared foods that provide a balance of nutrients are presented in a relaxed setting, children will consume an appropriate nutrient intake. Understanding and supportive help from parents and others who offer food to children lay the groundwork for the development of nutritionally sound and satisfying eating practices. Meals and snacks should be timed to foster appetite. Intervals necessary between meals and snacks may vary from one child to another; rarely can the clock be depended on to let one know appropriate intervals and times when it may be important for a child to eat.

Appetites may be satiated when energy needs are met, regardless of a child's need for nutrients. It is thus important that a food selection be provided that ensures that the foods consumed provide nutrients as well as calories. The food should be presented without comment and the child permitted to consume amounts that he or she desires without any conversation focused on what or how much is being eaten. Portions served should be scaled to the child's appetite. When the meal is over, food should be removed and the child should be permitted to leave the table.

Intervention for nutrition and feeding difficulties

Occasionally anxious or concerned parents need help replacing food sources of nutrients usually supplied by food refused or in estab-

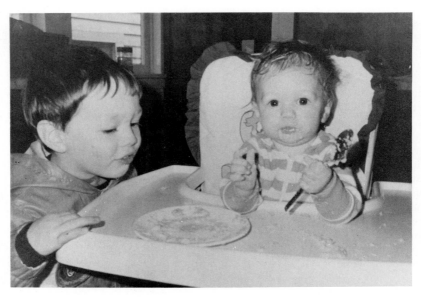

Figure 5-5 Children want to eat the same food as their siblings, even if it means regressing to baby food.

lishing limits to preschoolers' food intakes and feeding behavior. Of the commonly expressed concerns, limited intakes of milk, refusal of vegetables and meat, eating too many sweets, and limited intakes of food appear to cause the most problems. It is important to recognize that 1 oz of milk supplies 36 gm of calcium, and many children receive 6 to 8 oz of milk on dry cereal daily. Although they consume only 1 to 2 oz at a time, their calcium intakes may be acceptable when they consume milk with meals and snacks. When abundant amounts of fruit juice or sweetened beverages are available, children may simply prefer to drink them rather than milk. Other dairy products can be offered when milk is rejected. Cheese and yogurt are usually accepted. Powdered milk can be used in recipes for soups, vegetables, and mixed dishes.

Parents' perceptions of children's dislike of meat may need to be clarified. If preschoolers do consistently refuse all food sources of heme iron, their dietary intakes of iron should be carefully monitored. Parents concerned about children's excessive intakes of sweets may need help in setting limits on amounts of sweet foods they make available to their children. It may be important also to help parents convey their concern and the need to set limits on the availability of these foods to other family members, day-care operators, and teachers.

When vegetables are consistently refused, wars between parents and children should not be permitted to erupt. Small portions (1 to 2 tsp) should continue to be served without comment and should be discarded if the child does not consume them. Preschool behavior modification programs that included token rewards when children consumed vegetables and another that provided education about specific vegetables served at mealtime have been found to increase children's acceptance and intake of them.[32]

If children's food intakes are so limited that their intakes of energy and nutrients are compromised, parents may need help in estab-

lishing guidelines so that the children develop appetites. They should offer food sufficiently often that children do not get so hungry that they lose their appetite, yet not so often they are always satiated. Intervals of 3 to 4 hours are often successful. Very small portions of food should be offered, and second portions should be permitted when children consume the foods already served. Attention should always be focused on children when they eat and never when food is refused.

Group Feeding

Increasing numbers of children eat some of their meals outside the home. Preschool children of working mothers may be cared for and fed by babysitters or day-care workers. Kindergartens and preschools offer snacks and meals, and food experiences are often included as part of the learning exercises provided for children.

Day-care centers are licensed by state agencies that mandate the meal pattern and types of snacks to be provided for the children and the percentage of the RDAs that must be included in the menus. Licensed centers may receive financial assistance by entering into an agreement with the Food and Nutrition Service of the Department of Agriculture. Rates of reimbursement are variable based on family size, income, and number of children in the program. Meal requirements for children 1 to 12 years of age are shown in Tables 5-1 and 5-2.

In day-care centers or schools, breakfast needs to be provided for children who receive none at home. Snacks should be planned to complement the daily food intakes. Small portions of food should be served, and children should be permitted second servings of those foods they enjoy. Disliked or unfamiliar foods may be offered by the teaspoon, and the child's acceptance or rejection should be accepted without comment. Children who eat slowly need to be served first and should be permitted

Table 5-1   Required amounts of food to serve children age 1 through 12 for breakfast

Food Components	Age (Years)		
	1 to 3	3 to 6	6 to 12*
Milk, fluid	$\frac{1}{2}$ cup	$\frac{3}{4}$ cup	1 cup
Vegetables and fruits			
Vegetable(s) and/or fruit(s) or	$\frac{1}{4}$ cup	$\frac{1}{2}$ cup	$\frac{1}{2}$ cup
Full-strength vegetable or fruit juice or	$\frac{1}{4}$ cup	$\frac{1}{2}$ cup	$\frac{1}{2}$ cup
An equivalent quantity of any combination of vegetable(s), fruit(s), and juice			
Bread and bread alternates†			
Bread or	$\frac{1}{2}$ slice	$\frac{1}{2}$ slice	1 slice
Corn bread, biscuits, rolls, muffins, etc., or	$\frac{1}{2}$ serving	$\frac{1}{2}$ serving	1 serving
Cold dry cereal‡ or	$\frac{1}{4}$ cup or $\frac{1}{3}$ oz	$\frac{1}{3}$ cup or $\frac{1}{2}$ oz	$\frac{3}{4}$ cup or 1 oz
Cooked cereal or	$\frac{1}{4}$ cup	$\frac{1}{4}$ cup	$\frac{1}{2}$ cup
Cooked pasta or noodle products or	$\frac{1}{4}$ cup	$\frac{1}{4}$ cup	$\frac{1}{2}$ cup
Cooked cereal grains or	$\frac{1}{4}$ cup	$\frac{1}{4}$ cup	$\frac{1}{2}$ cup
An equivalent quantity of any combination of bread or bread alternate			

*Children age 12 and up may be served adult-size portions based on the greater food needs of older boys and girls but should not be served less than the minimum quantities specified in this section for children age 6 to 12 .
†Bread, pasta, or noodle products and cereal grains must be whole-grain or enriched; corn bread, biscuits, rolls, muffins, etc., must be made with whole-grain or enriched meal or flour; cereal must be whole-grain or enriched or fortified .
‡Either volume (cup) or weight (oz), whichever is less.

to complete their meals without being rushed to other activities. Teachers should eat with the children without imposing their attitudes about food on them.

A new setting provides an opportunity for children to have exposure to many new foods. Daycare centers, kindergartens, and preschools can provide an important educational setting for both children and their parents. Children learn to prepare food, how food grows, how it smells, and what nutrients it contains. Parents learn through participation, observation, and conversations with the staff. An organized approach to feeding children must include parents, teachers, and others who offer food to young children. Teachers and day-care workers can provide important information to parents about how children successfully consume food,

Table 5-2   Required amounts of food to serve children age 1 through 12 for lunch or supper

Food Components	Age (Years)		
	1 to 3	3 to 6	6 to 12*
Milk, fluid	$\frac{1}{2}$ cup	$\frac{3}{4}$ cup	1 cup
Vegetables and fruits[†]			
Vegetable(s) and/or fruit(s)	$\frac{1}{4}$ cup	$\frac{1}{2}$ cup	$\frac{3}{4}$ cup
Bread and bread alternates[‡]			
Bread or	$\frac{1}{2}$ slice	$\frac{1}{2}$ slice	1 slice
Corn bread, biscuits, rolls, muffins, etc., or	$\frac{1}{2}$ serving	$\frac{1}{2}$ serving	1 serving
Cooked pasta or noodle products or	$\frac{1}{4}$ cup	$\frac{1}{4}$ cup	$\frac{1}{2}$ cup
Cooked cereal grains or	$\frac{1}{4}$ cup	$\frac{1}{4}$ cup	$\frac{1}{2}$ cup
An equivalent quantity of any combination of bread/bread alternate			
Meat and meat alternates[§]			
Lean meat, poultry, fish or	1 oz	$1\frac{1}{2}$ oz	2 oz
Cheese or	1 oz	$1\frac{1}{2}$ oz	2 oz
Eggs or	1 egg	1 egg	1 egg
Cooked dry beans or peas or	$\frac{1}{4}$ cup	$\frac{3}{8}$ cup	$\frac{1}{2}$ cup
Peanut butter or	2 tbsp	3 tbsp	4 tbsp
An equivalent quantity of any combination of meat or meat alternate			

*Children age 12 and older may be served adult-size portions based on the greater food needs of older boys and girls but should not be served less than the minimum quantities specified in this section for children age 6 to 12 .

†Serve two or more kinds of vegetable(s) and/or fruit(s). Full-strength vegetable or fuit juice may be counted to meet not more than one half of this requirement.

‡Bread, pasta, or noodle products and cereal grains must be whole-grain or enriched; corn bread, biscuits, rolls, muffins, etc., must be made with whole-grain or enriched meal or flour.

§Edible portion as served.

the nutrients children need, and the foods that provide these nutrients. Parents offer important information to the centers about their children's food acceptance and needs. Parents and professionals need to positively reinforce each other to successfully provide food for children.

A study of 48 day-care and Head Start programs found that all participating children consumed appropriate intakes of nutrients. Total daily energy intakes were similar for all children regardless of whether one meal and one snack or two meals and two snacks were provided. In fact, when children consumed one meal and one snack in this setting, 82% of their energy intakes were provided, but when they consumed two meals and two snacks, 84% of energy intakes were provided.[33]

THE SCHOOL-AGE CHILD

The school-age period is one of relatively steady growth and few apparent feeding problems. A natural increase in appetite is responsible for normal increases in food intake. Because they spend their days at school, children adjust to a more ordered routine. They attempt to master physical skills, and they expend energy in organized sports and games. They also learn about food and nutrition as part of their curriculum at school. While they grow at their own genetically predetermined rate, the differences in height of children in the 10th and 90th percentiles are visible and of concern to those who are small or are late maturers, who compare their size to that of their peers.

School-age children are not without food and nutrition concerns. Unresolved conflicts from the preschool years may persist. Children in their early school years often continue to refuse a food that touches another on the plate or to demand a special arrangement of dishes and utensils on the table. Likes and dislikes have been established but are not necessarily permanent; however, they may become so if parents are so convinced that children will refuse a food that they do not offer it to them or if a food dislike is discussed so frequently that children become fully patterned into their food idiosyncrasies.

Undernutrition may have serious consequences for the school-age child. Undernourished children become easily fatigued, are unable to sustain prolonged physical and mental effort, and can not fully participate in learning experiences. The risk of infection is greater; therefore the child with limited nutrient reserves may have frequent absences from school. Hopwood and Van Iden[34] examined physical growth and school performance

Figure 5-6   Two 6-year-old girls whose birthdays are 1 week apart compare their height.

over a 10-year period in school-age children in Ohio. They found that unacceptable patterns of growth were accompanied by scholastic underachievement. In addition, the longer an individual child grew at a less than expected rate, the less able he or she was to achieve success in school.

Breakfast is an important meal. Children have to rise early to eat an unhurried and balanced meal and may have to prepare it themselves. Early morning school activities may make preplanning necessary. Some may find a glass of milk and fruit juice important before early sports activities. Studies have shown that when breakfast is consumed children have a better attitude and school record as compared with when it is omitted.[35] Pollitt, Leibel, and Greenfield[36] found that skipping breakfast affected problem solving in 9- to 11-year-old well-nourished children: there was an adverse effect on accuracy of response in problem solving but a beneficial effect on immediate memory in short-term accuracy.

Actually most children do eat breakfasts that contribute at least one fourth of the RDAs.[37] A larger percentage of children in the lower grades eat breakfast than of those in the middle and the upper grades. Reasons for skipping breakfast have been reported to be "not hungry," "no time," "on a diet," "no one to prepare food," "do not like food served for breakfast," and foods are "not available."[38] Morgan, Zabik, and Leville[37] found that children who consumed ready-to-eat cereals three or four times a week skipped breakfast less frequently than did children who ate non-ready-to-eat hot cereal.

A study of a school-age child's dietary habits and attendant psychosocial factors may reveal symptoms of obesity and anorexia nervosa. Intervention at this time is important, for intervention is more likely to be effective than later when the disorders are fully developed.[39]

As children explore the environment of school and peers they are likely to become influenced by these experiences. The credibility of parents is often questioned in the face of advice from teachers, peers, or peer's parents. The school-age child has more access to money, to grocery stores, and therefore to foods with questionable nutrient value.

Patterns of Food Intake

School-age children reduce the frequency of food consumption to four to five times per day on school days. They almost always want snacks after school, which they often prepare themselves. Although some increase the varieties of food they accept, many continue to reject vegetables, mixed dishes, and liver, and the range of food they voluntarily accept may be small. Sugar contributes 24% to 25% of calories in the diets of school-

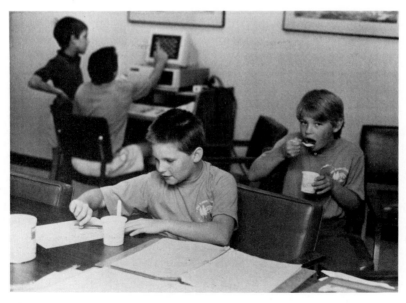

Figure 5-7 Children stop for a snack while completing their homework.

age children. Milk is the primary contributor. Sweetened beverages, fruit, fruit juice, cakes, cookies, and other desert items are also significant contributors.[39]

A common difficulty for parents is finding a time when children are willing to sit down and eat a meal. They frequently are so involved with other activities that it is difficult to get them to take time to eat. Often they satisfy their initial hunger pangs and rush back to their activities, returning later for a snack. They may become so engrossed in television programs that they demand to eat in front of the television set. In fact, some families have yielded to the pressure to not miss a favorite television program and have moved the evening meal from the dining room table to trays in front of the television. It frequently has been observed that children in such families become so engrossed in the shows that they lose interest in their food.

Snacking between meals and while watching television is an important factor in the school-age child's nutrient intake and food habits. Parents can take advantage of urges to snack by planning and providing appropriate foods and discouraging children from responding to advertised suggestions that they ingest sweet foods.

Patterns of Nutrient Intake

Increases in size are accompanied by steady increases in intakes of energy and of all nutrients. By the school-age years most children have established a particular pattern of nutrient intake relative to their peers.[29] Although wide ranges of intake continue to be observed, those who consume the greatest amounts of food, thus energy and nutrients, consistently do so, whereas those consuming smaller amounts of food maintain lesser intakes of food relative to their peers. Differences in intake between males and females increase gradually to 12 years of age and then become marked. Boys consume greater quantities of energy and nutrients than do girls.

School Meals

School feeding and nutrition education programs, when adequately implemented, provide not only important nutrients for children, but also an opportunity for them to learn to make responsible choices regarding dietary intake. Unfortunately, not all schools have provided well-prepared food or an optimum environment to encourage its acceptance. In some instances excessive food waste has been reported. In many instances schools have installed snack bars or vending machines that provide only sweet foods with high-energy and low-nutrient concentration that compete with the foods that provide a balance of nutrients. Factors believed to be responsible for food waste include unpalatability of the food, little choice in menus, children's low preference for vegetables, and the continuous availability of junk food in the school. Menus have been found to often provide insufficient iron and to offer no options for children who need to reduce their energy intakes to control obesity. Food waste has been found to be greater in elementary school programs than in high school programs. Less milk and a higher percentage of vegetables are returned than other foods.[40] Food handling has also influenced waste; on-site preparation, and service, results in the least food returns. Frozen preportioned and reheated lunches have been the least well accepted. Other factors believed to compromise children's food intakes include short lunch periods, long cafeteria lines, and a hurried, unsupervised atmosphere.

Successful programs have included students in menu planning and have prepared and served palatable, attractive food. Other programs have offered fast foods that comply with the National School Lunch Program (e.g., pizza, hamburger, milkshakes, and fruits).[41] Students have then had the option of selecting from the food available.

The fact that vending machines in schools (often viewed as money-makers for athletic and other school activities) have offered no choice but concentrated sources of sucrose has been a concern to many interested in dental health, control of obesity, and the development of sound food habits for all children. Sufficient concern has been created in some school districts that only machines that provide fruit, milk, nuts, and seeds have been made available to students. Initially, sales have been found to decrease, but ultimately they increase. One school discovered that they made a greater profit on apples than on chocolate bars.[42]

Since its inception in 1946, the school lunch program has been administered by the Department of Agriculture, which provides cash reimbursement and supplemental foods to feeding programs that comply with federal regulations. Federal regulations require that school lunches and breakfasts be sold at reduced prices or be given free to children of families that cannot afford to buy them. The lunch menus must be planned to meet the guidelines established for the National School Lunch Program. Table 5-3 shows minimum quantities of food required for the various age groups in a school lunch.

To provide variety and to encourage participation and consumption, schools are encouraged to provide a selection of foods. Senior high students may be permitted to decline up to two items. Students below the senior high level may decline up to two or only one item at the discretion of the local school food authority. Breakfast must include liquid milk, fruit or vegetable juice, and bread or cereal. Schools are encouraged to keep fat, sugar, and salt at moderate levels.

Current regulations require that schools involve students and parents in planning the school lunch program. They may be included in such activities as menu planning, enhancing the eating environment, program promotion, and related student community support activities.

Foods sold in competition with school lunch in snack bars or vending machines must provide at least 5% of the recommended dietary allowances for one or more of the following nutrients: protein, vitamin A, ascorbic acid, niacin, riboflavin, thiamine, calcium, and iron. This regulation eliminates the sale of soda water, water ices, chewing gum, and some candies until after the last lunch period. It should also encourage the offering of more fruits, vegetables, and fruit and vegetable juices in places that compete with the school lunch.

Children who do not participate in the school lunch program generally bring a packed lunch from home. Studies have indicated that, compared with the school lunch, these meals provide significantly fewer nutrients other than calories.[43] Little variety is seen in the lunches since favorite foods tend to be packed and repacked and lack of refrigeration limits the kinds of foods that can be carried.

Although elementary schoolchildren are making more decisions regarding food selection, supervision and supportive guidance may be necessary at lunchtime. Children may give priority to activities other than eating, often rushing through their meals. They may prefer to do without meals rather than reveal the fact that they must receive reduced price or free lunches. Some may refuse to eat many foods on the menu. Disposable aluminum foil trays and plastic spoons are not easy implements for children to use.

Children and their parents may need guidance in the selection of food to be consumed. Overweight and obese children may find it necessary to gain willpower to refuse the gravies and sauces and to ask for nonfat milk. As handicapped children enter the mainstream of education, careful planning with parents will be necessary to ensure that mealtimes at school provide appropriate foods and nutrients for these children.

Nutrition Education

Nutrition education during the school years is believed to be an important method of developing a nutritionally informed population, since the children are an impressionable and captive audience. Unfortunately nutri-

Table 5-3 School lunch pattern—approximate per lunch minimums

Components	Minimum Quantities				Recommended Quantities for Group V: 12 Years and Older; 7-12 +
	Group I: Age 1-2; Preschool	Group II: Age 3-4; Preschool	Group III: Age 5-8; K-3	Group IV: Age 9 and Older; 4-12	
Milk					
Unflavored, fluid lowfat, skim or buttermilk must be offered*	$\frac{3}{4}$ cup (6 fl oz)	$\frac{3}{4}$ cup (6 fl oz)	$\frac{1}{2}$ pint (8 fl oz)	$\frac{1}{2}$ pint (8 fl oz)	$\frac{1}{2}$ pint (8 fl oz)
Meat or meat alternate (quantity of the edible portion as served)					
Lean meat, poultry, or fish	1 oz	$1\frac{1}{2}$ oz	$1\frac{1}{2}$ oz	2 oz	3 oz
Cheese	1 oz	$1\frac{1}{2}$ oz	$1\frac{1}{2}$ oz	2 oz	3 oz
Large egg	$\frac{1}{2}$	$\frac{3}{4}$	$\frac{3}{4}$	1	$1\frac{1}{2}$
Cooked dry beans or peas	$\frac{1}{4}$ cup	$\frac{3}{8}$ cup	$\frac{3}{8}$ cup	$\frac{1}{2}$ cup	$\frac{3}{4}$ cup
Peanut butter or an equivalent quantity of any combination of any of above	2 tbsp	3 tbsp	3 tbsp	4 tbsp	6 tbsp
Vegetable or fruit					
2 or more servings of vegetable or fruit or both	$\frac{1}{2}$ cup	$\frac{1}{2}$ cup	$\frac{1}{2}$ cup	$\frac{3}{4}$ cup	$\frac{3}{4}$ cup
Bread or bread alternate (servings per week)					
Must be enriched or whole-grain—at least $\frac{1}{2}$ serving‡ for group I or one serving‡ for groups II-V must be served daily	5	8	8	8	10

From Food and Nutrition Service, Department of Agriculture: National School Lunch Program Regulations, Nov. 16, 1982, Federal Register.
* If a school serves another form of milk (whole or flavored), it must offer its children unflavored fluid lowfat milk, skim milk, or buttermilk as a beverage choice.
† The *minimum* portion sizes for these children are the portion sizes for group IV.
‡ Serving 1 slice of bread; or $\frac{1}{2}$ cup of cooked rice, macaroni, noodles, other pasta products, other cereal products such as bulgur and corn grits; or as stated in the *Food Buying Guide* for biscuits, rolls, muffins, and similar products.

tion is almost always a low priority to the educator. Few teachers have had basic nutrition information during their teacher training. Many have thought it to be a boring subject, difficult to integrate into an already crowded curriculum. Other reasons cited for ineffective nutrition education programs include lack of adequate research and resource materials and lack of specific curriculum guidelines that would be interdisciplinary and sequential.[44] Nutrition education activities have been a part of some programs of private sector groups, primarily the Dairy Council, and of some governmental agencies.

Because of concern that lack of adequate nutrition information was contributing to unwise food choices and to wasted food in the school lunch programs, Congress enacted the Nutrition Education Training Program in 1977. Administered by the Department of Agriculture, the program offered states grants to develop and implement a state nutrition education plan. Congress identified the following needs for this program in the NET legislation:[45]

1. The proper nutrition of the nation's children is a matter of highest priority.
2. The lack of understanding of the principles of good nutrition and their relationship to health can contribute to a child's rejection of highly nutritious foods and consequent food waste in school food service operations.
3. Many school food-service personnel have not had adequate training in food-service management skills and principles, and many teachers and school food-service operators have not had adequate training in the fundamentals of nutrition or in how to convey this information to motivate children to practice sound eating habits.
4. Parents exert a significant influence on children in the development of nutritional habits, and lack of nutrition knowledge on the part of parents can have detrimental effects on children's nutritional development.

5. There is a need to create opportunities for children to learn about the importance of the principles of good nutrition in their daily lives and how these principles are applied in the school cafeteria.

Funding, although minimal, has continued. The program has been authorized through 1989, with a minimum grant to states of $50,000.00.

During the program's most active phase, the states provided nutrition education for school lunch employees and teachers and developed curriculum guidelines and materials. Classroom activities that involved the cafeteria were developed in some schools.

When the effect of these programs was evaluated the programs were found to have a strong positive impact on nutrition-related knowledge. There was an increase in the number of children willing to select and taste new foods and in reported food preferences and food-related attitudes. However, the behavioral and attitudinal effects were neither as strong nor as consistent across grade levels as were the effects on knowledge. In grades 1 to 3 a positive impact was noted in self-reported measures of food preference and willingness of children to select unfamiliar fruits and vegetables when offered a choice during the school lunch.[46] In grades 4 to 6 children who participated in the programs were more willing to taste previously unfamiliar foods than were children who had not participated in the program. Although several programs noted a decline in food waste, no strong program-related effects were noted on overall food waste.[46] At the current level of funding, efforts are directed toward school food-service employee training, coordination of curriculum and food-service activities, and integration of nutrition into health education and other curriculums.

Other nutrition education programs have indicated that parental involvement in the nutrition education programs resulted in children who consumed a higher quality diet than in children in programs in which parents were not involved, an effect noted in kindergarten and the first grade but not in the upper grades.[47] The need to continue nutrition education programs is obvious. It is also important that we learn new methods of nutrition education that may have a greater impact on behavioral change in children.

As children prepare to enter adolescence, attitudes toward food will be well established. Between infancy and adolescence, nutrients and energy provide compounds necessary for growth. Reserves of some nutrients are accumulated that prepare children for stress and for their next stage of growth, the adolescent growth spurt. The knowledge of nutrition and attitudes toward food they acquire during this period provide a basis for the years when the decisions of food selection become theirs alone.

Summary

Children between 1 year of age and the onset of puberty grow at a steady rate. They acquire many new skills, learn much about the environment in which they live, and test the limits of behavior the environment will accept. All these factors influence their food and therefore nutrient intake. Parents need to provide appropriate foods and supportive guidance so that food patterns that support an appropriate nutrient intake are developed. The nutrition knowledge of the mother positively influences children's nutrient intake. Advertising and television programs also affect children's requests for and acceptance of food.

School feeding programs provide an opportunity for nutrition education, and children do learn from this nutrition education. The behavioral effects of nutrition education appear to be grade related.

Although most children appear clinically to be well nourished, groups exist within our population with both clinical and biochemical evidence of malnutrition. Nutrients most often consumed in inappropriately limited amounts are iron, vitamins B_6 and C, and calcium.

SUGGESTED LEARNING ACTIVITIES

1. Assess the nutrient intake of a preschool child.
2. Observe a preschool feeding program and describe the feeding environment.
3. Describe factors that influence food acceptability in the preschool child.
4. Describe appropriate snacks for school-age children.
5. Describe factors that influence foods acceptable to school-age children.
6. Plan a nutrition lesson for an elementary school class.
7. Plan a week's brown bag lunches for a school-age child that provide variety and are nutritionally appropriate.

REFERENCES

1. Centers for Disease Control: Ten-State Nutrition Survey, 1968-1970, DHEW Pub. No. (HSM) 72-8130-34, Washington, D.C., 1972, U.S. Department of Health, Education and Welfare, Health Services and Mental Health Administration.
2. Science and Education Administration: Nationwide Food Consumption Survey, 1977-1978, Preliminary Rep. No. 2, Food and nutrient intakes of individuals in 1 day in the U.S., Spring, 1977, Hyattsville, Md., 1980, U.S. Department of Agriculture.
3. Jones, D.Y., Nesheim, M.D. and Habicht, J.P.: Influences in child growth associated with poverty in the 1970's: an examination of HANES I and HANES II, cross-sectional U.S. national surveys, Am. J. Clin. Nutr. 42:714, 1985.
4. Windham, C.T., and others: Nutrient density of diets in the USDA Nationwide Food Consumption Survey, 1977-1978. I. Impact of socioeconomic status on dietary density, J. Am. Diet. Assoc. 82:26, 1983.
5. Owen, G.M., and others: A study of nutritional status of preschool children in the United States, 1968-1970, Pediatrics 53:597 1974.
6. Farris, R.P.: Dietary studies from a biracial population: intakes of vitamins in 10 and 13 year olds. J. Am. Coll. Nutr. 4:539, 1985.
7. Bowering, J. and Clancy, K.L.: Nutritional status of children and teenagers in relation to vitamin and mineral use. J. Am. Diet. Assoc. 86:1033, 1986.
8. Van Duzen, J., Carter, J.P., and Vander Zwaag, R.: Protein and calorie malnutrition among preschool Navajo Indian children, Am. J. Clin. Nutr. 29:657, 1976.

9. Owen, G.M., and others: Nutrition survey of White Mountain Apache preschool children in nutrition, growth, and development of North American Indian children, Pub. No. (N.I.H.) 72-76, Washington, D.C., 1972, Department of Health, Education and Welfare.

10. Zee, P., and others: Nutritional improvement of poor urban preschool children: A 1983-1977 comparison, J. A. M. A. 253:3269, 1985.

11. Fries, M.E., Crisley, B.M., and Driskell, J.A.: Vitamin B_6 status of a group of preschool children, Am. J. Clin. Nutr. 34:2706, 1981

12. Eppright, E.S., and others: Nutrition of infants and preschool children in the North Central Region of the United States of America, World Rev. Nutr. Diet. 14:269. 1972.

13. Eppright, E.S., and others: The North Central Regional study of diets of preschool children. II. Nutrition knowledge and attitudes of mothers. J. Home Ec. 62:327, 1970.

14. Caliendo, M.A., and others: Nutritional status of preschool children, J. Am. Diet. Assoc. 71:20, 1977.

15. Crawford, P.B., Hankin, J.H., and Huenemann, R.L.: Environmental factors associated with preschool obesity, J. Am. Diet. Assoc. 72:589, 1978.

16. Karp, R. and others: Parental behavior and the availability of foods among undernourished inner-city children, J. Fam. Pract. 18:731, 1984.

17. Laskarzewski, P., and others: Parent-child nutrient intake interrelationships in school children ages 6 to 19: the Princeton School District Study, Am. J. Clin. Nutr. 33:2350, 1980.

18. Eppright, E.S., and others: Eating behavior of preschool children, J. Nutr. Educ. 1:16, 1969.

19. Sims, L.S., and Morris, P.M.: Nutritional status of preschoolers, J. Am. Diet. Assoc. 64:492, 1974.

20. Lund, L.A., and Burk, M.C.: A multidisciplinary analysis of children's food consumption behavior, Technical Bulletin No. 265, St. Paul, 1969, University of Minnesota, Agricultural Experimental Section.

21. Harris, C.S. and others: Childhood asphyxiation by food: a national analysis and overlook, J. A. M. A. 251:2231, 1984.

22. Beal, V.A.: On the acceptance of solid foods and other food patterns of infants and children, Pediatrics 20:448, 1957.

23. Pelchat, M.L. and Pliner, P.: Antecedents and correlates of feeding problems in young children, J. Nutr. Ed. 18:23, 1986.

24. Huenemann, R.L.: Environmental factors associated with preschool obesity. II. Obesity and food practices of children at successive age levels, J. Am. Diet. Assoc. 64:489, 1974.

25. Lucas, B.L.: Nutrition in childhood. In Krause, M.V., and Mahan, L.K., editors: Food, nutrition, and diet

therapy, ed. 7, Philadelphia, 1984, W.B. Saunders Co.

26. Eppright, E.S., and others: The North Central Regional study of diets of preschool children. III. Frequency of eating, J. Home Ec. 62:407, 1970.

27. Frank, G.C., and others: Dietary studies of rural school children in a cardiovascular study, J. Am. Diet. Assoc. 71:31, 1977.

28. Farris, R.P. and others: Macronutrient intakes of 10 year old children, 1973 to 1982, J. Am. Diet. Assoc. 86:765, 1986.

29. Beal, V.A.: Dietary intake of individuals followed through infancy and childhood, Am. J. Public Health 51:1107, 1961.

30. Davis, C.M.: The self-selection of diet experiment: its significance for feeding in the home. Ohio State Med. J. 34:862, 1938.

31. Stuy, M. and Brown, J.E.: Do young children instinctively know what to eat? The studies of Clara Davis revisited, N. Engl. J. Med. 316:103, 1987.

32. Ireton, C.L. And Guthrie, H.A.: Modification of vegetable-eating behavior in preschool children, J. Nutr. Educ. 4:100, 1972.

33. Williams, S., Henneman, A., and Fox, H.: Contribution of food service programs in preschool centers to children's nutritional needs, J. Am. Diet. Assoc. 71:610, 1977.

34. Hopwood, H.H., and Van Iden, S.S.: Scholastic underachievement as related to sub-par physical growth, J. Sch. Health 35:337, 1965.

35. Tuttle, W.W., and others: Effect on school boys of omitting breakfast, J. Am. Diet. Assoc. 30:674, 1974.

36. Pollitt, E., Leibel, R.L., and Greenfield, D.: Brief fasting, stress, and cognition in children, Am. J. Clin. Nutr. 34:1526, 1981.

37. Morgan, K.J., Zabik, M.Z., and Leville. G.A.: The role of nutrient intake of 5- to 12-year-old chldren. Am. J. Clin. Nutr. 34:1418, 1981.

38. Singleton, A., and Rhodes, J.J.: Meal and snacking patterns of students, J. Sch. Health 52:529, 1982.

39. Morgan, K.J., and Zabik, M.E.: Amount and food sources of total sugar intake by children ages 5- to 12-years, Am. J. Clin. Nutr. 34:404, 1981.

40. Jansen, G.R., and Harper, J.M.: Consumption and plate waste of menu items served in the National School Lunch Program, J. Am. Diet. Assoc. 73:395, 1978.

41. Fast food staple for type A lunches, Sch. Food Serv. J. 31:19, 1977.

42. Crawford, L.: Junk food in our schools: a look at student spending in school vending machines and concessions, J. Can. Diet. Assoc. 38:195, 1977.

43. Emmons, L., Hayes, M., and Call, D.L.: A study of school funding programs. II. Effects on children

with different economic and nutritional needs, J. Am. Diet. Assoc. 61:268, 1972.

44. O'Donnell, N.L., and Alles, W.F.: School nurse demonstrates that mini-grant funding can improve elementary nutrition education, J. Sch. Health 5:316, 1983.

45. GAO/CED: What can be done to improve nutrition education? Gaithersburg, Md., 1982, U.S. Government Accounting Office, Document Handling and Information Services Facility.

46. St. Pierre, R.G., and Rezmovic, V.: An overview of the national nutrition education and training program evaluation, J. Nutr. Educ. 14:61, 1982.

47. Kirks, B.A., Hendricks, D.G., and Wyse, B.W.: Parent involvement in nutrition education for primary grade students, J. Nutr. Educ. 14:137, 1982.

6

Development of Food Patterns in Young Children

Miriam E. Lowenberg

OBJECTIVES

After studying this chapter, the student should:

1. Recognize differences between hunger and appetite.
2. Be aware of appropriate furniture and utensils for use when feeding young children.
3. Be aware of the factors to consider when writing menus for young children.
4. Have knowledge of appropriate foods and methods of preparation for young children.
5. Know common difficulties encountered by concerned parents when feeding young children.

Introduction

Investigations of child feeding began in the early 1900s and have continued throughout this century. Among those who will long be remembered for their contribution to our understanding of children's food behavior and child feeding are Arnold Gesell, Lydia Roberts, Icie Mary Hoobler, Virginia Beal, and Miriam E. Lowenberg, the author of this chapter. Dr. Lowenberg's studies have provided the information on which the philosophy of preschool feeding that has persisted throughout the last half of this century was developed.

Because of her interest in cultural food habits, Dr. Lowenberg later developed a course and co-authored a book, *Food and People*, emphasizing cultural influences on food patterns.[1]

This chapter presents Dr. Lowenberg's philosophy and approaches to feeding young children. It is a classic that anyone interested in food for young children must read, assimilate, and apply.

FOOD PATTERNS

Food patterns in the United States show distinct cultural characteristics that change as lifestyles change. Hurried small breakfasts, mid-morning coffee breaks, and light lunches followed by heavy evening dinners show modern adjustments to change. In the home, snacking is known to have increased as television has become an integral part of the day and night activities of the American family.

There are many different meal patterns in modern America. There are inner-city patterns of poor or rich families, suburban patterns, and rural patterns of nonfarm and farm families. The rich and the poor have throughout the ages had different food patterns. In fact, careful professional observers of young children eating in a group can often predict the home environment of an individual child.

The current enthusiasm for behavioral control of food intake points to a need to examine the day's program to learn when unneeded calories in food are taken. Researchers now believe that what happens during the first year of life, as well as during the preschool years, is of paramount importance. During the first 5 or 6 years of life it is undoubtedly easier to learn to like all foods than it will be later.

Presently the young child is introduced early to hamburgers and french fries when families eat out; attesting to this is one fast-food company's yearly sales—the highest in the restaurant industry. Eating out becomes a helpful respite for the young homemaker or working mother, and a pattern is established for the young child. When parents hope to establish a basic food pattern of meals enjoyed at home they must deal with the child's desire to eat out, even if the child only knows about it because other children talk about eating out.

Goals for the development of food patterns are the following:

1. Children should be able to eat in a matter-of-fact way sufficient quantities of the foods that are given to them, just as they take care of other daily needs. Preschool children who truly enjoy most foods but are able to eat without fuss those they do not especially like will be fortunate later.

2. Children should be able to manage the feeding process independently and with dispatch, without either unnecessary dawdling or hurried eating.

3. Children should be willing to try new foods in small portions the first time they are served to them and to try them again and again until they like or at least willingly accept them.

Professionals interested in guiding parents or prospective parents must know which patterns produce healthy children and adults. We must also believe that it is possible to set up a home environment to foster the development of desirable food patterns in young children. Often an impersonal professionally trained outsider can point out to parents how they can set up such an environment. It must be understood that food patterns begin to be formed from the day of an infant's birth. This reminds me of a healthy, happy young mother who telephoned from her hospital room to report the birth of a daughter 4 hours before. She said with joy that her baby had already tried to nurse; this mother, although still tired from the birth process, had already enjoyed the process of even feeble breast-feeding.

Those who are concerned about obesity as our chief problem of malnutrition wisely point out that prevention, the preferred cure, should begin early in infancy. Parents who give their newborns the privilege of deciding that they have had enough food are well on the way to solving this problem. It is believed that when an individual forms a pattern of quitting to eat at the first indication of satiety, the food intake regulatory mechanism is encouraged to continue to function. Of course, food that produces the growth of good body tissues must be provided so that more than calorie satiety is provided. This is an important part of early food patterning of a child.

The food patterns established in a home are reinforced by love of mother and father and therefore have far-reaching effects on lifetime patterns. No one has ever phrased the functions of parents more aptly than did C. Anderson Aldrich and Mary Aldrich[2] 40 years ago when they said:

> According to nature's plan then parents are meant to enter the feeding situation for three reasons:
> First, to provide the food,
> Second, to support a child's progress
> from simple to mature methods of eating, and
> Third, to make it easy for him to establish
> his own satisfying feeding habits.

Long ago I observed another principle that we need to emphasize with parents: It really is easier and quicker to change the food than it is to change the child. For instance, young children often have trouble swallowing dry food, and when extra milk is added to thin their mashed potatoes they seem thankful. Such methods are explained in detail later in this chapter.

To know what foods children like requires careful observations of young children while they are eating. Table 6-1 on pp. 146-147 gives approximate amounts of foods that one can expect the average child to eat.* *In no way are these amounts to be used to force a certain amount of food on any specific child.* If any child, however, habitually eats less than the amount in the chart, the reasons should be determined. As always, a particular child's food dislikes, his or her health condition, or specific family circumstances need to be considered.

CULTURAL PATTERNS

Many ethnic groups make up the population of the United States. Each ethnic food pattern, based on foods available and preferred, comes from the home country and is based firmly on tradition and often on long usage. Specific ways of cooking foods are always dependent on such factors as the fuel available, the time and the energy available for food preparation, and the interests and patience of the cook. For example, the generous use of rye breads and fish in the Scandinavian countries

is a result of the cool and short growing season, the long coastlines, and the Scandinavian people's knowledge of successful fishing. Even after such countries are able to import other foods, the preferred foods are still used as tradition dictates. The cause for the abundant use by Polynesian peoples of the coconut, tropical fruits and vegetables, and fish that are abundant in tropical waters is obvious.

The history of a people is written in their preferred foods. This explains why schoolchildren in North Dakota and in Georgia react in radically different ways to rice used as a vegetable. For instance, rice, which grew well in the American south from early colonial times, has become a preferred food in

---

*For 12 years I daily observed 20 nursery schoolchildren eating their noon meals. Later, for 2 years, the ideas generated by this observation were used in the daily feeding of 1000 children, mostly 18 months to 6 years of age, in two shipyard World War II nursery schools. My commission as chief nutritionist was to be in charge of feeding and nutritional development. Feeding for the 9 hours at nursery school was carefully planned, and mothers and fathers were also advised and helped to feed their children at home.

The knowledge gained while studying the eating patterns and food preferences of the college nursery schoolchildren for 12 years was used to teach college students about feeding young children. All food was measured onto the child's plate before it left the kitchen serving area; second helpings and leftover foods were measured and recorded. For 1 school year, the adult who ate at a table with two or three children was asked to record each child's reaction to each food and to the menu as a whole. They were to record: was a food too dry? too tough? too acid to be easily eaten? Were there other characteristics that made the food unsuitable? Were the combinations of foods acceptable and liked by the children? As these criticisms came in daily, corrections were made in the menus and recipes for the foods. During the following year the corrected menus and specific foods were again studied, and further corrections were made. During this study each day, a chart was made of the amounts of each food to be served to each child. The head teacher confirmed that when the children's appetites were closely studied a child's specific food intake could be accurately judged. Most thoughtful mothers can do this.

The advice in this chapter is based on the ideas gained from this meticulous study as well as on extensive tests of these ideas.

Table 6-1   Food pattern for preschool children

Food	Portion Size	Number of Portions Advised	
		Ages 2 to 4 years	Ages 4 to 6 years
Milk and dairy products			
Milk†	4 oz	3 to 6	3 to 4
Cheese	$\frac{1}{2}$ to $\frac{3}{4}$ oz	May be substituted for one portion of liquid milk	
Yogurt	$\frac{1}{4}$ to $\frac{1}{2}$ cup	May be substituted for one portion of liquid milk	
Powdered skim milk	2 tbsp	May be substituted for one portion of liquid milk	
Meat and meat equivalents			
Meat‡, fish§, poultry	1 to 2 oz	2	2
Egg	1	1	1
Peanut butter	1 to 2 tbsp		
Legumes—dried peas and beans	$\frac{1}{4}$ and $\frac{1}{3}$ cup cooked		
Vegetables and fruits			
Vegetables		4 to 5 to include 1 green leafy or yellow‖	4 to 5 to include 1 green leafy or yellow
Cooked	2 to 4 tbsp		
Raw	Few pieces		
Fruit		1 citrus fruit or other vegetable or fruit rich in vitamin C	1 citrus fruit or other vegetable or fruit rich in vitamin C
Canned	4 to 8 tbsp		
Raw	$\frac{1}{2}$ to 1 small		
Fruit juice	3 to 4 oz		

that part of the country, yet when first used in lunches in some schools in North Dakota, rice was rejected as an unfamiliar food. Another vegetable of historic importance to the southern United States is okra. This vegetable is said to have been brought by slaves from Africa, and its popularity has even withstood the memory of those sad journeys to which those slaves were subjected. Blends in Creole dishes could only occur where Spanish, French, black African, and American Indian influences came together. During the latter part of the twentieth century most Americans have come to prize their cultural backgrounds, cultural foods, and differences in food patterns.

In summary, two points should be emphasized. First, every ethnic diet must be based on nutritional adequacy, at least to some degree, for the group using it to survive. For example, the very poor and food-deficient Irish people of the nineteenth century, who had an extremely limited diet, could scarcely have cho-

Table 6-1   Food pattern for preschool children—*cont'd.*

Food	Portion Size	Number of Portions Advised	
		Ages 2 to 4 years	Ages 4 to 6 years
Bread and cereal grains			
Whole grain or enriched white bread	$\frac{1}{2}$ to 1 slice	3	3
Cooked cereal	$\frac{1}{4}$ to $\frac{1}{2}$ cup	May be substituted for one serving of bread	
Ready-to-serve dry cereals	$\frac{1}{2}$ to 1 cup		
Spaghetti, macaroni, noodles, rice	$\frac{1}{4}$ to $\frac{1}{2}$ cup		
Crackers	2 to 3		
Fat			
Bacon	1 slice	Not to be substituted for meat	
Butter or vitamin A–fortified margarine	1 tsp	3	3 to 4
Desserts	$\frac{1}{4}$ to $\frac{1}{2}$ cup	As demanded by calorie needs	
Sugars	$\frac{1}{2}$ to 1 tsp	2	2

* Diets should be monitored for adequacy of iron and vitamin D intake.
† Approximately $\frac{2}{3}$ cup can easily be incorporated in a child's food during cooking.
‡ Liver once a week can be used as liver sausage or cooked liver.
§ Should be served once or twice per week to substitute for meat.
‖ If child's preferences are limited, use double portions of preferred vegetables until appetite for other vegetables develop.

sen any two foods as nutritionally adequate as buttermilk and potatoes. The nutritional adequacy for a desirable state of health may point, in some ethnic patterns, to a need for supplementation with some other foods. Adding needed foods to this basic diet is often much easier than changing the *staple* food of a group. This, however, means that it is desirable to maintain the basic pattern with only the needed supplementation. American Indian children who have been taught to like the wild greens that their families eat, for instance, should be encouraged to follow these food patterns. Second, children who learn the cues of ethnic food patterns at an early age should be

allowed to make these patterns as permanent as possible in a new environment. Respect for differences in food patterns influences the way individuals view themselves and their worth.

POSITIVE REINFORCEMENT

Experience with helping young children form desirable feeding patterns show that positive reinforcement of desirable behavior is sound. (For further discussion of behavior modification, see Chapter 15.) Some 40 years ago it was found that children developed desirable feeding patterns when they felt successful and when negative behavior was ignored. It is wise to find out why a child does not like or does not readily eat a certain food or combination of foods. Often it is easy to change the food or menu.

There are many ways to help children eat successfully. Portion size is of paramount importance. When children are presented with less food than they normally eat they can accomplish the goal that the adult has set; they can then ask for second helpings. This allows them to receive adult approbation, which is a reward to them. If for some reason children cannot eat all the food that has been given to them, allowing them to set their own limit shows respect for them and lets them feel successful. However, when children restrict their food intake to much less than expected over a number of days, parents should investigate. Improving an environmental situation often corrects this low intake of food (see p. 151 for specific suggestions).

HUNGER AND APPETITE

Food is taken into the body to satisfy the primal urge of hunger. According to the physiologist Dr. Anton J. Carlson,[3] there are two unpleasant sensations that are involved in what we call hunger. The first is a generalized weakness and restlessness all over the body, which is probably caused by a need for more sugar in the blood. The second is a definite localized sensation of pains of tension in the upper part of the stomach. These pangs of hunger are comparatively brief and are followed by periods when hunger pain is not felt. The infant and the young child are thought to have frequent and severe hunger pains. In the infant these sometimes are severe enough to cause an outcry as they awaken him or her from sleep. Infants' stomachs have been observed to show feeble hunger contractions 1 hour after nursing and strong hunger contractions $2\frac{1}{2}$ to 3 hours after a feeding. The length of time the stomach shows in this way that it is ready for food varies with the individual infant. In the young child of 2 to 5 years of age these hunger pains

are somewhat less frequent or pronounced than in the young infant, but they are still quite definite. Normally, food taken into the body gives immediate pleasure to a child when it eases the pain of hunger. If nothing else interferes, food is associated with the easing of pain, and pleasure results from eating.

Hunger is quite different from appetite. Most authorities agree that although hunger is an unpleasant sensation, appetite is a pleasurable experience. Appetite is usually defined as the pleasant association of a food with past experiences with that food. Appetite, associated with the sight and odor of food, stimulates the flow of digestive juices and is therefore a vital part of good digestion, as has often been demonstrated in the clinic and laboratory.

Many people have searched diligently and long for foods that taste like those mother used to cook when they were children. No doubt her foods were good, but they were probably not incomparable. The remembered foods were eaten at times when the child was thoroughly happy, and, as a result, a strong appetite for them was created. As an individual grows older the zest for the same food may be lessened. There is only the memory of or the appetite for the former food. Thus appetites for certain foods are undoubtedly built up in children not only from the flavor, color, and texture of the food itself, but also from the many associations with the food.

It is normal for a young child to be hungry. To be persistently nonhungry is decidedly abnormal. The child who is not hungry should be taken to a physician who will carefully assess his or her physical well-being (looking possibly for a chronic infection) and his or her daily habits. This child may not get enough brisk exercise in the open air, or may need more sleep, a more regular diet pattern, sleep and rest, or a less stimulating environment.

If a child is in good health and is hungry, with a stomach calling urgently for food, food will be eaten to satisfy that urge rather than to satisfy whims. As has been so aptly said, hunger should control the child rather than the child hunger. This fact may be taken advantage of in many ways. New foods in very small portions may be served at the time of the day when the child is hungriest. It should be remembered that for a young child a new food is a step in the dark; children are generally not as adventuresome as adults. If a child eats the new food when hungry, it will probably leave a pleasant sensation, and the next time this food is served it will be recognized as a friend. Children learn to like a food by tasting it time after time, even though the first tastes are but a few tiny bites.

SETTING UP A FOOD ENVIRONMENT

In helping parents to understand why children eat as they do, it is well to direct their attention to the fact that *behavior is caused*. When causes of behavior are understood, a food problem is on the way to being cured. Parents who understand why children eat as they do can usually set up an environment that promotes a healthy appetite. Often an outside professional person can help a parent to discover these causes and to restructure the environment. Preparental education in which specific appetite problems are discussed can help prevent them. Part of this education must emphasize the requirements of a good food environment.

How does a parent help a child develop desirable food patterns? The following are suggestions:

1. The parents, as "gatekeepers," must recognize that the kinds of food available to the preschool child in the home are what they buy and provide. Many parents need to be shown that, in this, they are *really in command*. In a well-child clinic, a mother complained that her 3-year-old child was eating too many potato chips, yet she admitted that she was the one who bought them.

Of course, other family members must cooperate in not having foods of this kind available.
2. Often parents must decide which of their own food patterns they want to pass on to their children. Some parents need to be assured that they can change their own food patterns; they may even need to be helped to do this.
3. Feeding programs for groups of preschool children have proven again and again that the eating habits of young children can be repatterned under skilled guidance. This should give parents added confidence.

DEVELOPMENTAL PATTERNS

Children develop for the most part in an orderly pattern—physically, emotionally, and psychologically.

Eating is always dependent on the abilities of the eater. For instance, when normal infants are born they are able to root for a nipple and to suck vigorously to ingest milk. When infants are given a chance to satisfy their hunger in this manner, they attain their first success in eating. As parents discover the child's hunger patterns and provide foods to satisfy hunger, they set up the condition for successful eating.

DIFFICULTIES IN THE FORMATION OF GOOD FOOD HABITS AND WAYS TO AVOID THEM

When most infants are fed the first semisolid food, they often spit it out rather violently—not because they do not want the food but because they know only the sucking motion they have used thus far to ingest food (see Chapter 4). Now they try this motion again, and the semiliquid cereal or food spatters everywhere. They must learn an entirely new feeding technique. If they fail in the first efforts, a parent may be spattered and naturally quite upset. They have met their first feeding disaster. To laugh at these efforts is unwise because the infant learns to do this to make parents laugh.

Parents should prepare themselves in advance so that they can remain undisturbed by the incident.

Another difficulty enters into this situation—all the previous food has been liquid. Now, suddenly, here is a food with a new texture, as well as a new flavor that is different from the usual, mildly sweet milk. Difficulties may be avoided by giving the infant minute amounts of the new food, well moistened and thinned by the familiar milk, until the new food is easily accepted. Weaning begins right here. The infant is being weaned away gradually from an exclusively fluid diet.

In this discussion weaning is used to mean a general process involving, as far as food is concerned, any change in food flavor, texture, consistency, temperature, or method of feeding. Many feeding difficulties arise because the changes are expected to take place too abruptly or because adults fail to realize how difficult some of these tasks are for the infant and the young child. A child can and will learn these new things, but neither the parent nor child should become upset over failures at first. Nor must the child learn to get attention by spitting food out or by refusing it. The problem can be avoided by demonstrating the technique for spoon feeding.

At approximately 6 months of age, even before the first tooth appears, most infants make chewing movements with their gums. At this time infants should be given foods such as small strips of ovendried toast, which offer a chance for chewing at the same time as they soften to allow easy swallowing. It has been observed that when an infant is not given a chance to chew at this time, trouble in mastering this skill may occur later.

When the infant begins to gain the muscular ability to pick up small particles using the thumb and forefingers, particles of soft green beans or peas can be fed (see Chapter 4 for a more detailed discussion of this). These efforts, along with reaching for the bottle and later holding it, are the infant's first efforts to learn to feed independently.

The stage of developing independence at 9 to 18 months of age can either be exciting or distressing for parents. If parents understand that exploring everything new is very important to an infant, they can encourage this exploration by providing new textures and flavors in foods; this allows an infant to discover what a food such as oatmeal feels like. At this stage many infants have learned to crawl out from their former sitting position or to walk. It is no longer satisfying to them to just look at something; they now want to examine it. Wise parents take advantage of this new learning by providing a wide variety of food. They should not be discouraged at first if the child only feels a food before chewing it.

During the first year an infant has tremendous adjustments to make, only one of which is learning new foods and new methods of eating. In helping this infant to form good patterns, we will be most successful if we provide thoughtful and understanding guidance in the following ways:

1. Introducing new textures and flavors gradually
2. Enlarging the child's experience with as many individual foods in as many different forms as possible
3. Feeding individual foods and not mixtures so that the infant may learn to appreciate foods for their own flavors and textures
4. Observing at what time of day the infant takes the new food most easily and giving it then
5. Being patient with the first efforts and allowing the infant to learn to feed himself or herself; offering help when the infant becomes too tired to finish the process easily
6. Being understanding of the infant's efforts in each new feeding process

7. Above all, securing the entire family's cooperation.

The high level of nutritive need of the first year of life is superceded by a slower metabolic rate and a slower rate of growth; therefore the child does not need as much food per unit of body weight as before. What is eaten and how it is eaten are now more important than how much is eaten. To watch a young child grow increasingly independent in feeding himself can be as thrilling for a parent as watching the taking of the first steps from chair to chair. Perhaps in no other area of development in young children is progress more individual. Each child should be allowed to try new skills over and over with no record of failures unless development is obviously too slow to show any progress.

When parents understand what children are telling them in the way they eat, rebellion against food can be lessened and future food refusals can be reduced. For instance, the realization that the 2-year-old child may have a sporadic appetite, which should not be the cause for undue alarm, may prevent the long-lasting influence of battles over food.

SPECIFIC SUGGESTIONS FOR SETTING UP A FOOD ENVIRONMENT

Perhaps no arrangements for eating are more important than those that afford physical comfort to a child. Children should always feel secure on a sturdy, well-balanced chair with their feet well supported on the floor or other structure. They should be able to reach their food easily without straining their muscles. This also provides a better opportunity to eat without spills, although wise parents also prepare table surfaces and floors for children's spills. Dishes and utensils, as well as table arrangements, can foster success in eating. It is desirable to give the child sturdy and as

nearly unbreakable utensils as possible so that spills and breaking utensils will not give a sense of failure. Also it is important not to laugh at the child, because if parents laugh at a child's mistakes the child may gain an undue feeling of being the center of attention.

When children's chairs are being purchased, these should be "tried on" as clothing is. Some chairs, for instance, are designed to fit a child's torso and are much more comfortable than are perfectly straight chairs.

Sometimes children, who for some months have eaten at the family table, may suddenly be happier eating at their own small table with a parent nearby. Some mothers even find it possible to eat a quiet noon meal with the child at a small table.

Colorful table arrangements intrigue young children and are worth the trouble to provide. When children have developed some skill in eating, they will appreciate eating from the family's best china. Parents who show confidence in a child's accomplishment are usually rewarded by the child's care in handling prized possessions. These children who have had help in gaining skill in successful eating are easy to recognize as one observes families eating together in restaurants.

Forks and spoons should be chosen for their suitability for young hands. The spoon, which is the first eating implement a child uses, should have a round shallow bowl and a blunt tip that allows the child to shove food from the plate. A handle that is blunt, short, and easily held in the child's palm is desirable; at this age a child uses the hand as a mass of muscles. Only after 5 or 6 years of age is control of the finer muscles of the fingers accomplished. Forks with short, blunt tines are best adapted to the child's palm. Although some parents report that their children enjoy sharper tines with which they can spear food, sharp tines can be dangerous.

Glasses that sit firmly on the table and are small enough for children's hands to encircle are best for 2- to 4-year-old children. Small delicate handles on cups are difficult for small hands to maneuver.

The shape and weight of the dishes is also very important. The young child delights in pouring his or her own milk. Interesting, squat pitchers with broad handles from which the child can easily pour milk are recommended. Parents can be encouraged to experiment with dishes and utensils for their children and to look for those that satisfy children's needs.

FOODS CHILDREN LIKE

Patient observation and long experience in feeding young children, as well as in counseling parents, have given me an insight into what children want in their food. When this knowledge of children's preferences is combined with the knowledge of nutrients, children can be adequately and happily fed. The results of these observations are discussed on the following pages.

Menus

Simplicity in menus is very important. At the same time there must be variety to allow young children to learn to know many foods, since variety in foods is a good foundation for an adequate diet.

The following outline gives a general meal pattern that should satisfy nutrient needs in a hungry preschool child.

A. Breakfast
 1. One high-protein food
    a. 1 egg *or*
    b. 2 oz of muscle meat *or*
    c. 3/4 to 1 oz of cheese *or*
    d. 1/2 cup of cereal, cooked, *or*
    e. 1 cup of dry cereal with 4 to 6 oz milk
 2. Bread with butter or margarine (1 slice whole grain or white enriched bread, plus 1 tsp butter

 3. Milk, 6 to 8 oz
 4. Fruit—preferably one serving of citrus
    a. 4 oz of orange juice *or*
    b. 1/3 to 1/2 medium-sized grapefruit *or*
    c. 1 medium-sized orange
B. Noon meal
 1. One high-protein food (See breakfast for list of high-protein foods)
    a. 1 serving of a thick soup or stew *or*
    b. 1 serving of a casserole dish of a protein food in a starchy base
 2. Vegetables
    a. 1 cooked (see Table 6-1 for amounts)
    b. 1 raw (see Table 6-1 for amounts)
 3. Bread (1 slice whole grain or enriched white bread with 1 tsp butter)
 4. Milk, 6 to 8 oz
 5. Dessert
    a. Simple dessert based on a combination of milk, eggs, and fruit *or*
    b. Serving of fruit
C. Evening meal
 1. One high-protein food
    a. 2 oz meat *or*
    b. 1 oz cheese *or*
    c. 1 egg *or*
    d. Combinations of these and vegetables
 2. Vegetables
    a. 1 or 2 cooked *or*
    b. 1 raw
 3. Bread and butter (1 slice whole grain or enriched white bread with 1 tsp butter)
 4. Milk, 6 to 8 oz
 5. Dessert (see noon meal, dessert)
D. Snacks between meals or at bedtime These should provide some of the needed nutrients and be low in sugar and fat so that they do not interfere with the appetite for the following meal; use, for example, any of the following:
 1. Fruit juices with a cracker or a piece of bread *or*

2. Small pieces of fruit *or*
3. Small pieces of raw vegetables *or*
4. Small pieces of cheese with a small piece of bread or cracker

Combinations of Food

Most children eat most easily those foods with which they are familiar. It is advisable that a very small portion of a new food be introduced with a familiar and popular food. If the child only looks at the new food or just feels or smells it at first, this is a part of learning to accept it.

Dry foods are especially hard for children to eat, as is discussed later in this chapter. In planning a menu, always carefully balance a dry food with one or two moist foods. For instance, it is wise to put a slice of meat loaf (relatively dry) with mashed potatoes and peas in a little cream sauce.

Combinations of sharp, rather acid-flavored foods with mild-flavored foods are popular with young children.

Ease of Manipulation

The ease of eating food with the unskilled and seemingly clumsy hands of a young child is very important. Many small pieces of foods such as cooked green peas of beans are difficult for a child to spoon up. These can be mixed with mashed potatoes to make for easier eating.

When a 2-year-old child eats a bowl of thin soup, many trials are made before it is finished. Although it is advisable to serve young children soups occasionally, one must realize that the process of spooning it is tiring. Two things may be done to make soup easier for a child to eat. It may be drunk from a cup, or the soup may be made slightly thicker so that it does not spill from the spoon easily. I suggested a two-way soup to a prominent soup company. The company promoted a canned soup that was to be thinned, preferably with milk, and then strained so that a child could spoon up the solid portion and drink the liquid. Soup for young children should be either spoonable or drinkable. Later, the child may have soup to be eaten with a spoon when he or she is able to manage a spoon without spilling its contents.

Many foods can be prepared so that a child can eat them with the fingers. Hard-cooked eggs may be served in quarters, cooked meat can be cut in small strips, and cooked green beans can be served as finger foods. Children have been observed to like oranges that have been cut in wedges (skin and all) much better than peeled and diced oranges. Young schoolchildren prefer simple pieces of raw vegetables with no salad dressing to mixed-up salads, which are much more difficult to eat. It is best to serve cottage cheese or similar foods separate from the lettuce leaf on a child's plate. Creamed foods served on tough toast are difficult for children to manage.

The size of pieces of food for children must be given serious consideration. Handling silverware and conveying food to the mouth at this early age is a greater task than many adults realize. Pieces of carrots that slide across the plate and are too small to remain on the fork or cubes of beets so large that they must be cut into bite-size pieces exhaust the patience of a 2- or 3-year-old child. Most foods served to young children should be cut into bite-size pieces. When the child is 4 years of age and older, the skills to cut up some foods may have been developed. If, however, much difficulty in managing is noticed, small pieces should usually be served, accompanied by occasional encouragement to cut up some foods. Canned pears and other soft fruits are usually easily cut into bite-size pieces.

Stringy spinach or tomatoes are a trial for anyone to eat. Much can be done with a handy pair of food shears in the kitchen to make these foods easier to eat. Finger foods, such as pieces of lettuce or toast, should be used in meals where some of the foods are difficult to handle.

Small sandwiches—that is, a large one cut into four squares—are popular with young children.

Texture

I have found it wise to serve one soft food (for easy eating), one crisp food (to allow easy chewing and enjoyment of the sounds in the mouth), and one chewy food (to use emerging chewing skills without having too much to chew) in each meal for young children.

Some children can fall into the habit of rejecting all foods of a certain texture; this limits the kinds of foods the child tries to eat. See pp. 156–157 for suggestions on how to handle this problem.

Pieces of meat are hard for young children to eat because the teeth of 2- or 3-year-old children do not grind meat as easily as adult teeth do. This explains why children often prefer hamburgers or frankfurters and why thrice-ground meat is often popular with nursery school children. Most children's meat can be served as ground meat. When parents want steaks, a roast, or a pot roast, the mother can cook a small portion of ground meat from the freezer for the young child. Ground meat should be cooked only long enough for the color to change to brown. It should not be allowed to become dry with a hard crust, which is hard for a child to eat. Some children may prefer moderately rare meat, which is even more moist.

Flavor

In general, young children reject strong flavors. Many children, however, do seem to like pickles, some spicy sauces, and beer, preferences which may seem to contradict this. In general, it has been found that children like food that is mildly salted, with about half as much salt as is used in adult recipes. Because some authorities now believe that all of us would profit by taking less salt, this may be a good health habit to foster (Chapter 11). In general, sharp spices such as pepper and acids such as vinegar should also be used sparingly on children's food.

Strong-flavored vegetables such as cabbage and onions are more popular with young children when served raw. If these vegetables are cooked, it is recommended that they be prepared in excessive amounts of water so that some of the strong flavor can be thrown away. Of course, water-soluble nutrients are lost if the water is discarded, but teaching children to eat these foods is most important at this time in their lives. A mild-flavored cream sauce also helps to make these vegetables more palatable. This was shown in a nursery school when some children asked for very mild-flavored creamed onions after they had eaten dessert.

Because sharply tart fruits are often rejected by young children, such fruits should be diluted with those of mild flavor. Tart oranges were found to be popular when mixed with cooked peaches or bananas. The rule of one tart, one mild, and one crisp is good to follow. The crisp fruit may be small unpeeled pieces of apples.

In general, when helping children develop desirable food patterns, keep the natural flavor of the food so that only small amounts of sugar are needed. The use of a little honey is also recommended because it is sweeter than an equal amount of granulated sugar and less can be used.

Color

Children have a natural interest in color in their foods, and teaching them to appreciate the lovely fresh color of foods is a worthy aim. Young children are delighted when they may choose one of several different colored desserts. Green, orange, yellow, and pink are popular colors in food (Figure 6-1). Children in nursery schools rarely failed to comment on the food to which a tiny sprig of parsley had been added or to notice bits of hidden color such as tomato, carrot, or parsley in sandwiches.

Cakes, cookies, and candies containing molasses, dried fruits, and nuts provide other

Figure 6-1   18-month-old twins enjoy finger-feeding one another.

nutrients in addition to calories. Natural fruit juices have more of the needed nutrients than sweetened, colored, and artificially flavored drinks. Because the water that fruit juices contain is also desirable for children, strong-flavored juices should be diluted, giving additional water to the child.

SPECIFIC FOOD PREPARATION

Children should be considered when the family plans meals. Many parents do, of necessity, vary their life-styles when they are raising their families, so the importance of food-patterning during this period is emphasized. Young children can be taught that just as adults wear different clothes than children, so there are adult-type foods and drinks. Children often prefer an orange or a serving of fruit to the cherry pie that is being served to adults.

Foods can be made soft enough in texture for young children by adding extra milk to a dry, starchy food.

If the parents prefer strong-flavored vegetables, a small portion for the young child can be rinsed under the hot water faucet before it is served.

A young child may prefer food served at room temperature. In fact, preschool children often appear frightened by hot food. They also often stir hard ice cream until it is soupy and less sharply cold.

While the father serves dinner at the table, the mother may prefer to dish the preschool child's food in the kitchen. This can serve two purposes: (1) young children's hunger makes them impatient participants at a meal, so rapid service of food is desirable, and (2) the mother can easily regulate the amount of food served or can make any sudden changes. Fathers sometimes have more difficulty serving small enough portions to a child than mothers do.

Table 6-1 has been devised from my many years of careful observations of how much the average child can eat easily. Some pediatricians who believe that children should not be forced to eat a specific amount of any food object to setting up such expectations in a chart. Yet mothers often need some help in the amount of food the *average* child can eat easily to get the needed nutrients. Such goals may also prevent mothers from expecting their children to eat more than their children want. These average portion sizes may be too large for a new food, for a disliked food, or for a nonhungry child. Of course, the hungry child can have extra servings.

FOOD DISLIKES

It is safe to allow every person to have at least one or two food dislikes. Unless a child is on a medically prescribed diet, no one food has to be eaten assuming that a family can afford a varied diet.

Some food dislikes, as has been previously discussed, have unusual causes. One woman reports that sugared oranges always have a flavor of castor oil to her, though she enjoys oranges without sugar. When she was young she was given doses of the then strong-flavored castor oil with sugared oranges to cover its flavor. Though she knows that she only imagines the castor oil flavor in the oranges, she says that even now she thinks "What has been on my spoon, castor oil?" The association of sugared oranges and castor oil has survived with her over many years.

Substitutions for liquid milk, which children sometimes dislike, can temporarily be made. Powdered milk (4 tbsp substituted for 8 oz of fluid milk) can be added to foods, and cottage or cheddar cheese can be used.

When children are in control of their appetite and hunger, they sometimes refuse all foods. This can be handled by structuring the environment in which they eat. One cold, winter day in a nursery school when we were weary of preparing food for nonhungry children, we decided to give them a shock. On the usual array of dishes, we placed only 1 tbsp

of vegetable meat stew in the soup bowl. No other food was in evidence in the entire dining room, no baskets of sandwiches, no pitchers of milk, no trays of dishes of desserts. When the children took one look, they at once exclaimed "Where's our dinner? Is this all of our dinner?" Rather slowly, second servings were brought in from the kitchen. The food records showed that more food was eaten that day than any day for several weeks before.

Telling a child that we know he or she doesn't like boiled potatoes and can have more green beans often encourages a good appetite. However, when a child rejects many foods, for example, all vegetables or all meat, the parents should try to find out the reasons. Adequate substitutions may need to be made. For instance, in hot summer weather, fruits can replace cooked vegetables in a child's diet if the family budget can tolerate the extra cost. This serving of fruit sometimes stimulates failing appetites.

At times parents may need to seek professional help from someone who understands children both from closer observation of many children eating, as well as from knowing the findings of research in the area. My observation and research have shown me the importance of the following:

1. Belief that changes can occur in a child's eating patterns is of primary importance. Eating is one of the pleasures of life. The individual who likes foods he or she needs to eat for the adequate nutrition of the body is fortunate.
2. The goals set by someone counseling parents about children's eating should be easy to accomplish. Success in following the advice of professional people promotes confidence and positively reinforces the child who succeeds in eating what is presented. When a food dislike is firmly established before the parent seeks help, it will probably not disappear suddenly; only gradual correction can be expected. Progress may not be consis-

tent, and temporary failures to reach the goal must be expected. Often the best methods of correction are progressive. For instance, to help a child learn to eat food with texture, a mother can gradually add coarser textured food to those that are usually eaten.

3. Parents should accept a child's strong dislike for a particular food and should substitute another food that provides the same nutrients. Often a temporary release of pressure concerning eating a specific food causes the child to try it later. A mother who was looking at her 3-year-old son's noon meal food consumption record in a nursery school said "But he never eats eggs at home and this noon he had seconds!" That is exactly the reason why a parent enrolling a child is not asked about the child's food dislikes, only about the foods that make the child ill. Another mother said to her son as she looked at the school records, "But you don't like turnips!" Whereupon her son answered, "Yours are black. They are white at nursery school. I like them white!"

4. Children are good judges of well-prepared food. Sometimes classes in food preparation for parents or prospective parents would be the best approach to handling children's food dislikes.

5. Sometimes the war over children's eating becomes so sharp that withdrawing one of the combatants is the only solution. Someone other than the parent feeding the child temporarily may be a solution to the problem.

6. Because children are usually rhythmic in all they do, the satisfaction of their hunger should also be kept rhythmic. This means that meals served at the same time each day generally promote a good appetite. Fatigue, the most defeating factor in children's appetites, is thus avoided. I have found again and again that starving a child to get the child to eat does not promote good eating.

COMMON PROBLEMS

Healthy, hungry children will eat if they are given a calm atmosphere in which to eat. This is the first and most important consideration.

One of the most common problems, that of fatigue, has just been discussed. Sympathy should be extended to the child who, eating at a tearoom in a large store after a morning's shopping, just looks at the food and cries when urged to eat. The child probably needs to rest more than he or she needs to eat.

When a child is regularly more hungry at a certain time of day than at other times, this should be accepted. Perhaps the greater hunger at the evening meal is caused by having rested while watching a favorite television program before dinner. Sometimes healthy outdoor running, followed by a quiet rest, restores a lagging noontime appetite. It was found that nursery school food costs increased when the children played outdoors in a warm Iowa March after a cold and confining February.

Some of the earliest eating skills learned by a young child are those of chewing and swallowing. Each of these is accomplished to a great extent by trial and error. Some impatient parents worry over this slow progress.

Swallowing seems to be difficult for some children. They tend to swallow only after the food is thoroughly chewed and finely ground. In fact, some children hold food in the cheeks like chipmunks, and some children eat their dessert and still have the vegetable in their cheeks. The fact that some children apparently gain more enjoyment from filling their mouths full of food than from taking small mouthfuls makes learning to chew and swallow a bit complicated for them. These children may almost appear helpless as they sit with packed mouths. Encouraging them to take small bites and to chew and swallow each mouthful has been successful in some cases.

No discussion of children's food problems would be complete without a discussion of the so-called vegetable war. Sometimes this may be created at first by a generally disgruntled parent who really wants to have the child reinforce his or her own belief that all vegetables are horrible. Perhaps a father associates cooked vegetables with his mother with whom there was always a clash. Histories of American colonial times tell of husbands who refused their wives the money to buy seeds for green leafy vegetables because they considered these foods fodder. This was, of course, in the "previtamin days. " This idea of fodder appears too often in the history of food patterns. Yet we also find in these histories stories of gathering wild greens for use during the so-called hunger weeks of spring when the food preserved for winter was either all gone or too spoiled to be used. It is also interesting to observe in tropical countries of Asia and Africa the vast array of what are to us strange-looking green leafy vegables that are bought eagerly from native markets.

The rejection of some kinds of foods can easily be passed down from parents to their children. Sometimes a dislike for the usually popular milk can be directly accounted for in this way. The labeling of salads as "women's food" may also have caused some boys to reject them.

All of these influences, although subtle, are definitely effective in the development of food prejudices. Being branded as someone who does not like carrots often prevents a child who would later like to try them from doing so. When we begin to understand the basis of a food prejudice, we are on the way to counteracting it.

However, many children do like vegetables. Some raw vegetables are preferred, but well-cooked vegetables are accepted also. Of course, I am assuming here that strong acrid odors and unpleasant flavors are not present in these cooked vegetables. When a person, coming in from outdoors and the fresh air, smells unpleasant cooking odors in a poorly ventilated kitchen, a prejudice may precede the actual meal. Sometimes better selection at the market of tender young root vegetables is necessary to prevent the unpleasant "woodiness" in root vegetables.

Another specific food problem concerns the child who is exceptionally fond of sweet foods; often parents who are very fond of such foods have patterned the child to be overfond of them. Sweet foods used as rewards or as special treats also reinforce the child's desire for sweets. The use of cake for a birthday celebration is too well grounded in American tradition to be uprooted, but we should recognize that a wonderful birthday cake reinforces the value of a sweet food. One child asked whether fruit cake (always served in his home at Christmas time) was Christ's birthday cake.

Summary

In no other area are family influences more strong than in food preferences. The association of mother's food and her love last over years and may supersede all outside influences. Studies have shown that of all meal patterns, Sunday dinner meal patterns change most slowly when a family moves to a new country. A father's influence on a child's food preferences was shown in one study in which children were found to dislike the foods that the father disliked. [4] The principle reason was that since mothers did not serve the food fathers disliked, these foods were unfamiliar to the children and they refused them when they were served later.

Modern parents, buffeted by their children's faith in television advertisements for food as well as by the sweets offered in vending machines at school, sometimes lose faith in their role as the "home gatekeeper. " They may need professional bolstering to reinforce their faith in themselves so that they actually do control the food in their homes and in their children's lives.

To assist children to develop desirable food patterns, I recommend the following:

1. All foods should be well prepared and attractive in color, flavor, and texture, so that the child will approach the meal and eat it happily. Children appreciate and enjoy an attractive plate and often comment on foods being "pretty"; they eat with greatest enthusiasm when there is a variety of flavors and textures in the meal.
2. The environment for eating should be suited to the abilities and comfort of the young eater. This includes appropriate tables and chairs as well as suitable dishes and implements.
3. A child should be expected to have a good appetite and to be hungry when in good health physically and emotionally.
4. Appetite will be fostered if the child is hungry and happily excited over the fact that it is mealtime.
5. Pleasant associations with the food are fostered if the meal can be eaten successfully with reasonable effort. Fatigue often defeats children's desire for food. They should come to the meal rested, and the eating process should not be tiring.

SUGGESTED LEARNING ACTIVITIES

1. During observation of a preschool feeding program, identify food preferences of the children.
2. Describe factors in the environment at mealtimes that influence children's food acceptance.
3. Discuss appropriate portions for 2- and 5-year-old children.
4. How can parents facilitate a child's acceptance of new textures?
5. Describe appropriate tables, chairs, and utensils for feeding utensils for young children.

REFERENCES

1. Lowenberg, M. E., Todhunter, E. N., Wilson, E. D., Savage, J. R., and Lubawski, J. L.: Food and people, New York, John Wiley and Sons, 1979.
2. Aldrich, C. A., and Aldrich, M. M.: Feeding our old-fashioned children, New York, 1946, Macmillan, Inc.
3. Carlson, A. J.: The control of hunger in health and disease, Chicago, Ill., 1916, University of Chicago Press.
4. Bryan, M. S., and Lowenberg, M. E.: The father's influence on young children's food preference, J. Am. Diet, Assoc. 34:30, 1958.

7

Factors That Shape Food Patterns in Young Children

Cristine M. Trahms

OBJECTIVES

After studying this chapter, the student should:

1. Be aware of taste preferences of infants and young children.

2. Be aware of adult and peer influences on children's food acceptance.

3. Recognize social and family influences on food patterns of children.

4. Know the effect of television on food preferences and intake of children.

5. Be aware of the role of learning in the development of food preferences, regulation of food intake, and ability to distinguish between food and inedible substances.

Nutrition educators have long been curious about the forces that shape food habits and consequently health status. It has been generally accepted that patterns of food choices are developed early in life and that parents are influential in shaping food-related behaviors. The traditional manner of counseling parents has been to provide nutrition information and hope for a concomitant increase in knowledge and change in attitudes and behaviors related to nutrition and food choices. Guidance on shaping food-related behaviors has been primarily based on observation and common sense principles.

It is very difficult to define terms related to food behavior, such as food choices, food preferences, dawdling, and coaxing, and then to measure the intervening and confounding variables that may affect food behavior. Parents clearly no longer, if they ever did, have the single significant impact on the food choices of their young children.

Currently, the interaction of factors that shape food choices is being evaluated. These factors include nutrition attitudes and knowledge of parents and child-care providers, economic and social status of the family, ordinal position of the preschool child, siblings, peers, and media advertising. It is difficult but necessary to incorporate both an assessment of individual nutritional adequacy and an evaluation of food habits in an effort to assess the effect of food preferences on long-term health status.

In this chapter, some of these factors will be discussed in the light of recent research. This section is an afterword to Dr. Lowenberg's discussion of earlier research and the practical aspects of the development of the food habits of young children.

Factors that have recently been evaluated for the young child are texture, taste, familiarity of food, preferences of the child compared with those of parents and other significant adults, and interaction patterns of parents and children around food. The limitations of these reports are the usual limitations found when dealing with a complex set of interacting factors. However, these reports do point a direction for clinical practice and suggest important considerations in developing multidimensional research models that build a solid base for that practice.

PHYSIOLOGICAL BASIS OF TASTE

Brillat-Savarin noted in his 1825 book *The Physiology of Taste*, "It is no easy matter to determine the precise nature of the organ of taste. It is more complicated than it would appear at first sight."[1] The nature of taste is still largely unknown. It is an essential part of our lives, influencing our food choices and our willingness to consume enough of specific foods to provide adequate nourishment. Some aspects of taste are believed to be innate to the human organism, whereas others are believed to be developed by physical maturation and experience. Recent work with infants and young children has endeavored to measure these almost unmeasurable aspects of taste. Willingness to ingest food is affected by a series of factors that include the sensory attributes of food, as well as immediate hunger, nutri-

tional status, prior experience with the food, and beliefs and feelings about food.

It is believed that preference for sweet tastes is innate to the infant.[2] However, this preference may be modified in early life. Beauchamp and others[3] demonstrated that to maintain the newborn level of preference for sugar water it must be offered to the infant. Without this exposure in the early newborn period, the relative acceptance of this beverage diminishes.

Aversion to bitter tastes appears at an early age, and reactions to salty taste are initially neutral.[2] This indifference for the taste of salt shifts to relative preference for salt at about 4 months of age when the taste interacts with other tastes in foods. Younger children and infants prefer a saltwater solution. However, preschoolers reject this solution, favoring instead relatively high levels of salt in foods that are usually associated with a mildly salty taste. For example, preschoolers prefer a much higher level of salt in soup than do most adults.[4]

DEVELOPMENT OF FOOD PREFERENCES

Innate tastes are only one aspect of food preference. Infants and young children often favor foods because they are offered or because their parents and peers enjoy them. For preschool children, sweetness and familiarity are primary enhancers of choice; familiarity becomes less important with older children.[5] Preference rankings made by preschool children are highly correlated with consumption,[6] and the preferences of children can be strongly influenced by their peers. Fear of a new food can be diminished by increasing exposure to the food.

It would also seem that the food preferences of young children would be significantly influenced by the adults who provide their care and thus their food. Child-parent preference associations would be expected to be strong because of intimate social contact inside the

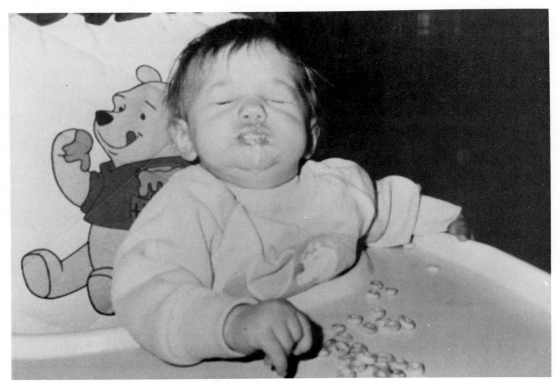

Figure 7-1 Infants recognize sour and bitter tastes and make their dislikes known.

family. However, the evidence is contradictory. One study suggests that both mother and father influence a child's food preferences equally, possibly because of the high priority given to the father's preferences in the family menu.[7] Another study shows that unrelated adults of the same subcultural group, such as day-care teachers, exert an influence equal to that of parents in development of food preferences.[8] In a comprehensive evaluation of family resemblance in food patterns, mother-child choices were similar, whereas father-child choices had no relationship. Parent–older child similarities in food choices were stronger than parent–younger child similarities (Figure 7-2). The food preferences of young children were more similar to those of their siblings than to those of their parents,[9] perhaps because children in a given family generally accept a narrower range of foods than the adults accept.

LEARNED RESPONSES THAT AFFECT FOOD INTAKE

The role of learning in the process of regulation of intake, food preferences, and differentiating food from nonfood substances is important. Young children must learn to differentiate food from nonfood substances. It has been demonstrated that the young child learns by experience to place "foods" into edible foods and inedible categories, such as disgust (feces), danger (poisons), inappropriate (grass, sticks), and unacceptable combinations (catsup on cookies). The youngest

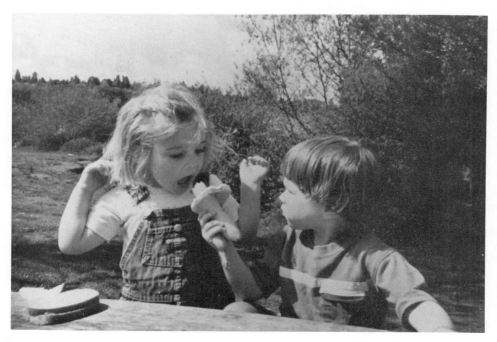

Figure 7-2   Siblings exert an influence on food preferences.

children had a high to moderate level of acceptance of all categories of food and nonfood items offered. Fortunately, the acceptance of dangerous and disgusting substances decreased with age. However, almost all of the children accepted combinations that were unacceptable to adults (e.g., hot dog with chocolate sauce).[10]

Young children must also learn to differentiate hunger from other cues, since the failure to learn to discriminate among various cues can lead to inappropriate eating and perhaps intake regulation disorders. Birch found young children show clearer evidence for caloric compensation than adults. Nearly all of the children studied (95%) ate less at lunch following a high-caloric density preload than a low-caloric density preload. Only 60% of the adults had this same pattern.[11]

A significant learned food behavior is the response to the parent admonition to eat speci-

fic foods "or else!" A preschool child usually knows that foods presented as the means in the contingency are the ones that are usually disliked (e.g., "Eat your spinach before you can have more french fries"). When a food is placed as the means component of a contingency to increase the consumption of a particular food, the consumption of that food increases while the contingency is in effect. However, the consumption of the food is actually reduced after the contingency is removed.[12]

EXTERNAL CONTROLS OF FOOD PREFERENCES

"Attempts to externally control the child's intake reflect an implicit assumption that children are incapable of self-regulation and the attempts at control often have effects counter to those intended."[11] It is feared that external control strategies may lead the young child to see that external cues, such as the amount of food remaining on the plate, rather than the internal cues of hunger and satiety are important to the regulation of food intake.

Satiety is specific to particular foods and influences both the choice of a food and the amount of a food that is eaten; this specificity can lead to a greater intake when a variety of foods is available. Food intake in humans increases as the variety of foods offered at a meal increases.[13]

SOCIAL INFLUENCES ON DEVELOPMENT OF FOOD HABITS

Social influence is one of the most important aspects of food acceptance and rejection. An estimated 50% of all people have conditioned taste aversions. The relationships between food rejections and other personality variables such as anxiety, instability, and poor self-concept have been questioned. Mothers of 2- to 7-year-old children were asked, "Is there anything about your child's current eating behavior that bothers you?" The most frequent response was finicky behaviors; the most common food listed was vegetables. Mothers were also concerned about eating habits, especially dawdling and messiness. Even with cautious interpretation there was a relationship between the feeding problems score and psychological-behavioral problems. For example, greater acting-out, toileting problems, and fearfulness were reported for children who had higher feeding problems scores.[14]

CATEGORIZATION OF FOODS

How children themselves categorize foods is a facet of food choice that has been only recently evaluated. Children aged 5 to 11 years were asked to separate food into groups by whatever criteria they chose to use.[15] The children, regardless of age, used some common characteristics to divide foods into categories, such as sweet versus nonsweet foods, meal entrees versus drinks, and breakfast foods.

None of the children used nutrient terminology to classify foods into groups. (e.g., protein foods), nor was dislike of a particular food used as a basis for classification. The cognitive stage of the children indicated the ability of the child to sort foods into groups and followed guidelines established by Piaget.[16]

The younger children who are classified as preoperational in Piaget's terminology used concrete features to classify foods (e.g., sweet taste or liquid versus solid). They also used the occasion of eating as a basis for classification (e.g., meal entrees versus breakfast foods). As cognitive development increased, so did the basis for food classification. Those children in Piaget's concrete operational category were able to classify foods in more than one category and by more than one characteristic (e.g., both amount of processing and plant or animal origin). All of the children formed a sweets group, 50% a fruits group, 50% a vegetable group, about 50% a drinks group, about 25% a dairy group, and 20% a breads and cereals group.[15] It may be reasonable to use these spontaneous notions about food groups as the basis for nutrition education even when the goal is to foster a more sophisticated understanding of nutrition.

NUTRITION KNOWLEDGE OF CARE-GIVER

Nutrition knowledge of parents and other care-givers would seem to be an important factor to consider in the shaping of the food preferences of children. The degree to which knowledge of nutrition is incorporated into family meal planning appears to be related to positive attitude toward self, problem-solving skills, and family organization, in spite of a professed concern by all mothers interviewed about the total diet offered to young children and importance of mealtime with children.[17] The ordinal position of the preschool child in the family appears to influence choices of specific foods regardless of equivalent knowledge of nutrition between groups of mothers.[18] When preschool children were the youngest children in a family, mothers were found to be less susceptible to children's requests for new products. They were willing, however, to accommodate that preference when the preschool child was the oldest child in a family.

Day-care teachers would, presumably, also have an impact on the development of food preference in young children. In a survey, day-care teachers reported that they knew little about nutrition, but they thought it was important.[19] Since young children are very responsive to early influences, the role of the day-care teacher in shaping positive food-related attitudes needs to be strongly supported by the nutrition community.

INFLUENCE OF FAMILY

In a recent review, Hertzler[20] encouraged the development of a broader conceptual framework for studying children's food behavior and urged that the family unit be included in the research model.

The influence of the family unit on changing food-choice patterns to manage obesity has been reviewed. [21] Families are, as a unit, well-organized and supportive. Families also provide appropriate role models and reinforcements that are most likely to bring about appropriate food habit changes.

The child-parent interactions have an important influence on food consumption. There appeared to be differences between the interactions of thinner children and their mothers and fatter children and their mothers both in food and nonfood situations.[22] The thinner children and their mothers talked more with each other, ate less food and more slowly, and in general had a more positive, supportive relationship than the fatter children and their mothers. This type of study begins to look at the broader construct of family units as related to food and eating and needs to be further researched.

Obviously, children respond to the social environment when they make food choices for themselves. Birth, Zimmerman, and Hind[23] demonstrated that preferences for foods were enhanced when foods were offered as a reward or with brief positive social interactions with adults.

NUTRITION EDUCATION

The overt shaping of food choices and food behaviors by educational strategies happens less specifically than we would like for optimal nourishment. Results suggest that healthy snack choices increased in school in the training setting. However, without a strategy for promoting generalization of healthy snack choices such as cueing, little generalization across settings occurred even at school. Furthermore, generalization to healthy snack choices at home was achieved only when individualized procedures to program it were organized and implemented. Unfortunately, even with cueing the change was not permanent. After withdrawal of the reinforcement procedures, snack choices eventually returned to baseline levels.[24] It is obvious that knowledge of healthy eating alone may not be sufficient to change the children's eating behavior. Parental involvement in the nutrition education programs has been more successful in changing food choices and eating behaviors. Kirks and Hughes[25] have demonstrated that the diets of young children whose parents concomitantly received nutrition education were better than those of children whose parents were not directly involved (Figure 7-3).

INFLUENCE OF MEDIA ON THE FOOD BEHAVIORS OF YOUNG CHILDREN

In addition to the many familial, cultural, and psychosocial influences on children's food habits, mass media have an impact on children's requests for and attitudes toward food. Of the forms of mass media, television has the

Figure **7-3** Food patterns are influenced by nutrition education activities such as making bread.

greatest impact on children because it reaches many children before they are capable of verbal communication.[26] Children spend more time in front of the television set than they do in any activity other than sleeping. Children from low-income families watch more television than do children from moderate- to high-income families. [27] It has been estimated that the preschool child watches television for 26.3 hours per week, and 6- to 16-year-old children watch for 25 hours per week.[28]

The average child watches 3 hours of television advertising per week and 19,000 to 22,000 commercials per year.[29]

Kindergarten children often are unable to separate commercials from the program and frequently explain them as part of the program.[30] Younger school-age children (5 to

10 years of age) watch commercials more closely than do older children (11 to 12 years of age). [31] Older children are conscious of the concept of commercials, the purpose of selling, and the concept of sponsorship and are less likely to accept advertisers' claims without question. They perceive that television commercials are designed to sell products rather than entertain or educate. Children in second grade have been found to have a concrete distrust of commercials based on experiences with advertised products, and children in sixth grade have been found to mistrust all commercials.[30]

It has been pointed out that certain attributes of food are promoted as superior to others. The main characteristics presented positively are "sweetness," "chocolatey," and "richness."[32] Many food manufacturers, in other words, deemphasize the physiological need for nutrients and encourage selection on the basis of sweet flavor. Exposure to such messages may distort a child's natural curiosity toward other characteristics of food, such as the fresh crispness of celery or apples.

There has been ongoing concern about the influence of television on the growth and health of young children. It has been demonstrated that television influences the eating habits and thus the nutritional status of children in three significant ways: (1) television advertising influences family food purchases and the snacking patterns of young children; (2) the use of food as depicted by television programs shows food being used for many activities other than the satisfaction of hunger; (3) the few overweight children used on television programs suggests that inappropriate use of foods has no impact on health or nutritional status.[33] Dietz and Gortmaker outline other aspects of television watching and television advertising that are of concern: (1) the relationship between increased television watching and increased snacking; (2) the consumption of foods advertised on television increases with increased viewing time; (3) increased viewing time is directly associated with the number of attempts by the young child to influence the supermarket purchases of the parent. The foods advertised on weekend children's programming are usually high–caloric density foods, that, if purchased and consumed without an increase in activity, can lead to inappropriate weight gain and poor food habits. The larger intake of highly concentrated sweet and fat foods plus the decrease in activity that is associated with excess television watching has led to an increase of obesity among children in the United States.[34]

Parents must set limits on their children's requests for advertised food and may need support in their efforts to do so. They may need guidance in principles of behavior modification (Chapter 15) and reassurance that it is to the child's advantage to learn that not all advertised products are a part of every child's meal pattern.

Other advertising also influences children's food requests. Box tops and prize offers lead to increased demand for and consumption of certain foods. Door-to-door sales of candy and cookies for charitable causes may adversely influence the distribution of the food dollar and encourage consumption of foods that provide sugar but few nutrients.

Summary

The feeding relationship between the child and the parent or care-giver is an important one. The tempo of parent-child interaction gives the child cues on how much and how fast to eat. The shaping of this tempo and pattern ultimately affects nutritional status and overall well-being. Young children are shaping patterns for a lifetime. They are developing a sense of food as nourishment, as well as an appropriate sense of food's uses in comfort, sociability, and satisfaction.

The child has innate taste. Adults are responsible for enhancing the sense of taste or defeating it by setting the tone of the interaction around food. Clearly adults must be mindful of the nutrient needs of children. Satter[35] states that the parent or care-giver is responsible for what is offered; the child is responsible for how much to eat. Although there are still many unanswered questions about the formation of food preferences, it is clear that preferences are a major determinant of food selection. If allowed free choice, children select sweet foods over nonsweet, more nutritious foods. Giving children free access to highly preferred but nutritionally weak foods encourages the development of nutritional problems during childhood and beyond.

To exert a maximum influence on the health and well-being of young children, nutrition educators must attend to the influences

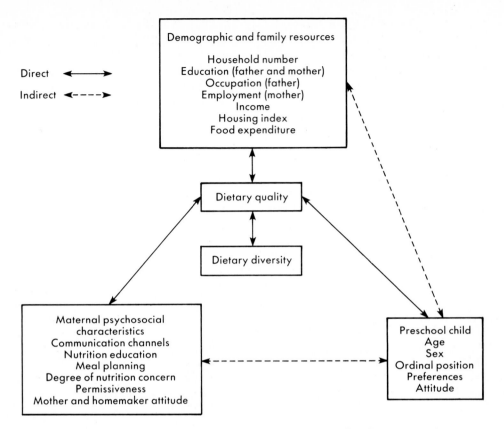

Figure 7-4 Factors related to child's dietary status. (From Caliendo, M.A., and Sanjur, D.: J. Nutr. Ed. 10:69, 1978.)

that shape the food preferences and eating patterns of young children. These influences are dynamic and multidirectional. Figure 7-4 indicates one approach to describing these influences. Young children are shaped by their particular family unit in several ways. Effective nutrition work with young children and their families requires nutrition educators to forge strong ties with the social scientists.

SUGGESTED LEARNING ACTIVITIES

1. Ask a group of 3-year-old children and a group of 4-year-old children to separate a group of edible and nonedible items from two containers. Describe the differences in the age groups.
2. Describe the effectiveness of food contingencies in getting a child to accept a specific food.
3. Plan and implement a nutrition education program for children 5 to 6 years old.
4. Watch children's television for 1 hour and describe the food commercials presented during that hour.
5. If you were asked to provide a diet of 1000 kcal/day for a very overweight 2-year-old

boy (weight: 40 pounds, greater than 95th percentile; NCHS, height: 90th percentile), what factors would you need to consider in relation to the family unit and eating environment?

6. If you were a nutrition consultant to a preschool that provides morning and afternoon snacks for the children and provides milk at lunch although children bring their own lunches
   a. What easy, nourishing snacks that can be linked to activities for the children would you recommend?
   b. What basic concepts do you consider important in developing guidelines or in-service education for parents who prepare their children's lunches?

REFERENCES

1. Brillat-Savarin, A.: The physiology of taste, New Haven, Conn, Leete's Island Books.
2. Lawless, H.: Sensory development in children: research in taste and olfaction, J. Am. Diet. Assoc. 85:577, 1985.
3. Beauchamp, G. K., and Cowart, B. J.: Congenital and experimental factors in the development of human flavor preferences, Appetite 6:357, 1985.
4. Cowart, B. J., and Beauchamp, G. K.: The importance of sensory context in young children's acceptance of salty tastes, Child Dev. 57:1034, 1986.
5. Birch, L. L.: Dimensions of preschool children's food preferences, J. Nutr. Educ. 11:77, 1979.
6. Birch, L. L.: Preschool children's food preferences and consumption patterns, J. Nutr. Educ. 11:189, 1979.
7. Burt, J. V., and Hertzler, A. A.: Parental influence on the child's food preference, J. Nutr. Educ. 10:127, 1978.
8. Birch, L. L.: The relationship between children's food preferences and those of their parents, J. Nutr. Educ. 12:14, 1980.
9. Pliner, P., and Pelchant, M. L.: Similarities in food preferences between children and their siblings and parents, Appetite 7:333, 1986.
10. Rozin, P., and others: The child's conception of food: differentiation of categories of rejected substances in the 16 months to 5 year age range, Appetite 7:141, 1986.
11. Birch, L. L., and Deysher, M.: Conditional and unconditioned caloric compensation: evidence for self-regulation of food intake in young children, Learning and Motivation 16:341, 1985.
12. Birch, L. L., Marlin, D. W., and Rotter, J.: Eating as the 'means' activity in a contingency: effects on young children's food preferences, Child Dev. 55:431, 1984.
13. Rolls, B. J.: Experimental analysis of the effects of variety in a meal on human feeding, Am. J. Clin. Nutr. 42:932, 1985.
14. Pelchant, M. L., and Pliner, P.: Antecedents and correlates of feeding problems in young children, J. Nutr. Educ. 18:23, 1986.
15. Michela, J. L., and Contento, I. R.: Spontaneous classification of foods by elementary school-aged children, Health Educ. Q. 11:57, 1984.
16. Bybee, R. W., and Sund, R. B.: Piaget for educators, 2nd ed., Columbus, Ohio, 1982, Charles E. Merrill Publishing Co.
17. Swanson-Rudd, J., and others: Nutrition orientations of working mothers in the North Central region, J. Nutr. Educ. 14:132, 1982.
18. Phillips, D. E., Bass, M. A., and Yetley, E.: Use of food and nutrition knowledge by mothers of preschool children, J. Nutr. Educ. 10:73, 1978.
19. Gillis, D. E. G., and Sabry, J. H: Daycare teachers: nutrition knowledge, opinions, and use of food. J. Nutr. Educ. 12:200, 1980.
20. Hertzler, A. A.: Children's food patterns—a review. I. Food preferences and feeding problems. II. Family and group behavior, J. Am. Diet Assoc. 83:551, 1983.
21. Hertzler, A. A.: Obesity—impact on the family, J. Am. Diet. Assoc. 79:525, 1981.
22. Birch, L. L., and others: Mother-child interaction patterns and the degree of fatness in children, J. Nutr. Educ. 12:17, 1981.
23. Birch, L. L. Zimmerman, S. I., and Hind, H.: The influence of social-affective context on the formation of children's food preferences, J. Nutr. Educ. 13:115, 1981.
24. Stark, L. J., and others: Using reinforcement and cueing to increase healthy snack food choices in preschoolers, J. Appl. Behav. Anal. 19:367, 1986.
25. Kirks, B. A., and Hughes, C.: Long-term behavioral effects of parent involvement in nutrition education, J. Nutr. Educ. 18:203, 1986.
26. Somers, A. R.: Violence, television, and the health of American youth, N. Engl. J. Med. 294:811, 1976.
27. Reid, L. N., Bearden, W. O., and Teel, J. E.: Family income, TV viewing, and children's cereal ratings, Journalism Q. 57:327, 1980.
28. Television, 1976, North Brook, Ill., 1976, A. C. Nielson Co.

29. Choate, R.: Statement presented before the House Sub-committee on Communications of the Committee on Interstate and Foreign Commerce, U.S. House of Representatives, Washington, D.C., 1975, U.S. Government Printing Office.

30. Blatt, J., Spencer, L., and Ward, S.: A cognitive developmental study of children's reactions to television advertising. In Rubinstein, E. A., Comstock, G. A., and Murray J. P., editors: Television and social behavior, vol. 4, Television in day to day life: patterns of use, Washington, D.C., 1972, U.S. Government Printing Office.

31. Ward, S., Levinson, D., and Wackman, D.: Children's attention to television commercials. In Rubinstein, E. A., Comstock, G. A., and Murray, J. P., editors: Television and social behavior, vol. 4, Television in day to day life: patterns of use, Washington, D.C., 1972, U.S. Government Printing Office.

32. Gussow, J.: Counternutritional messages of TV ads aimed at children. J. Nutr. Educ. 4:48, 1972.

33. Palumbo, F. M., and Dietz, W. H.: Children's television: its effect on nutrition and cognitive development, Pediatr. Ann. 14:793, 1985.

34. Dietz, W. H., and Gortmaker, S. L.: Do we fatten our children at the television set? Obesity and television viewing in children and adolescents, Pediatrics 75:807, 1985.

35. Satter, E. M.: The feeding relationship, J. Am. Diet. Assoc. 86:352, 1986.

8

Nutrition and the Adolescent

Betty Lucas
Jane Mitchell Rees
L. Kathleen Mahan

OBJECTIVES

After studying this chapter the student should:

1. Recognize the variability in total nutrient needs among teenagers.

2. Be aware of the need to use maturational stages rather than age as a basis for evaluating nutrient and energy needs.

3. Be aware of psychological and environmental influences that affect food intake.

4. Be aware of concerns of nutrient intake during adolescence.

5. Be aware of nutritional problems often identified during adolescence.

The adolescent period is a unique stage in the process of growth and development. A rapidly changing time of growing up, it is characterized by a wide variability in norms of growth, increasingly independent behavior, and the testing of adult roles. Adolescence lasts nearly a decade and has no specific beginning or end. This critical period of human development occurs at the physiological, psychological, and social levels. Changes do not occur simultaneously but at varying rates. Thus a teenager may be at several age levels at the same time: chronological, physical, psychological, and social. Although adolescence may be defined as the teenage years between 12 and 20, physical maturation and changes in nutrient requirements actually begin at younger ages and extend into the third decade.

Teenagers assume greater responsibility for decision making in their lives than do younger children. Peer and social pressures require them to choose between drinking or not drinking, smoking or not smoking. Adolescents often determine their own food intake. Because their food choices are a reflection of many factors, including family eating patterns, peer and media influences, appetite, and food availability, the nutritional quality of adolescents' diets is often determined by social and psychological influences.

This chapter focuses on the growth and maturation of the adolescent, nutrient needs, factors that influence food intake, and the usual nutritional concerns of this population.

PHYSICAL GROWTH AND PUBERTY

The velocity of physical growth in adolescence is second only to the rate of growth during infancy. Approximately 20% of adult height and 50% of adult weight is gained during this period. Therefore there is a high demand for energy and nutrients to support optimal growth. After the relatively latent growth period of childhood, adolescent growth is characterized by an increase in cell number, cell size, and reproductive maturity. Completion of adolsecent physical growth is usually signaled by slowing of growth, completion of sexual maturation, and closure of the epiphyses of long bones. This is a general guide, however, and does not apply to other parameters of growth, such as psychological and social development.

Up to approximately 9 years of age, males and females grow in height and weight at the same rate, with males being slightly larger and heavier. The prepubescent growth period begins about 2 years earlier in females than in males. At this time females temporarily are taller and have a larger limb muscle mass than do males. As pubertal growth proceeds, the male develops more muscle and the skeleton enlarges, particularly in the shoulder region. In the female there is a smaller increase in muscle, but a larger increase in fat. At the beginning of the prepubertal period, many children normally store excess fat. If a child has not been fat during earlier years, however, this fat will probably diminish gradually in 1 to 2 years.

The most rapid phase of adolsecent growth is known as the growth spurt, and its highest point is called the peak. Growth velocity decelerates from birth until the pubertal growth spurt, at which time the increased growth velocity of a 14-year-old boy is comparable to that of a 2-year-old child. The average peak velocities of height and weight are shown in Table 8-1. Although the peak velocity age occurs later in males, it is more intense and results in more tissue accumulation. Findings from the National Health Examination Survey (NHES) suggest that American adolescents attain their peak height velocity earlier than do British adolescents: three quarters of a year earlier for boys and one quarter of a year earlier for girls.[1] The NHES data, however, are based on a cross-sectional study and cannot be interpreted as longitudinal data.

In females, the height spurt signals the beginning of puberty, with pubic hair and breast development being the first notable changes. Menarche occurs at the end of the growth spurt, approximately 9 to 12 months after peak height velocity is attained. The average age for menarche in the United States is about 12.8 years, although the normal range is from 10 to 16 years of age.[2] The earlier the onset of menarche, the greater the peak velocity of growth and the less time that elapses between peak velocity and menarche. Early-

Table 8-1 Average peak velocities of height and weight

	Height	Weight
Males		
Peak velocity	10.3 cm/year	9.8 kg/year
Peak velocity age	14.1 years	14.3 years
Females		
Peak velocity	9.0 cm/year	8.8 kg/year
Peak velocity age	12.1 years	12.9 years

Adapted from Tanner, J.M., Whitehouse, R.H., and Takaishi, M.: Arch. Dis. Child. 41: 454, 1966.

maturing females do not necessarily become taller, but they do complete their growth spurts more quickly and at younger ages. These females have more subcutaneous fat, even from childhood years, and a greater predisposition to obesity.

Frisch[3] has proposed the theory that a critical body weight or fat composition is necessary to achieve menarche. A minimal level of fatness needed for the onset of menstrual cycles is apparently 17% of body weight as fat, and about 22% of body weight as fat is minimal to maintain regular ovulatory cycles. This theory has been supported by epidemiological data as well as by observations of females with anorexia nervosa, ballet dancers, and well-trained athletes with minimal fat stores who develop amenorrhea or delayed menarche.[4] Others, however, have shown that this hypothesis is limited in its applicaton to all adolescent females. Other factors determining onset or delay of menarche include skeletal development, strenuous physical activity, and stress.[5]

In males, secondary sexual changes (pubic hair, voice changes, and penis and testicular growth) indicate the beginning of the growth period. The height spurt occurs toward the end of the growth period. Males actually lose limb fat at the the peak height velocity, probably because of testosterone action, whereas females maintain a positive balance of fat without loss of limb fat. The state of puberty is usually determined by using the Sexual Maturity Ratings.[6] (See Chapter 1.)

Even though it is commonly assumed that full stature is attained by 18 to 20 years of age, growth in length can continue for another decade. This growth is small (1 to 3 cm) and is believed to be primarily vertebral. In relation to skeletal growth, it must be remembered that stature is not an indicative measure of skeletal mass. At 10 years of age approximately 80% of maximum stature has been attained, but only 50% of adult skeletal mass has been gained. Skeletal mass can increase into the fourth decade, about 4% for males and 6% for females after 18 years of age.[7] The continued increase in both skeletal length and mass indicates the need for ongoing calcium retention for a longer period than has been commonly accepted.

Sex differences in body composition begin in infancy but are most dramatic by adolescence. Percent of lean body mass rises in adolescents, especially in males, who finish growth with 1.5 times the lean body mass of females. Fat content is higher in the female after approximately the twelfth year, and by the end of the second decade it is 1.5 to 2 times the male value. Correspondingly, the female has a lower percentage of body water than does the male. Because of these significant sex differences in the body composition of the adolescent, total body weight alone is not a valid measure with which to assess growth or to predict nutrient requirements.

Over the last century or more, growth records throughout the world have indicated secular trends in growth. These reports show that children are growing taller and weighing more with each generation. In addition, there has also been evidence for earlier sexual maturation, but this has stabilized in recent decades.[8] This early maturation is primarily responsible for children being taller and weighing more at one particular age. There is a shorter growth period and earlier cessation of growth. For example, a 10-year-old boy in 1875 might have been only 50% of the way through his growth period, whereas a 10-year-old boy today might be 60% to 65% mature. The eventual adult size has not, however, increased as dramatically as the growth rate. Greulich[9] has compared growth parameters of American-born Japanese children in 1956 with data 15 years later and found little difference in heights and weights. This and other evidence suggests that growth trends have reached a plateau in developed countries in the past 30 to 40 years.

These factors of puberty—rapid physical growth, sexual maturation, and changes in appearance and body shape—have a significant impact on the adolescent's self-esteem, body image, and personality. Because of the wide variability of rates of growth and their timing, there are no norms for adolescent growth in conjunction with chronological age. Tanner refers to this varying rate of maturation as the adolescent's growth "tempo."[10] Our culture does dictate some standards, variable though they may be, and adolescents continually compare themselves to these standards or to their peers. No other age group is as concerned and sensitive about their bodies or as devastated by criticism and comparison as are adolescents. This is particularly true of the obese adolescent and the early or late maturer. It is not unusual to find these adolescents with distorted body images making inappropriate food choices and thus compromising optimal growth.

ENERGY AND NUTRIENT REQUIREMENTS

Since no period of growth is less predictable than adolescence, nutrient allowances are only estimates and should not be applied to individuals. Indeed, most of the allowances have been extrapolated from data on young children and adults. Basically, the highest nutrient and energy demands occur at the peak velocity of growth, thus paralleling the growth rate. Requirements, then, should be determined by sex, age, stage of puberty, and current growth parameters.

Energy

The 1980 recommended dietary allowances use the age groups of 11 to 14 years of age and 15 to 18 years of age, but include a range of kilocalories for each group and sex. Thus, the range of energy intake for 11- to 14-year-old females is 1500 to 3000 kcal; for 15-to 18-year old males, it is 2100 to 3900 kcal;[11] These allowances represent an increase of 85% to 150% from minimum to maximum kilocalories, a wide range. These allowances have limited use for an individual, since they do not take rate of growth into consideration.

Heald, Remmell, and Mayer[12] compiled, from previous studies, energy intake data on 2750 females and 2200 males between 7 and 20 years of age. For males, average energy intakes increased steadily to 16 years of age, when the intake reached 3470 kcal, paralleling accelerated growth. From 16 to 19 years of age, energy intake decreased by approximately 500 kcal. In females the rise in energy intake increased to 12 years of age, when total kcal reached 2550, followed by a gradual decline to 18 years of age, when intakes averaged 2200 kcal. Although decelerated growth rate was probably the major factor in decreased energy consumption, physical activity, which was not differentiated, may have been a factor.

In a longitudinal study conducted by Hampton and others,[13] there was great variation in energy intakes from day to day for each individual, but more consistent intakes from week to week. According to body fat class, the lean females and average males consumed more kilocalories than did the other groups.

Age or weight alone is not a useful predictor of energy needs. Using a single measure, height in adolescents best expresses energy requirements because it usually correlates well with physiological development. Data from the longitudinal Child Research Council study give estimated intake percentiles of 7 to 19 kcal/cm for females and 11 to 23 kcal/cm for males, all healthy, growing adolescents 11 to 17 years of age.[14] Calculation of energy per median height from the RDAs shows similar variance. An intake of 23.6 kcal/cm is estimated for an 11- to 14-year-old male consuming the maximum 3700 kcal; an intake of 7.4 kcal/cm is estimated for a 15- to 18-year-old female consuming the minimum 1200 kcal.[11]

Physical activity and other life-style habits are also key factors in considering energy needs. Adolescents may have widely varying and erratic caloric intakes and still continue to show optimal growth. It is possible that an internal mechanism exists for conserving energy in times of low intake or for eliminating excess energy.

Protein

Reports indicate that protein in the adolescent diet ranges from 12% to 16% of total energy intake.[12,13] Males consistently consume more total protein than do females. As with energy, total protein intake increases steadily in males up to approximately 16 years of age, whereas females have their highest intakes at 12 years of age.

Balance studies have found that a positive nitrogen balance was sustained only when the energy requirement was satisfied and when 15% of total kilocalories was derived from protein.[15] In the 1980 recommended dietary allowances, protein represents only 6.7% to 8.8% of kilocalories during adolescence.[11] Eating practices and food patterns of teenagers, however, usually result in higher protein consumption.

An important consideration is that a restricted energy intake during the rapid period of growth compromises lean body mass accumulation and nitrogen retention despite a seemingly adequate protein intake. Without enough kilocalories, protein is used for energy instead of growth needs. This can occur in adolescents dieting to lose weight or athletes attempting to make a specific weight class.

In the United States, since reported intakes of protein usually exceed the recommended dietary allowances, some individuals question whether persons living in the United States receive too much protein. Hegsted[16] has proposed that there is no strong evidence to support a substantial increase in protein requirements for adolescents. Similarly, the FAO/WHO Expert Committee[17] recommends progressively decreasing levels of safe pro-

tein intakes from childhood to adulthood. The actual amount of protein intake will increase with growth, but the amount per kilogram decreases with age. However, some adolescents (e.g., those adhering to extreme reducing diets, those from lower socioeconomic classes, and those eliminating all animal products from their diets) are at risk of suboptimal intakes of protein.

Minerals

Calcium

In the adolescent, calcium needs depend on growth velocity, bone structure and size, and absorption rate. Individual growth variability also influences calcium requirements; the unusually tall adolescent and the early maturer or late maturer vary considerably in their needs. Because calcium is absorbed more efficiently at lower levels of intake than at higher levels of intake, numerical recommendations have limited use. The amount of calcium needed to maintain a positive balance during growth is thought to be affected by previous intake, explaining the absence of problems in areas of the world where the daily intake is a minimal 200 to 300 mg of calcium.

In relating calcium requirements to skeletal weight, the largest gains occur in females between 10 and 14 years of age and in males between 12 and 16 years of age. Calcium retained as bone is approximately 100 mg/day in preschool years; however, this doubles for adolescent females and triples for adolescent males during peak periods of retention.[8] For example, a 14-year-old male may require 600 to 1200 mg of calcium/day, depending on absorption rates of 50% or 25%.

Recommended allowances are usually designed to meet the needs of the adolescent who is growing at the fastest rate, and levels less than that may be quite adequate for some adolescents. A recent preliminary study, however, found that a mean calcium intake of 1500 mg/day was needed for maximal calcium retention in 14-year-old girls.[18] This data indicates that a calcium intake higher than usually reported may be needed at periods of rapid growth to reach peak bone mass and to protect against osteoporosis in later years.

Those adolescents who are at risk of limited calcium for growth are probably males with unusually rapid rates of bone growth, late-maturing females who are concerned with caloric restriction, and adolescents eliminating milk products from their diets. A low calcium/phosphorus ratio as a result of excess dietary phosphorus or a reduced calcium intake may also compromise optimal calcium status, but this is still a controversial issue. The intake of phosphorus-containing additives used in food processing may add 500 to 1000 mg of phosphorus/day above that found naturally in food. Many of the foods that contain this added phosphorus, such as carbonated beverages, are popular with teenagers.

Iron

Iron is significant because it is frequently marginally adequate or deficient in adolescents. Although females are assumed to be most at risk, data from the HANES survey showed that the greatest prevalence of low hemoglobin and hematocrit levels was among boys.[19] In a review of 12 studies with approximately 1300 females and 1000 males, the average iron intakes were 9.6 to 13.5 mg/day for females and 14.0 to 18.7 mg/day for males.[20]

The higher requirement for iron in adolescence is directly related to rapid growth, which is accompanied by increases in blood volume, muscle mass and respiratory enzymes. For females, menstrual iron losses after menarche also increase the need for this mineral, but these losses vary widely in adolescents, and are likely correlated with iron absorption. Because of their increased need but often limited intake of iron, adolescents are particularly susceptible to iron deficiency anemia.

There is little sex difference in iron requirements of children until females begin puberty, at which time their requirements are higher. By 15 years of age requirements for both males and females rise sharply. For females this increase is directly related to menstrual losses. In the males the increase in tissue mass plus the rise in hemoglobin levels, which is probably caused by androgen activity, result in higher requirements.

As with other requirements, chronological age is a poor predictor of iron needs. Daniel[21] has shown that differences in hematocrit values of males are more significant when correlated with sex maturity rating than when correlated with age. The same investigator demonstrated that iron intake increases consistently in both males and females as they progress in maturity stages. He found that intake was greater for males than for females at each maturity rating and that white adolescents had slightly greater intakes than did black adolescents. Following the same trend, iron stores, as measured by transferrin saturation, were consistently higher in males than in females but did not correlate with dietary intake of iron.[22]

Zinc

This mineral is an essential component in dozens of enzymes systems, including those that contribute to protein synthesis and bone mineralization. Zinc deficiency results in growth retardation, decreased taste acuity, sexual immaturity, anorexia, and impaired wound healing. Severe zinc deficiency was first described in Middle Eastern adolescent males who exhibited dwarfism and hypogonadism.[23] Their diets were high in *phytate* and fiber, which interfere with zinc absorption. Following treatment with zinc and an improved diet, these males showed increased growth and sexual maturation.

In both sexes there is an increase in zinc retention that parallels the increase in lean body mass. Increasing evidence suggests that this population is one of the groups most at risk for marginal intakes, and that poor zinc status may compromise growth potential.[24, 25]

Vitamins

Little satisfactory data are available to establish vitamin requirements for the adolescent, and most recommended amounts are extrapolated from other age groups. Many of the vitamin allowances are the same as those in adulthood because of the higher growth demand. Although most needs are met by usual foods, mild vitamin deficiences are not uncommon in this age group, resulting both from a poorly chosen diet and from the increased metabolic requirements during the growth spurt. Vitamins most commonly reported at low or marginal intakes include vitamin A, folic acid, and vitamin B_6.[26,27] In addition to identifying food sources of vitamins, the dietary assessment should also consider any supplements taken by the adolescent, especially large doses of the fat soluble vitamins A and D.

As with other nutrients, vitamin requirements are best correlated not with age but with growth demands. Using folate as an example, Daniel, Gaines, and Bennett[28] have shown that sexual maturity is a more significant factor than age in dietary intakes of folate. They found that males had higher intakes of folate than did females and that these values increased with maturity levels for both sexes. Plasma folate concentrations were, inversely, higher for females than for males, decreasing with maturity in both sexes. This paradox may represent the greater needs for folate during rapid cell growth, especially in males who may double their muscle mass during adolescence.

In summary, the energy and nutrient requirements of adolescents are directly related to the rate and stage of growth, the highest demand being at the peak velocity of growth.

Care should be taken in interpreting common recommendations based on age groups and in comparing individuals to those standards.

FACTORS INFLUENCING FOOD INTAKE

The adolescent is not only maturing physically but is also progressing in social and pyschological parameters. He or she is striving to achieve the developmental tasks between childhood and adulthood. The changes and experiences each encounters affect his or her living pattern and, ultimately, his or her food intake and nutritional status.

Newly acquired independence and decision making result in adolescents spending more time outside the home, thus making independent food choices. It is not unusual for these choices to be made on the basis of sociability, enjoyment, and status, rather than on nutrient content. Activities of school, sports, part-time jobs, interest groups, and peer activities may result in the adolescent being away from home from early morning until after the evening meal. Adolescent life-styles and independence often result in irregular eating patterns, such as skipped meals and increased frequency of snacks.

Body Image

Because of the multiple changes that are occuring simultaneously during this period of growth, adolescents are usually anxious and dissatisfied with their body images. This bodily overconcern is a normal preoccupation; that it may be distorted and unrealistic does not make it any less important to the adolescent. One study demonstrated this paradox well. It revealed that 70% of the females studied wanted to lose weight but that no more than approximately 15% were actually obese. On the other hand, 59% of the males wanted to gain weight, although only 25% were lower than average in fatness.[29]

Studies also indicate that adolescents are dissatisfied with their body dimensions. For males there is the desire for larger biceps, shoulders, chest, and forearms. Females, conversely, desire smaller hips, thighs, and waists.[29,30] Numerous clinical experiences with adolescents further document this phenomenon.

The body image is further influenced by advertising and mass media, which dictate the "in" look, clothing styles, and other elements of being accepted. In attempting to conform to cultural ideals, adolescents may compromise their own well-being, including optimal nutrient intake.

Perhaps the strongest influences on the adolescent are peer pressure and the desire to fit in. These influences may come from the immediate peer group or may include respected adults and national idols. This desire to be accepted may be manifested in such dietary practices as embarking on a weight-reducing scheme, espousing vegetarianism, indulging in alcohol, or altering diet to complement a muscle-building program. Any harmful results depend on the practice and how it is carried out, but the initial decision to change is often the result of others' influence rather than health reasons.

Family

As adolescents move toward independence and autonomy, family influence on eating habits diminishes. The parental influence shifts from instructing to advising; the teen can take it or leave it. Because of cognitive development, which allows teenagers to think in abstract terms and question parental rules, they question inconsistencies between what parents recommend and what they actually do, including eating habits. This can be very irritating to parents as their teens refuse to accept their word as given.

In a survey of adolescents, 77% believed that eating at least one meal a day with family members was important; however, 90%

stated that their parents put more importance on the family meal than they did. Of the 23% who rated it as unimportant, the main reasons given were lack of time, indifference, and family conflict.[31]

Most teens and their families enjoy positive family relationships and are satisfied with how they get along. However, for those who are not satisfied, poor family relationships can affect eating habits. One study found that adolescent girls who scored high on family relations had better diets, whereas those whose families were critical of their eating habits skipped more meals.[32] Adolescents whose parents are authoritarian and rigid often use food as a vehicle to express rebellion against parental authority. This can lead to erratic and bizarre food practices such as binges, strong food aversions, food refusals, bizarre diets, fasting regimens, and missed meals. The same behavior can also be exhibited by teens with very permissive parents who are attempting to force their parents to set some limits on the teens' behaviors. Teens who eat with their families on a regular basis usually eat better and have more adequate diets.[33]

Peers

During adolescence the influence of peers becomes stronger as that of the family weakens. A study of 766 young adolescents showed that the youths spent more than twice as much time with peers than with parents during a weekend.[34] Adolescents with poor parental relationships are more susceptible to peer group control and influence over their behavior. The peer group becomes a source of self-esteem and behavioral standards, and appears to be even more important the greater the antagonism toward and emotional distance from parents. The peer group defines what is socially acceptable in terms of learning, dress, entertainment idols, language, and food and drink choices. Implied meanings of foods can be determined by the peer group.

Eating is an important form of recreation and socialization with friends; foods eaten usually need to meet the approval of the peer group. This can be a problem for teens with chronic illnesses that require diet modification, and they may face considerable social pressures and risk alienation and isolation by following the diet. In general, the peer group usually has a negative influence on the eating habits of adolescents and it seems that adolescents whose diets are poorest are those who eat alone or with their friends most of the time.

Media

Media consist of radio, films, television, magazines, newspapers, and books. The influence of media comes not only from its content but also from the advertising messages that usually accompany it.

From an economic standpoint adolescents are a unique and coveted market. Because they usually have an allowance or are earning money and yet do not have to pay for fixed expenses such as housing, food, or health care, they usually have more discretionary money to spend than their parents. Advertisers take advantage of the adolescent's need for self-esteem, desire to be attractive and popular, need to be accepted, and admiration of heroes and idols to sell their products. For example, television advertising aimed at youth depicts a life of fun, popularity, and success as associated with a particular soft drink.

It is estimated that children between 6 and 16 years of age watch about $24\frac{1}{2}$ hours of television per week—an average of $3\frac{1}{2}$ hours per day. This time decreases to about $2\frac{1}{2}$ hours per day or $17\frac{1}{2}$ hours per week for 17- to 18-year old persons.[34,35] During this time they are exposed not only to the commercial advertising that accompanies the programming but also the nutritional messages from the programs themselves. In addition to observational learning during program watching, adolescents may attempt to emulate the behavior of their favorite stars and pick up cues regarding foods and eating.

Kaufman[36] analyzed the food-related messages in ten popular prime-time television programs. She found that 65% of the references to food in programs were to beverages and to sweets. Results showed that television program characters frequently snacked on foods of low-nutrient density, rarely ate a balanced meal, ate on-the-run, and used food primarily for the satisfaction of social and emotional needs.

Way[37] did a similar analysis of 101 hours of prime-time television programming. She found that there was an average of 7.67 food-related behaviors per hour of programming. Program characters (only the main characters were recorded) ate away from home about twice as often as at home. Overall, the number of food-related behaviors that involved more nutritious foods was almost equal to those involving less nutritious foods; however, the foods actually eaten by television characters were more often less nutritious, but the foods purchased, requested, prepared, or served were most often more nutritious. Comedies more often showed behaviors involving less nutritious foods than did dramas.

Magazine reading increases during adolescence and the popular magazines become a source of information on food and nutrition. Among consumers in general, magazines are a main source of nutritional information, but the information is not always reliable. However, a review of popular magazine articles discussing weight control showed that in general the articles were fairly accurate, optimistic, supportive, and sympathetic. They conveyed the message that weight control is an individual responsibility that requires continual effort and that the outcome will most likely be positive.[38] This is a good message for adolescents to read in contrast to much of the advertising in these same magazines, which promotes rapid weight loss by questionable means. In summary, there is a wide range in the quality of nutrition information in popular magazines that adolescents read, and the nutrition professional should try to educate the adolescent in basic methods for evaluating the reliability of articles.

Fast Foods

The presence of fast food in fast-food restaurants, convenience stores and vending machines has increased tremendously within the past decade. This rapidly growing industry is having a large impact on the American diet and on eating patterns, including those of adolescents.

Story[33] describes fast-food restaurants as having a great appeal for adolescents for several reasons. Fast-food restaurants are a prime employer of adolescents and provide a socially acceptable and casual place to "hang out" with friends. The food is inexpensive and convenient, and the service is fast. Ordering requires a minimum of decision making, and the food offered is the kind adolescents like, is in a standard and familiar form, and can be eaten without utensils or plates. In short, fast foods fit the adolescent's life-style.

In general fast foods tend to be calorically dense; high in fat (many selections have more than 50% of calories as fat), sugar, and sodium; and low in fiber, vitamin A, ascorbic acid, calcium, and folate. Therefore, if they form the mainstay of an adolescent's diet, they could have a negative impact on the diet's nutritional value. Whether they do or do not depends on the frequency with which they are consumed and the nutritional value of the fast-food selections. For example, if the adolescent chooses servings from the salad bars, which are increasing in popularity, the nutrient contributons of a fast-food meal will most likely improve. If the limitations and potential problems of excessive fast-food intake are explained to teens, they can then make more appropriate selections from fast foods that will build to an overall nutritionally sound diet.

REPORTED INTAKES AND EATING PATTERNS

Intakes of adolescents tend to be more variable than those of younger children or adults for the various reasons mentioned previously. Over the years studies have indicated that adolescent diets are lowest or deficient in calcium, iron, ascorbic acid, folic acid, vitamin B_6, and vitamin A.[26,27] Because females often reduce their energy intakes, they are most at risk for suboptimal intakes.[39] On the other hand, it is not uncommon for the same proportion of adolescents, primarily males, to exceed the recommended allowances for these same nutrients.

Meal Skipping and Snacking

Teenagers generally have the reputation of being meal skippers, and this is documented by reports as well as by numerous clinical interviews. Breakfast and lunch are the meals usually missed.[33,40] According to the 1977-1978 Nationwide Food Consumption Survey (NFCS), 19% of teenage girls and 11% of teenage boys (12 to 18 years of age) missed breakfast.[41] On the other hand, teenagers tend to eat often, and snacking is characteristic of the adolescent life-style. However, even though adolescents in general eat more frequently than adults, this snacking behavior is not so different from that of adults. From the NFCS is was found that 56% of teenagers (12 to 18 years of age) ate four or more times in the day as compared with 46% of the adults (19+ years of age).[41]

The NFCS also reported on the snacking patterns of 1424 adolescents. Almost half of the snacking occurred in the evening with less in the afternoon and the smallest proportion in the morning. The peak periods for snacks were from 8 PM to 10 PM (27% of snacking occasions) and 2 PM to 4 PM (20% of snacking occasions.)[42] Generally, adolescents eating less than three times a day have poorer diets than those eating more frequently.[13]

The snacking habits of teenagers have long been maligned, with parents and professionals alike being concerned about the 'empty calorie' foods being consumed. Various studies, however, have shown that this between-meal eating contributes significantly to the total nutrient intake.[13,43,44] The most limiting nutrients provided by snacks are vitamin A, calcium, and iron; low intakes of these nutrients also occur in the overall adolescent diet. Thus, although the nutrient density of snacks is less than that of meals, snacks can make a significant contribution to meeting total daily nutritional needs. Observation, on the other hand, shows that some teenagers consume large amounts of energy-laden, low-nutrient snack foods. The most frequently reported snack item for teenagers in the NFCS was soft drinks.[42] Given the choices available from vending machines, school stores, and neighborhood grocers, it is not unusual for the adolescent to end up with a snack that is high in kilocalories, sucrose, fat, and salt but that provides minimal nutrients. This combination of frequent snacks and sucrose consumption is significant in the high incidence of dental caries in adolescence.

Irregular eating patterns, common during adolescence, are especially prevalent in middle and late adolescence. This pattern reflects an increasing need for independence and time away from home. Although there are exceptions, adolescents who eat regular meals and snacks tend to have better nutrient intakes than do irregular eaters. Rather than stressing regular meals and elimination of snacks, teens and their families should be directed into choosing nutritious snacks and having quality foods convenient and available for snacks and quick meals.

Nontraditional Eating Patterns

Adolescents are going through a period of development in which they are forming values and testing their newly acquired independence, which may be manifested in unusual eating patterns for a variety of reasons. The obese teenager may try the latest reducing diet with hopes of a quick cure, and the young athlete may ingest protein supplements and vitamins in the hopes of improving his or her performance. Both individuals are subject to nutrition misinformation, which may be harmless or which may compromise growth.

Some young people may adopt nontraditional eating patterns such as vegetarianism or eating only organically grown foods. Motivation for these dietary changes may include asserting independence, a particular philosophy or religion, an ecological or environmental concern, rebellion against parents, pressures to conform or fit a cultural ideal, or a genuine interest in health. Any detrimental effects of these dietary practices on the optimal nutritional status of adolescents will depend on the particular diet, the volume and variety of foods it includes, and the length of time it is practiced. Specific nutrients likely to be at risk in vegetarian and other nonmeat diets are discussed in Chapter 9.

Fad diets for weight reduction are often tried by adolescents and can be detrimental to their nutritonal intake and health. These diets or diet products are attractive to teens if they are dissatisfied with their bodies and yearn for miraculous transformations. Adolescents' vulnerability and anxiety about their physical appearance make them easy prey for promoters of special diets and diet supplements.

NUTRITIONAL ASSESSMENT

The assessment of an individual's nutritional status includes anthropometric, biochemical, clinical, dietary, and environmental data. These aspects are covered in detail in Chapter 2. Some special considerations, however, apply to assessing adolescents.

Height and weight measurements for all children are plotted on the NCHS growth grids, and over time a growth pattern is discerned. This information shows whether teens are staying "in channel" or whether the rate of growth is decreasing or increasing.

The common practice of using the percentile designations to determine an ideal, or desired, weight is inappropriate. For instance, if a 15-year-old female who is at the 90th percentile for height is also at the 90th percentile for weight, she is overweight. The growth curves reflect the demographic distribution of adolescents in this country, with upper percentile weights skewed up. To appropriately determine a weight-for-height relationship in adolescents, the original NCHS data from which the growth grids were derived must be used.[1] For each sex and age (from 12 to 17 years), a range of weights (5th to 95th percentile) is given for each 2 cm increment of height. Generally, a range of weight for height between the 25th and 75th percentile is considered normal.[26]

Other anthropometry includes upper arm circumference and triceps fatfold, which can be used to estimate arm muscle area and arm fat area. These indirect measures of body composition are important in establishing a nutrition plan or to reassure adolescents and their parents. Also, determining the stage of sexual maturity is necessary for a comprehensive assessment, to estimate energy and nutrient needs, and to develop appropriate nutrition plans.

Interviews to obtain dietary and nutritional environment data must encompass the breadth of the teenager's life-style, including family, school, peers, cultural influences, personal interests, and economic factors. Finally, some assessment of the adolescent's feelings about his or her nutritional concern and his or her attitude toward food and nutrition helps the nutritionist in developing counseling strategies.

NUTRITIONAL CONCERNS

Eating Disorders

Eating disorders account for a large number of nutritional concerns during adolescence. The physical symptoms of teenagers with the disorders range on a spectrum from the skeleton-like thinness of the terminally starving person with anorexia nervosa to the hugely overfat condition of the morbidly obese person (100% above ideal body weight), as shown in Fig. 8-1. Although it is easy to focus on the outward appearance of these conditions, the underlying psychological characteristics must also be studied to fully understand the development and treatment of eating disorders. Understanding the relationship between human development and eating habits is necessary in this regard.

From infancy, interaction, first with the parents, and then with an expanding environment, influences the child's development according to the particular characteristics of the individual. In families in which interactions are disturbed, eating habits are among the patterned behaviors that are vulnerable to maladjustment.[45] If the needs of the child are misinterpreted throughout childhood by parents and caregivers, a severe distortion of the eating function may be built up by the time the child reaches adolescence. This is particularly true in the case of individuals whose inherent characteristics predispose them in some way to an eating problem.[46]

Parents of adolescents with eating disorders have been found to be so intrusive in the lives of their children that the children have not been free to develop autonomy. Children and parents are enmeshed in a system of overdependence, which is destructive. The families are rigid in their approach to life, unable to foster creativity in problem solving among their children. They, in fact, demonstrate a lack of ability to resolve conflicts, attempting instead to ignore serious problems.[47]

Within this family milieu children are unable to develop into normal independent beings. Maladaptive eating behaviors are among the outstanding manifestations of developmental problems for certain adolescents. It is thought that misuse of food (rather than other psychosomatic problems such as alcoholism) is the mode of expression in families in which food, weight control, or fitness is emphasized in some way.[47]

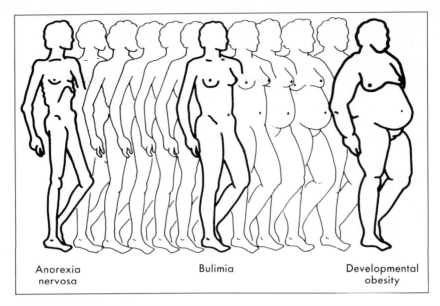

Anorexia
nervosa

Bulimia

Developmental
obesity

Figure 8-1   The spectrum of eating disorders. Underlying psychologic characteristics are held in common, whereas physical conditions vary across the spectrum. (From Rees, J.M.: Eating disorders. In Mahan, L.K., and Rees, J.M., editors: Nutrition in adolescence, St. Louis, 1984, The C.V. Mosby Co.)

The rapid development of body image during adolescence accounts for much of the psychological component of eating disorders in some teenagers. Adolescents along the spectrum are generally unable to view themselves without distortions, their problems being similar to those of all adolescents as described earlier but to an exaggerated degree.[46,48]

Obesity

Obesity is probably the most common nutritional and general health problem among adolescents in developed countries. Although the prevalence is not known, estimates of obesity range from 10% to 20% depending on the population studied and the obesity criteria used. From a public health view, it is disconcerting that the prevalence of adolescent obesity has increased by nearly 40% in the past two decades.[49] The prognosis for these teenagers is poor: 80% of them will remain obese as adults and be resistant to treatment.[50] This is an important fact to consider in helping obese adolescents set realistic goals.

Characteristics.   Although there is no typical obese adolescent, certain physical characteristics seem to persist. These include earlier maturation, greater muscle mass, and earlier menarche. This is especially true for those who have been obese through the growing years.

The physiological processes that are associated with long-term obesity have been operative for over a decade in many overweight adolescents. Their overweight status is often maintained by fat cell hypertrophy and hyperplasia, increased lipoprotein lipase levels, decreased thermogenetic potential, insulin insensitivity, and inherent genetic traits.[48,51] The longer the overweight status has persisted, the more difficult it is to overcome these effects since they affect the body's use of energy in a way that has been described in the "set point" theory.[52] Theoretically the set point is defended by the channeling of energy to maintain a certain rather narrow range of body weight. It is therefore difficult to achieve the energy deficit necessary to decrease body fat. At present decreasing dietary energy intake and increasing energy output through activity are the only means for accomplishing this deficit.

Since adolescents are, in general, sensitive about their bodies, teenagers are especially affected by the social rejection of and derogatory attitudes toward the obese in our culture. In our society, which admires and merchandises slimness, obese teenagers are under constant pressure to change their bodies to conform with social norms. Obese girls have traits in common with other minority groups, such as

obsessive concern (with overweight and food), passivity, withdrawal, and self-contempt. They are actually discriminated against: in reality obesity does affect attractiveness, popularity with the opposite sex, ability to obtain a job, college acceptance, and other practical life situations. These teenagers may experience so much humiliating rejection and poor self-esteem that they become socially isolated.[53] In addition, their consistently low level of activity requires less energy. This combination of emotional and environmental factors often leads to more severe obesity. A vicious cycle ensues whereby food and eating may be the only outlets for frustration and depression (Figure 8-2).

Food practices and activity patterns.   In considering the food practices of obese adoles-

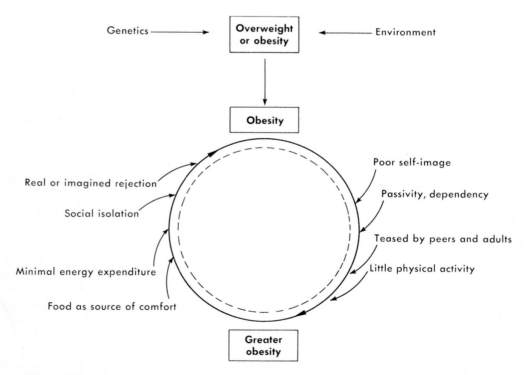

Figure 8-2   Factors that contribute to obesity. (Courtesy Betty Lucas, Clinical Training Unit, Child Development and Mental Retardation Center, University of Washington, Seattle, Wash.)

cents, one should remember that they may not be consuming excessive energy. Studies have shown that the energy intakes of some obese adolescents are equal to or lower than those of nonobese adolescents.[13,48] There is a tendency for obese teenagers to eat less frequently and to skip more meals, especially breakfast. Expressions such as "I'm not hungry in the morning" and "Eating breakfast makes me sick" are common. Often an accompanying pattern is the frequent or continuous eating from after school until late in the evening.

Another major factor is the inactivity of obese adolescents as compared with adolescents of normal weight. This has been demonstrated by activity records and motion picture sampling.[48,54] Since inactivity is often accompanied by reduced energy intake, it is not surprising that inactivity is a strong predictor of a poor quality diet.[39] It is not hard to imagine why body-sensitive overweight teenagers decline to participate in sports and activities that make them feel awkward, embarrassed, and exhausted. In addition, many obese adolescents are eliminated from participation in organized sports because of poor performance. Because they expend less energy, they may eat less than normal weight adolescents and yet still gain weight or at least maintain their weight. This seeming self-denial without results often causes feelings of frustration and hopelessness in the individual.

Treatment. It has been estimated that the odds against an overweight adolescent becoming an average weight adult are 28 to 1.[55] Despite these discouraging statistics, there is a large demand for adolescent weight control programs from parents, teachers, health professionals, and teenagers themselves. Adolescence can certainly be a critical period of influence in the establishment of positive health attitudes and practices. On the other hand, not recognizing the complex make-up of the obese adolescent or establishing unrealistic treatment plans can subject both the adolescent and the helping professional to feelings of failure and discouragement.

In most cases conventional methods such as structured diets or parental control have produced poor results. Anorectic drugs are usually contraindicated because of their ineffectiveness and because of the potential for abuse. Surgery has not been considered a reasonable option because of its high postoperative morbidity and unknown effects on growth. Gastric bypass has been done with a limited number of adolescents and should only be considered for those who are sexually mature, who are morbidly obese, and who have not been successful in previous reducing attempts. Even then, outcomes have been mixed.[56]

A less invasive treatment is the protein-sparing modified fast, which is used in an inpatient setting and requires biochemical monitoring.[48,56] This method should be used to treat sexually mature adolescents only if life-threatening complications develop and if a change in environment for the adolescent is assured following dismissal from the hospital. Neither gastric surgery nor fasting lead to long-term maintenance of a lower weight without an altered eating pattern and life-style changes that are supported by family and health professionals.

Behavior modification techniques have been used extensively in the treatment of adult obesity. This therapy can be useful in working with teenagers, but success depends on the motivation, maturity and family support of the adolescents. Programs that have included physical activity and behavioral components, as well as diet, have demonstrated more success, but few long-term follow-up studies have been done.[57] A behavioral approach alone seems to have limited application to the situation of the obese adolescent.[58]

Assessment. To determine the best therapeutic approach for the obese adolescent, a myriad of factors must be considered. One clinical asssessment tool that addresses the complexity of the problem is shown on pp. 16-17.

Table 8-2 Clinical assessment of eating disorder

	Date	Date	Date	Date
Motivation Appropriateness of weight goals Desire to change unhealthful habits Insight into problem				
Emotional psychological status Depression Locus of control Body image Self-esteem Oral expression Coping skills Compulsivity Perfectionism Independence				
Mental function Intellectual ability School performance Attitude toward school Ability to articulate				
Family characteristics Eating disorders Other diseases Natural or other parent Intrusiveness Enmeshment Rigidity Conflict resolution Role of food Exercise patterns Perceptions of problem Attempts to intervene Willingness to participate in therapy				

Table 8-2—cont'd.

	Date	Date	Date	Date
Social relationships Friends Social habits Social skills Attitude of peers				

Eating behavior
Knowledge/acknowledgement
  of nutritional needs
Meal pattern
Bizarre eating habits
Personal philosophy toward
  eating
Nutritional adequacy
Control over food supply				

Physical status Signs of bulimia Signs of starvation Terminal signs of starvation Thyroid status (obesity) Resting heart rate (HR) Exercise to reach 60% maximum (HR)				
Growth and adiposity Weight/height/age percentile Triceps skinfold/age percentile Arm muscle area/age percentile Weight/height history Growth velocity Maturational stage Age				
Physical activity Exercise patterns Hobbies/interests Personal feeling about exercise				
Plan				

From Rees, J. M., Williams, S. R., and Worthington-Roberts, B.S., eds.; Nutrition throughout the life cycle, St. Louis, The C.V. Mosby Co, 1988.

By assessing these factors, preferably through an interdisciplinary team process, a treatment approach can be planned to meet the needs of the individual.

Those adolescents who have poor self-esteem, who are signfiicantly depressed, and who are dependent and immature will generally require intensive counseling before they can deal with the weight problem. Those individuals who are more motivated and relatively unencumbered by the severe psychological aspects will probably have success with a program that includes dietary guidance, physical activity, behavioral components, and supportive counseling. Reports indicate that such a combined approach can be effective, both in clinical and in school settings.[59,60]

Clinical management. Successful treatment of the obese adolescent usually involves several health professionals and requires both an understanding of adolescent development and counseling skills. The ideal program incorporates decision making and goal setting by the adolescent and is realistic in its time frame.

Goals for treatment must acknowledge the adolescent's pubertal stage. For those in their growth spurts, weight can be maintained or slowly increased over time, allowing for changes in the ratio of lean body mass and fat. Both teenagers and parents must understand that weight gain is expected in periods of growth. For those who have completed their growth spurts, the plan will probably include actual weight reduction by loss of fat. Regular anthropometric assessment, including skinfolds, help determine the composition of any weight loss.

Most obese adolescents benefit from nutrition education because they have tried various types of diets or have acquired misinformation regarding obesity. Too often they are not aware of the basic concepts of energy balance (consumed versus expended). They may have the idea that a calorie is only negative and undesirable. They should learn about the physiological processes involved in body weight gain, maintenance, and loss. Activities such as keeping food records, assessing activity patterns, trying new recipes, calculating energy values, analyzing popular fad diets, or checking labels at the supermarket give adolescents a feeling of responsibility and accomplishment. A key to counseling is to assist teenagers in using food in positive and appropriate ways and to help them develop alternate coping skills to replace the misuse of food. The professional can help them to focus on food behaviors they would like to change gradually at their own speed and to consider options for handling feelings and food-oriented situations. They should, in all cases, be encouraged to make their own decisions. Role playing is often an effective tool in this regard.

Physical exercise is often given little credit in the treatment of obesity in general. For the adolescent, activity should be encouraged and reinforced as a permanent aspect of his or her life-style. In many cases it provides an alternative to eating as well as a means to increase energy expenditure with or without restriction of energy intake. Regular exercise yields positive changes in body composition, such as decreases in body weight and relative fat, increases in lean body mass, and cardiovascular benefits.

It is vital to encourage activities that the teenager enjoys. The activities should be relatively inexpensive and feasible and should have potential for continuing on into adulthood. Popular activities include bicycling, swimming, skating, walking, running and tennis. For the signficantly obese, care should be taken to assess the teenager's abilities and to program a slow, consistent increase in exercise. Actual fitness testing has been used in clinical settings to plan realistic exercise programs for obese adolescents and to engage their interest and motivation. This testing evaluates strength, flexibility, endurance, and cardiorespiratory function. The steps of assessing fitness levels and planning subsequent activity programs are outlined on p. 19.

Fitness: Testing and Planning Improvement Programs

1. a. Have client sit quietly and relax for 3 to 5 minutes.
   b. Take pulse for 10 seconds.*
   c. Record *resting heart rate* (RHR):_____

2. a. Find intensity of exercise required to reach *training heart rate* (THR)†immediately after exercise.
      THR for teens: 20 to 22 beats/10 seconds
      Stop with the exercise that achieves 20 to 22 beats/10 seconds. This is the exercise to use initially in the improvement program.

↑	Run for 5 minutes
Intensity increases	Jog for 5 minutes
	Jog for 2 minutes—walk for 2 minutes—jog for 2 minutes
	Walk uphill or upstairs for 2 to 3 minutes
	Walk for 5 minutes at a more rapid pace
START	Walk for 5 minutes at a moderate pace

   b. Monitor pulse return toward RHR after each exercise level—it should be below 16 beats/10 seconds

   Immediate _____→ 1 minute _____→ 2 minutes _____→ 3 minutes _____→ 5minutes _____→

3. *Improvement program:* To maintain THR for 15 minutes 4 to 5 days/week:
   a. Work with client to design an individualized program that is comfortable for him/her
   b. Plan 5-minute warmup—move at level below the level that maintains THR
   c. Exercise at intensity that maintains THR
   d. 5-Minute cool down—back to warmup speed—client should not sit or lie down immediately.
   e. Use a combination of exercise levels and types, if necessary
   f. If the client is ill, he/she should begin after illness at lower intensity and return slowly to intensity achieved before illness.

4. a. Retest every 3 to 4 weeks.
   b. Increase intensity of exercise to maintain THR.
   c. Client can increase time spent doing the exercise by 5-minute increments, up to 30 minutes.
   d. When client has reached jogging level and maintained it for 6 to 8 weeks, increase THR to 22 to 25 beats/10 seconds.
   e. Client can use any aerobic activities (e.g., jogging, bicycling, skating, or dancing) or combinations that the client prefers.

Developed by Scott. B., and Rees. J., Adolescent Program, University of Washington Seattle.
* 10-Second time segment is easiest to measure and use.
† *Maximum heart rate* (MHR): ≈ 200 beats/minute for persons under 20 years of age (Cumming, G.R., Everatt, D., and Hastman, L.: Bruce treadmill test in children: normal values in a clinic population, Am. J. Cardiol. **41**:69, 1978). THR is 60% of MHR for persons with poor initial fitness, 75% for of MHR for persons who are fit (i.e., 60% of 200 =120 beats/minute =20 beats/10 seconds [20 to 22 beats/10 seconds for normal variation]).
Note: Contraindications for testing and initiating fitness program are revealed by routine medical history and physical examination.

Although psychotherapy alone has not been recommended, teenagers with significant weight problems will be able to make changes only when they are presented within the context of a therapeutic relationship. The psychological aspect is usually a component of the total weight management program; for some teens, it may be the major focus and may take a significant length of time. In some situations, family therapy is essential to help the adolescent from a dysfunctional family make progress.

Group treatment is commonly used for many adolescent difficulties, including obesity. It ranges from intensive treatment in a summer camp to weekly sessions in a school or clinical setting. The specific goals of group sessions may include the acquisition of nutrition information, the use of behavior modification tools, physical activity, social skills improvement, emphasis on a positive image, and the development of peer relationships. Success by group treatment cannot be measured by weight loss alone; psychosocial parameters must also be evaluated. For some adolescents, willing attendance at group sessions, initiating a conversation, or reporting a personal achievement to the group will be a big step. The group leader plays a critical role. He or she should have an understanding of adolescent development in general, an awareeness of the varying complexity of the obese teenager, and skills in group process. Camps and other groups that provide only for short-term weight loss are detrimental and should be avoided.

Although some common characteristics exist, there is no typical overweight teenager. Programs may vary with the individual, but in all cases attention should be given to the adolescent's diet, activity, and feelings. Figure 8-3 illustrates a teaching tool developed to help instruct and motivate adolescents.

Outcome. Because of the poor prognosis for many obese teenagers to achieve ideal weight, the professional working with them should help them avoid setting unrealistic

BE SIZEWISE
Don't Lose Your Balance.

Nourishment	Activities	Feelings
Be good to your body—give it what it needs	Do interesting things—quiet as well as energetic	Learn to know and like yourself
Don't starve or stuff yourself	Take time to relax everyday	Have realistic goals for yourself
Know what's in the food you eat	Don't let eating be your only recreation	Don't substitute food for love and companionship
	Do some strenuous activity every day	Build satisfying relationships with your family and friends
	Share active and quiet time with friends	Get help for problems you can't cope with alone

Figure 8-3 Be Sizewise—materials for clinicians, educators, and teenagers. (© American Heart Association of Washington.)

goals or believing that they can accomplish the impossible. For these individuals obesity should be considered a chronic condition. Treatment goals should include working toward the adolescent's acceptance of his or her body as it is and focusing on developing healthy life-style practices. Once obese individuals maturely accept their condition, ongoing modification of eating patterns and activity patterns can be emphasized.

Despite poor prognosis and lack of long-term success of obesity treatments, program efforts for obese adolescents usually yield positive changes, although they may be small and difficult to measure. But for the individual teenager, these effects can be signfiicant by enhancing his or her present situation or by providing information and skills that can be put into practice at a later time. Most importantly the adolescent's self-esteem can be enhanced.

Anorexia nervosa

Anorexia nervosa is an eating disorder with serious underlying developmental and psychological disturbances. It occurs most commonly among females, and the symptoms are usually manifested in adolescence. The initial symptoms include amenorrhea, weight loss, compulsive physical activity, and dietary restriction. In many cases, everyday events or remarks critical of their bodies appear to precipitate the weight loss. It may seem to be a response to real or imagined obesity. Initially, the weight goals may be reasonable, but with success these individuals are reinforced both externally and internally to continue losing weight. When weight goals are reached, new lower ones may be established. Dieting becomes a primary focus of the lives of those with anorexia nervosa, described by Bruch[46] as "a relentless pursuit of thinness."

Anorexia is actually a misnomer for this disorder. Patients do not lack hunger, but rigidly deny and control it. As outlined by Bruch,[46] a pattern of denial occurs: denial of thinness, hunger, fatigue, and personal effectiveness.

Characteristics. The disorder may be characterized by progressive or significant weight loss and avoidance of any fattening foods. Anorectic young women may alternate binge eating with dieting. They are usually very clever at concealing their gorging of food, self-induced vomiting, and heavy use of laxatives. There is a dramatic increase in hyperactive behavior and compulsive exercise patterns. The hyperactivity may begin as routine physical exercise but may increase, as the disorder progresses, to compulsive jogging and calisthenics, denying the need for adequate rest, even to the inability to sit down for more than a moment. Significantly, the physical activity is usually done alone.

These individuals are often preoccupied with food and will prepare energy-laden dishes for their families but limit themselves to a taste or nothing.

Aspects of nutrition are also of great interest to them, and in fact most are more knowledgeable of nutrition than their peers. However, this nutritional knowledge may be distorted, and the individual may be unable to practically conceptualize the information. The bizarre eating habits of individuals with anorexia nervosa may be well hidden, so that family and friends often deny any problems and do not seek help until the disorder becomes severe.[61]

Psychodynamic features of the anorexia nervosa syndrome include a distorted body image, fear of physical maturation and adulthood, and a tremendous dependence/independence conflict. Even when the disorder has progressed to the point of emaciation, these anorectic women will deny reality, insisting that they are normal or even overweight. The apathy, preoccupation with food, and inability to think coherently observed in starving individuals can be recognized in the disturbed personality of the starving anorectic person. There is a pattern of doing exceptionally well academically by setting high goals and studying excessively but withdrawing from peer relationships in preference for a self-imposed isolation. Their ability to function realistically in a school or work setting, however, may be significantly compromised. Family histories of patients with anorexia nervosa reveal psychopathology among families, as well as a higher prevalence of obesity and anorexia nervosa. Some evidence also suggests an increased incidence of perinatal complications in these individuals.[62] Classically, the family is very achievement oriented and successful at economic, social, and academic levels, but parents may experience significant hidden marital discord. The parents' need to control and the anoretic person's need to please form a basic conflicted relationship that demands resolution for the patient with anorexia nervosa.

It is well to remember that not all individuals with anorexia nervosa exhibit the classical characteristics. Approximately 5% to 10% are male; some individuals do not manifest symptoms until later adulthood; and other patients do not show dramatic weight loss or all the common psychological behaviors.

Pugliese and others[63] report that males as well as females often severely restrict food intake out of fear of fatness. Those who were referred to an endocrinology clinic for growth retardation responded to education by normalizing their eating habits so that growth resumed. They represent a group in our culture who do not have true eating disorders but lack understanding of the positive nature of weight gain as they develop mature bodies.

In recent years, there have been numerous studies of the metabolic and endocrine abnormalities often associated with the nutritional crisis of this disorder, focusing primarily on pituitary and hypothalamic function.[48] Hormonal secretion patterns have been shown to be essentially those of the prepubertal state. Hypothalamic function and physical symptoms such as edema, postural hypotension, bradycardia, and hirsutism parallel those seen in other cases of starvation. At this time it appears these alterations are the effects rather than the causes of the voluntary starvation.[48]

With the continual weight loss and semistarvation, the nutritional status of these individuals deteriorates. Fluid and electrolyte imbalances can result from induced vomiting and purging. Long-term debilitation results in death in a small percentage of cases.

Treatment. Treatment and management of anorexia nervosa is varied, and depends on the stage and severity of the disorder. Most programs include nutritional, medical, and psychological support. Although early intervention may prevent a nutritional crisis, cases of severe debilitation require hospitalization and refeeding. It is not unusual for the patient to sabotage treatment attempts by hiding food, performing surreptitious exercise, or attaching weights to her body before stepping on the scale. But with support, a positive response can usually be developed. Satisfactory weight gain by a patient in an institution cannot be interpreted as success. Although it is essential that the underlying developmental problems be resolved, a hospital stay and subsequent weight gain can be the first stage of a comprehensive program.

Comprehensive interdisciplinary inpatient treatment programs usually include an initial psychiatric assessment, a refeeding program with bed rest, and ongoing individual and family psychotherapy. Emphasis is placed on the psychological environment, which is accepting and supporting of the patient. After attaining normal weight, the patient is allowed more freedom while ongoing counseling is provided in the hospital setting.

Outpatient management is used for the recovering anorectic or for those who have not deteriorated to a crisis state. Successful intervention strategies continue to require a comprehensive, interdisciplinary approach, with good communication and coordination between professionals.[48] The time period required may be several years.

Behavior modification, in which weight gain is required to earn certain privileges or activities, has been criticized for its lack of long-term evaluation and its focus on only tangible measures.[64] Critics believe that it tends to undermine the patient's individuality, which is essential for ultimate treatment success. Many experts, however, believe that behavior modification techniques can be usefully incorporated into eclectic treatment protocols.

Long-term individual and family psychotherapy is the basic component of treatment. A high success rate has been reported if patients and their families are treated within 1 year of the onset of the syndrome.[65]

Assessment. A thorough knowledge of anorexia nervosa is necessary for the identification and assessment of teenagers with this disorder. Taking a history using the assessment guidelines on pp. 186-187 enables the professional to decide whether the patient is just beginning to physically manifest the disorder, is near or at a crisis, or is in the recovery period. Weight-for-height proportion, along with the presence or absence of signs of significant starvation, will be an important indication of the physical state. Food habits, exercise patterns, use of laxatives and diuretics, induced vomiting, and distorted beliefs about body image and food intake must be explored. Patient and family psychological assessment are necessary to establish the degree of disturbance in perceptions and relationships, as well as the ability to respond within the bounds of a therapeutic relationship.[66]

Clinical management. The nutritional component of management varies greatly depending on the stage of the disorder. If the patient is not at a physical crisis point, the goal will be to help her establish a psychotherapeutic relationship and to provide nutritonal guidance within the context of the patient's ability to respond. During a crisis, refeeding will be managed in a manner that blends with the overall philosophy of the inpatient program. It is usually possible to obtain sufficient cooperation from patients so they can take food by mouth.[67] A concentrated fluid dietary preparation may be prescribed as medicine if other food is refused. Invasive procedures such as **parenteral** or **enteral** nourishment are reserved for life-threatening states. Following a crisis or in the event a crisis is avoided, the patient will need guidance in developing realistic nourishment and exercise patterns as well as an understanding of physiological needs.[61]

Outcome. Common features of anorexia nervosa are the strong resistance to treatment and the high incidence of relapse or partial recovery. Some of these patients manifest varying degrees of the symptoms in adulthood. Very few follow-up evaluations have been conducted on the long-term outcome of the various treatment modes used for anorexia nervosa. Hsu, Crisp, and Harding[68] in England reported on the outcome of a follow-up study of 100 patients. The time lapses ranged from 4 to 8 years after the initial clinic visit. All but 12 of the patients had been involved in refeeding programs and/or psychotherapy. Using the criteria of near-normal weight, regular menstruation, and satisfactory psychosexual and psychosocial adjustments, 48% had a good outcome. Poor outcome was associated with longer duration of illness, lower body weight during illness, onset at a later age, presence of vomiting, compulsive overeating, anxiety when eating with others, poor social adjustment in childhood, and disturbed parental relationships. The low mortality (2%) in these severely ill patients supports the use of weight gain and psychotherapy. Though follow-up criteria have been inconsistently used by researchers, a compilation of results reported from 1954 to 1978 indicate that though weight-for-height proportion improved in about three fourths of the patients described, menstrual cycles were often unsatisfactorily maintained and psychosocial maladjustment was common.[69] Health care professionals should watch for symptoms (often well disguised) in vulnerable individuals and attempt to intervene early. Whether the person with anorexia nervosa is treated as an inpatient or an outpatient, the goals of management include (1) maintaining a positive nutritonal state, (2) achieving physical and developmental maturation, and (3) providing therapy for the patient to work out underlying conflicts and emotional disorders.

Bulimia

Bulimia, referring to the gorging and vomiting first described in anorexia nervosa, is now recognized as a separate syndrome (bulimia nervosa) in the spectrum of eating disorders. The term is applied to individuals who combine periodic gorging/binge-eating (eating excessive amounts of food) with self-induced vomiting and abuse of diuretics and laxatives but who nevertheless maintain normal weight. Separate studies report that bulimic symptoms affect 19% of college women and 5% of high school students.[70,71]

Unfortunately, there is a growing practice among normal teenagers to use vomiting as a form of weight control. It may be socially reinforced on athletic squads or when groups of adolescents or young people such as college students live together. Although this is not a practice to be encouraged, it is not classified as bulimia unless it is an obsession, which signifies interrupted development.

Bulimia is at present thought to arise under similar patterns of familial disturbance as anorexia nervosa.[72] Bulimic persons may have previously been obese or have experienced classical anorexia nervosa. They are often older than the average anorexic person when seen for treatment.

Characteristics. Physically, bulimic persons are usually near normal weight for their height. This attests to the fact that they retain sufficient nourishment to sustain themselves though vomiting and purging frequently. Individuals may, for example, follow the practice of vomiting only snack-type foods that they have eaten following regular meals. Bulimic persons differ in the practices they follow. In fact, some will define eating one cookie as a binge because of their distorted attitudes about foods and their physiological needs. They experience dental damage, swollen parotid glands, and irritation of the throat as the result of exposure of unprotected tissues to acidic vomitus.[48] Rectal bleeding may be caused by excessive use of laxatives. Electrolyte imbalances and the development of fistulas in the esophagus are more rare and serious consequences requiring hospitalization.[73]

Psychological characteristics most prominently seen are an overriding sense of guilt and a linkage between self-worth and the ability to maintain a body size close to the "ideal."[48,74] The preoccupation with these issues and the physical activities of eating and ridding herself of the food fill the day of the bulimic person to the extent that it interferes with her ability to succeed in an educational or professional setting.[75] Nevertheless, the bulimic person will often appear to be very attractive and to lead a busy and successful life as compared with her peers. Bulimic persons are prone to problems of impulse control including abuse of drugs and alcohol, shoplifting, and outbursts of anger. Bouts of binge-eating and vomiting are often attempts to deal with unwanted feelings.

Treatment

Assessment. Major areas to be included in the nutrition assessment include weight history, dieting behavior, binge-eating episodes, purging behaviors, and eating and exercise patterns.[76] With some individuals this requires several visits, whereas others welcome disclosure to rid themselves of guilt. It is now well accepted that most bulimics have adopted a severely restricted philosophy toward eating, so that both physically and psychologically they are driven to binge. A physical examination is necessary to detect any truly significant symptoms and to assure those of normal physical status that they have done no permanent damage to themselves. A psychological assessment will be necessary to determine the nature of the personality disorder.[75]

Clinical management. An electrolyte imbalance requires aggressive management, usually in a hospital setting. Otherwise, key changes in bulimic behaviors will be facilitated by skillful techniques on the part of the nutrition counselor in conjunction with individual and family psychotherapy.[76] Guilt is often alleviated by the opportunity to discuss specific practices. If a great deal of anxiety is provoked by discussion of dietary habits in detail, it is best to postpone direct intervention until the individual is ready. It is usually unworkable to attempt to control vomiting and lose weight at the same time, although many bulimic persons will declare these goals on entering treatment. To succeed, cessation of vomiting must be a primary goal. Following the realization that she can control her vomiting, the bulimic person will gradually be able to control her eating, primarily by learning to provide herself with sufficient nourishment. Because the behavior is commonly based on faulty ideas about physiological needs, the chance to learn within a trusting relationship allows her to formulate new concepts about foods.[75] Cognitive restructuring techniques have been used with good results.[77] These methods can also be applied to facilitate her adoption of goals regarding weight for height, which are more reasonable in terms of her natural physiological makeup. Weight-for-height standards should be presented without an authoritarian stance to the bulimic person who exhibits readiness. A range of weights for a particular height such as those available by including the 25th through the 50th percentile of the HANES detailed tables[1,78] should always be used to demonstrate the wide range that is normal. The speed at which cognitive and behavioral goals can be accomplished will be determined by the gains bulimic persons make in psychotherapy. Successful psychotherapeutic

group treatment protocols have incorporated all elements mentioned above.[74-77]

Outcome. Improvement in both psychological and physical states of bulimic persons in treatment have been reported.[74-77] Incorporation of strategies directed toward the nutritional and developmental aspects of the disorder based on experience with anorexia nervosa appears to be an important aspect of positive outcomes seen to date.

Pregnancy in Adolescence

Although the overall birth rate in the United States has been declining, this is not the case for the adolescent age group. An estimated 1 million teenage pregnancies occur annually; two thirds result in births.[79] Most of these young women are unmarried and most keep their babies.

Teenage mothers have more complications during pregnancy and give birth to a higher percentage of stillborn infants and low birth weight infants than any other age group. The American Academy of Pediatrics[80] states that an increase in low birth weight infants and preeclampsia are the two major complicatons related to the teenage pregnancy itself. The incidence of births of babies weighing less than 2500 gm is significantly higher among all adolescents, but especially among those who give birth before they are 15 years of age.[79] Low gynecological age (time interval since menarche) is associated with a higher incidence of births of low birth weight infants.[81]

Some of the adverse effects of teenage pregnancy are believed to be related to socioeconomic status and other environmental factors that are difficult to isolate. In a study by Zuckerman and others,[82] pregnancy outcomes were compared between adolescent and nonadolescent women independent of numerous health and social differences. The only statistically significant difference between the two groups was that infants of adolescent mothers weighed 94 gm less than infants of nonadolescent mothers.

The authors demonstrated that several health and social factors (including low pregnancy weight gain, low prepregnant weight, and marijuana use during pregnancy), but not adolescent status itself, were associated with adverse infant outcome.

The pregnant teenager characteristically does not receive early prenatal care, thus increasing her risk for a poor outcome. A subsequent pattern of dropping out of school and thus decreasing future employability, having no financial independence, and often having little emotional support creates a poor psychosocial milieu for the adolescent.

Teens are particularly at nutritional risk when pregnancy occurs before their own growth is completed. The question of whether pregnant adolescents, especially younger teens, are also growing rapidly in height and weight has not been answered. Some data has shown that increases in stature and weight for the period of pregnancy was less than that expected, despite the observed higher pregnancy weight gains.[83] Hormonal changes may be involved in slowing growth during pregnancy.

Another nutritional risk factor is that nutrient stores may be minimal at the time of conception because of recent rapid growth, poor eating habits, and dieting attempts. Studies indicate that many pregnant adolescents receive inadequate amounts of nutrients and that they have lower blood nutrient levels.[84] The multiple nutrient demands of adolescent growth and pregnancy, combined with a poor food intake, do not predict an optimal outcome of pregnancy.

Generally, the nutrient needs of pregnant adolescents are estimated by adding the recommended dietary allowances for pregnancy to the allowances for 15- to 18-year-old females.[84] These nutrient levels may be an overestimation for some individuals, depending on changes in nutrient absorption, hormonal alterations, or decreased physical activity. But unless the adolescent is obviously mature, the additive allowances of adolescence plus pregnancy are probably the best guides in planning diets for this group. Each individual should be assessed for current intake and life-style. Many pregnant girls decrease their levels of physical activity and thus may not require all the energy allowed. Iron and folic acid needs are increased substantially during pregnancy; these nutrients are often found marginally in adolescent diets. A prenatal supplement therefore is usually standard practice to cover the increased needs.

For many young teenagers, it may be normal and appropriate for weight gain to exceed 25 to 30 pounds, especially if the women are average weight or underweight. One study reported the average term weight gain of 80 adolescents to be 37 pounds, with females of younger chronological and gynecological age gaining less than older, more mature females.[85] In addition, some data suggest that although these young women lose weight easily in the postpartum period, their weight usually stabilizes at a higher level than their prepregnant weight.[85] These two trends, more prenatal weight gain and a higher postpartum weight, seem to indicate continued physical growth and maturation during the pregnancy.

Pregnant teenagers are just as likely as other teenagers to have patterns of meal-skipping, poor snacks, overconcern about weight, and limited food choices.[86] Professionals working with adolescents to improve prenatal nutritional status and the subsequent pregnancy outcome should be cognizant of the patient's life-styles and habits as they affect eating behavior.

The psychosocial factors imposed on the pregnant adolescent can cause her to be in a situation where she is alone, has no emotional support, has little or no money to buy food, and does not seek prenatal care. A team of health care providers with expertise in multiple areas is best suited to meet her needs. Comprehensive programs have been developed that include prenatal care, nutritional guidance, psychological counseling, family planning, continued schooling, and parenting and infant care. In practical terms, however, programs such as these are not found consistently in all localities and they generally struggle for financial and program support. This type of program, if available in a community, however, is the most appropriate resource to optimize the outcome for both the teenage girl and her baby.

Sports and Athletics

Most adolescents participate in a variety of physical activities. These may range from the organized, competitive sport and daily training to weekend skiing and bicycle trips. Regardless of the type of sport, optimal nutrition is a basic requisite for training and maintaining good physical performance. It is probably not coincidental that Olympic gold medal winners come from those countries with a high level of nutritional status.

As with the nonathlete, the diet of the athlete must supply optimal amounts of energy, protein, water, fat, carbohydrates, vitamins, and minerals. Energy is needed for growth plus extra expended energy. In most situations appetite is the guide for food intake. Carbohydrate is the best source of this extra energy with emphasis on complex carbohydrates. Extra protein is not needed; even during a muscle building program, adequate protein is provided by usual intakes. Vitamin and mineral supplements are not needed for the teenage athlete who is receiving enough energy and a varied diet. One exception may be the female adolescent athlete, who is more at risk for iron deficiency and anemia.[87] Some athletes who limit their food intake tend to have low intakes of several nutrients, as well as energy. Adequate hydration is a primary concern for the adolescent athlete; fluids should be replaced before, during, and after exercise. For each pound of weight lost through exertion, one pint of water should be drunk.

Despite the influence of good nutrition, dietary practices alone cannot be counted on

to supply the winning edge. It is not unusual for adolescent athletes to emulate the professional star, including following a "winning" diet or accepting an endorsement of a food supplement. Adolescents competing in sports in which minimal body fatness is desired (e.g. gymnastics, wrestling, distance running, and ballet) may compulsively control food intake or use other methods to lose weight to an unhealthy and dangerous degree. This can lead to amenorrhea, anorexia nervosa, or bulimia. Coaches and trainers, who work closest with the athlete, may allow or encourage undesirable dietary practices because they lack nutrition expertise or they hope that the practice will improve performance. Many dietary practices relating to foods included or excluded in the athlete's diet are often based on psychological reasons or superstitions rather than on physiological and nutritional soundness.

Ideally, more nutrition education should be available to coaches, trainers, and others who greatly influence the young athlete. Because adolescents are developing lifelong eating habits, it is desirable that those adults guiding them should reinforce positive dietary practices. More specifics of nutrition and sports are discussed in Chapter 10.

Substance Use and Abuse

Tobacco, alcohol, and marijuana are the substances most used and abused by the adolescent age group.[88,89] These substances are often referred to as "gate-way drugs": drugs that lead to other drug use. Hard or addictive drugs are used by a smaller percentage of teenagers. The use of these substances presents significant problems in the public health, social, and family spheres.

Alcohol

Increased attention has been given to the problem of alcohol consumption in adolescents. The decision to drink or not to drink is made in the teen years. It has been reported that more that 90% of high school students have had at least some experience with alcohol by 18 years of age, and most have their first exposure under parental supervision between 12 and 15 years of age.[89,90] Currently, alcohol use among females is almost as high as among males.

Alcoholism or problem drinking in the adolescent age group has been difficult to define, because most definitions and classifications of alcoholism have been based on adult males. In most cases adolescent drinkers are identified by higher rates of alcohol-related problems such as school difficulties, psychological problems, arrests, or delinquency. Young people tend to drink less regularly than do adults, but they consume larger amounts at a time (i.e., binge drinking).[89]

The degree of nutritional risk for drinking adolescents depends on the frequency and amount of their alcohol consumption. It is known that alcohol has deleterious effects on nutritional status in more than one way. The alcoholic beverage, which has almost no nutritional value, may displace food that provides nutrients for growth. The B vitamins, especially thiamine and niacin, are needed for alcohol metabolism in the liver. Ethanol provides energy, at 7 kcal/gm, but significantly dilutes the nutrient content of the diet, making the individual at risk for nutritional deficiencies. In addition, continued alcohol consumption has a direct toxic effect on the gastrointestinal mucosa, interfering with digestion and absorption.[91] This adverse effect occurs independently of the malabsorption that can result from alcoholic cirrhosis. The nutrients most likely to be deficient are pyridoxine, folic acid, thiamine, and vitamin B_{12}. In many cases of chronic alcoholism, the malnutrition that exists is a result of both an inadequate diet and the alcohol's direct action on the gut.

A recent survey of adolescent males found that those who were alcohol and marijuana abusers reported significantly more symptoms of poor nutrition (i.e. muscle weakness, bleeding gums, tiredness) but not significant differences in biochemical measures.[92] Although all reported adequate nutrient intake, the abusers ate more snack food and had lower intakes of milk, fruits, and vegetables. The lack of identifiable nutrition deficiencies may be related to the length of exposure to these substances, approximately 1 year. A continued pattern of dependency on snack foods and substance abuse leads to severe nutritional problems in later life.

For the pregnant adolescent who consumes alcohol, there is the risk of producing a child with fetal alcohol syndrome.[91] More subtle effects on the offspring may be caused by the alcohol itself or by the combination of alcohol and a marginal diet.

Nutritional status evaluations of adolescents should not neglect the area of alcohol consumption. Some individuals may initially withhold this information, in which case the interviewer should adopt a nonthreatening approach. Those adolescents who have significant alcohol problems obviously need comprehensive programs of counseling and rehabilitation, but it is appropriate that nutritional therapy and education be a component of such treatment. Programs for education about and prevention of alcohol-related problems are needed, starting at the elementary school level.

Tobacco

Cigarette smoking continues to be popular in the teenage years despite evidence of its negative health effects. A 1985 national survey of high school seniors reported that 30% smoked regularly, with a higher percentage of smokers being female.[89] Reduced plasma vitamin C levels have been reported in smokers, but the effect of smoking on vitamin C needs is unclear.[33] Of recent concern is the increased use of smokeless tobacco by children and adolescents. Complications of regular use of this ubstance include periodontal disease, dependence, oral cancer, and hypertension.[93]

Drugs

Drug use by teenagers may run the gambit from caffeine to illegal narcotics. The kind of drug and as its frequency of use or abuse will determine the detrimental effects on nutritional status and overall health.

Caffeine. Carbonated beverages provide most of the caffeine in teenage diets, but coffee and tea are also contributors. Soft drinks were the most frequently reported snack items in the Nationwide Food Consumption Study.[42] Although moderate amounts of caffeine can have positive stimulant effects, larger amounts can result in nervousness, agitation, gastric distress, and sleep problems. Because food habits in adolescence set the stage for adult eating patterns, teenagers should be encouraged to use caffeine-containing beverages in moderation. Although the soft drink industry is now making caffeine-free beverages available, these beverages may still displace milk, fruit juice, and other fluids that provide nutrients.

Marijuana. Marijuana is a substance often used by many adolescents as an alternative to, or in combination with, alcohol. Although it is illegal, it is readily attainable and socially accepted in many peer groups. Controversy exists as to its harmful effects compared with other drugs, especially when used infrequently. The more detrimental effects are seen with heavy, long-term use.[94]

Marijuana causes changes in mental sensations and alters perceptions of time and space.[94] Sensory organs are affected, with an increased appetite and enjoyment of eating, expecially sweets, reported by users.[95] Whether this is a direct effect of marijuana or an environmental effect is not clear. No specific marijuana-nutrient interaction has been identified but limited research has been done in this area.

Although many people believe that moderate marijuana use is benign, the social milieu of purchasing and using an illegal substance can have serious consequences for an adolescent. With chronic use the most critical consequences are the negative effects on the adolescent's emotional and cognitive maturation.

Hard drugs. Included in this category are heroin, cocaine, PCP, morphine, and LSD. Although used by a small percentage of adolescents, these are the addictive drugs that are routinely abused by their users. Their use in adolescence is associated with a downward life-style—poor school performance or drop-out, deteriorating family interactions, isolation, and illegal activities such as theft to obtain money to purchase the drug.

Because of their habit, drug abusers are faced with a multitude of problems including poor health and nutrition. Their nutritional status is often negatively affected because of (1) money used for drugs instead of food, (2) depressed appetite, (3) irregular life-style and eating habits, (4) hepatitis and other infectious diseases that cause anorexia and increased need for nutrients, and (5) the simultaneous use of alcohol or other drugs.

A comprehensive drug treatment program is almost always needed to help the young person get free of the drug dependency and regain control of his or her life. Good nutrition is certainly an important part of that treatment. Nutritional assessment identifies the critical areas and provides information for counseling and educating the adolescent regarding food choices for optimal health.

Acne

Problems of poor complexion, blackheads, and pimples are dreaded by all adolescents of both sexes. Many experience these problems to some degree during puberty, and a small percentage are affected by a full-blown case of the clinical disease, acne vulgaris. Although teenage acne is subject to fads and fallacies regarding cause and treatment, there is nothing mysterious about the phenomenon. Acne is not caused by eating chocolate, french fries, or carbonated beverages, despite popular thought to the contrary. The sebaceous glands of the skin are under hormonal control, chiefly that of androgens; thus the rapid acceleration and increase of hormone production are directly related to the skin changes.

There is no rationale for recommending a specific diet in the treatment of acne, although any food that seems to be aggravating for an individual should be limited. Medical treatment of acne vulgaris involves both topical and systemic medications. Retinoic acid (a vitamin A acid) is sometimes used as a topical agent in difficult cases, but its use requires physician supervision.[96] Large doses of vitamins, however, will not alleviate the symptoms of acne and may lead to toxicity of fat-soluble vitamins. Some studies have suggested that zinc supplementation improves severe acne. A level of 135 mg of oral zinc daily reduced the mean acne score by 85%. [97] The mechanism for this zinc response is unknown.

In preventing or lessening the symptoms of acne, a basic diet providing optimal nutrients helps ensure healthy skin, but again, specific foods should not be eliminated unless they are suspect for the adolescent. An optimal diet combined with good skin care will not prevent the superficial signs of acne but will help lessen the severity of the symptoms.

COUNSELING AND NUTRITION EDUCATION

Adolescents in the United States are not experiencing dire results of malnutrition, despite the fact that some of them do not receive optimal nutrition. This realization is significant when considering methods and approaches to nutrition counseling and education for this age group.

According to Piaget's theory of cognitive development, 11 years of age and beyond is the formal operations period.[98] At this stage, there is expansion of abstract thinking and deeper understanding of scientific and hypothetical processes. The concept of nutrients functioning at biochemical levels can be grasped, yet knowlege as to wise food choices may be overshadowed by peer and social influences.

Counseling

Providing nutritional counseling to adolescents can be challenging, frustrating, and rewarding. Counselors who work with adolescents must be knowledgeable of the developmental stages of adolescence, including the physical, social, and emotional. A positive aspect of working with many teenagers is their interest in nutrition as it affects their bodies, even though their information sources may not be completely reliable.

Establishing rapport with the adolescent is a first priority, one that often takes time and patience. Past experiences with adults may make it difficult for the adolescent to initially trust the helping professional. Emphasis on making the adolescent comfortable, showing a genuine interest in him or her as a person, and allowing flexibility in the session will result in more productive counseling. A wide variety of counseling approaches can be successful, depending on the characteristics of client and counselor, but either extreme of authority figure or buddy is not likely to work.

Initial assessment should be made as to whether dietary practices are beneficial, neutral, or harmful. The positive aspects of a dietary regimen can be emphasized. Reinforcement can certainly be given to the adolescent who has decreased consumption of concentrated carbohydrates and packaged snack items in favor of more fruits, vegetables, and whole grains.

In the case of unhealthy dietary patterns, concrete supportive data are more likely to be accepted by questioning adolescents than are superficial answers. The pregnant teenager will more likely accept the idea of an optimal weight gain if she understands the various components of weight gain and why each is essential for a healthy baby. Likewise, the overweight adolescent may be willing to give up a fad diet if the counselor helps him or her analyze its nutritional quality and long-term consequences.

The counseling relationship should encourage the adolescent to participate mutually with the counselor in setting goals, although the professional needs to make sure the goals are reasonable and attainable. Parents should be included when they can be supportive. Specific counseling techniques are described in detail in other sources,[99] but the following guidelines can assist the professional in working with the adolescent:

1. Supportive counseling. This should be provided on a consistent basis and is often long-term.
2. Setting realistic goals. These may include specific goals for weight change (gain, loss, or maintenance), changes in activity, or altering food-related behaviors. Goals should be short-term and developed in a gradual but progressive manner.
3. Positive reinforcement. Initially this will be provided by the counselor and others supportive to the adolescent. Eventually the adolescent can learn to reinforce himself or herself.
4. Patience. This requires the counselor to accept periods of silence, to listen actively, and to reassess after a period of regression. Too often the professional is ready to give up and conveys this to the adolescent as failure.

Because some adolescents do not seek health care through established avenues, successful nutrition counseling and education have been demonstrated by rap sessions and team efforts in free clinics, youth centers, and other places accepted by the adolescents.[100] An initial appeal to their desire to be healthful persons will help in establishing a good rapport.

Since adolescent nutrition issues are multifaceted, nutrition counseling is most successful when it is a component of an interdisciplinary health care team. In some communities, the team may be the result of coordination and communication between various agencies and professionals.

Implications for Nutrition Education

Adolescents are generally interested in how their particular diet affects them, but their

Figure 8-4   Nutritionist counsels adolescent on an appropriate diet.

knowledge of nutritional concepts and facts may be limited or erroneous. This reveals a definite need for innovative nutrition education approaches to the adolescent. Leverton[101] points out some positive aspects in reaching adolescents: (1) they get hungry, (2) they like to eat, (3) they want energy, vigor, and the means to compete and excel in whatever they do, and (4) they have many good food habits that were established in childhood. Primary assets such as these yield access points to reach the adolescent at his or her own level of interest and readiness. By respecting the adolescent's ideas about food, it is easier for the health professional to emphasize the positive aspects and to build on them.

In addition to their roles in the family, adolescents also have significant roles as students and consumers. At school, a well-designed nutrition curriculum incorporated with relevant subjects can provide a base of knowlege. In a larger sense the school can be a nutrition laboratory, providing practical experience not only in science and health classes, but also in the lunchroom and at the vending machine. As consumers, teenagers are increasing their power in the marketplace but are also the targets of sophisticated advertising. To make rational food choices, they need practical information about food labeling and purchasing, nutrient density of foods, and how to analyze advertisement messages.

Today's teenagers will usually respond to nutrition information in terms of growth and development, even in physiological parameters. With respect to future parenthood, it is obvious that the female should understand the impact of long-term nutrition on the outcome of pregnancy. However, since the father's food preferences are the most influential factor in family food choices, appropriate nutrition education for the male adolescent is just as vital.

Practical experience has shown that visual aids or other media developed specifically for adolescents lead to stimulating discussion and an increased interest in many areas of nutrition.

Some novel and successful attempts at getting a nutritional message across to teenagers have included the use of a fantasy comic format and a radio/television media campaign using prizes and contests.[102,103] Newer techniques used in the classroom include computer-assisted learning programs and the use of games and tournaments that emphasize team effort.[104]

It should be remembered that food is only one part of the exciting and rapid journey to adulthood, and that nutrition education can be incorporated along with many aspects of adolescents' life-styles and at various stages of readiness. In completing their own growth and maturity, adolescents are nearing the time when they will influence and make decisions regarding the food habits and nutritional status of the next generation.

SUGGESTED LEARNING ACTIVITIES

1. Analyze a typical menu from two different fast-food establishments for energy and major nutrients. What deficiencies and excesses exist? How would you correct them?
2. Ann is 14 years of age and pregnant. What other information would you need (i.e. physiological, environmental, social, emotional) to adequately counsel her regarding nutrition for an optimal pregnancy?
3. Obtain 5-day food records from three adolescents. Assess the records in terms of frequency of eating, meals skipped, types of snacks chosen, times of day eaten, and location eaten. How do these data compare with the NFCS reports?
4. Perform a fitness test on an overweight adolescent. Working with the individual, design a program of appropriate aerobic activities to maintain the training heart rate.
5. Prepare a 40-minute talk on eating disorders for a high school health class; include the concepts of nourishment, activities, and feelings.
6. Review several magazines popular with teenagers and young adults. What is the

focus of the health-nutrition-diet articles? What image(s) do the advertisements convey?

7. Prepare a talk for a wrestling team and coach regarding the critical nutritional factors needed for both good health and optimal performance.

REFERENCES

1. Height and weight of youth 12-17 years, Vital and Health Statistics, Series 11, No. 124, Washington D.C., 1973, Department of Health, Education and Welfare, U.S. Government Printing Office.
2. McMahon, B.: Age at menarche, DHEW Pub. No. (HRA) 74-1615, Supt. of Documents, Washington, D.C., 1973, U.S. Government Printing Office.
3. Frisch, R.E.: Critical weight at menarche, initiation of the adolescent growth spurt, and control of puberty. In Grumbach, M., Grave, G., and Mayer, F., editors: Control of the onset of puberty, New York, 1974, John Wiley & Sons, Inc.
4. Vandenbroucke, J.P., van Laar, A., and Valkenburg, H.A.: Synergy between thinness and intensive sports activity in delaying menarche, Br. Med. J. 284:1907, 1982.
5. Ellison, P.: Skeletal growth, fatness, and menarcheal age: a comparison of two hypotheses, Hum. Biol. 54:269, 1982.
6. Tanner, J.M.: Growth at adolescence, ed. 2, Oxford 1962, Blackwell Scientific Publications, Ltd.
7. Garn, S.M., and Wagner, B.: The adolescent growth of the skeletal mass and its implications to mineral requirements. In Herald, F.P., editor: Adolescent nutrition and growth, New York, 1969, Meredith Corp.
8. Wyshak, G., and Frisch, R.E.: Evidence for a secular trend in age of menarche, N. Engl. J. Med. 306:1033, 1982.
9. Greulich, W.W.: Some secular changes in the growth of American-born and native Japanese children, Am. J. Phys. Anthropol. 45:553, 1976.
10. Tanner, J.M.: Issues and advances in adolescent growth and development, J. Adol. Health Care 8:470, 1987.
11. Food and Nutrition Board: Recommended dietary allowances, ed. 9, Washington, D.C., 1980, National Academy of Sciences, National Research Council.
12. Heald, F.P., Remmell, P.S., and Mayer, J.: Caloric, protein, and fat intakes of children and adolescents. In Heald, F.P., editor: Adolescent nutrition and growth, New York, 1969, Meredith Corp.
13. Hampton, M.C., and others: Caloric and nutrient intake of teenagers, J. Am. Diet. Assoc. 50:385, 1967.
14. Beal, V.A.: Nutritional intake. In McCammon, R.W., editor: Human growth and development, Springfield, Ill., 1970, Charles C. Thomas, Publisher.
15. Johnston, J.A.: Protein requirements of adolescents, Ann. N.Y. Acad. Sci. 69:881, 1958.
16. Hegsted, D.M.: Current knowledge of energy, fat, protein, and amino acids needs of adolescents. In McKigney, J., and Munro, H., editors: Nutrient requirements in adolescence, Cambridge, Mass., 1976, MIT Press.
17. Report of a Joint FAO/WHO Ad Hoc Expert Committee: Energy and protein requirements, World Health Organization Technical Series No. 522, FAO Nutr. Meet. Ser. No. 52, Geneva, 1973, World Health Organization.
18. Matkovic, V., and others: Influence of calcium on peak bone mass: a pilot study, J. Bone Min. Res. 1(Suppl 1): Abstract no. 168, 1986.
19. Abraham, S., Lowenstein, F.W., and Johnson, C.L. Preliminary findings of the first health and nutrition examination survey. United States, 1971-1972: Dietary intake and biochemical findings, Washington D.C., 1974, Department of Health, Education and Welfare.
20. Bowering, J., Sanchez, A.M., and Irwin, M.I.: A conspectus of research on iron requirements of man, J. Nutr. 106:985, 1976.
21. Daniel, W.A.: Hematocrit: maturity relationship in adolescence, Pediatrics 52:388, 1973.
22. Daniel, W.A., Gaines, E.G., and Bennett, D.L.: Iron intake and transferrin saturation in adolescents, J. Pediatr. 86:288, 1975.
23. Prasad, A.S., Halstad, J.A., and Nadimi, M.: Syndrome of iron deficiency, dwarfism, and geophagia, Am. J. Med. 31:532, 1961.
24. Greenwood, C.T. and Richardson, D.P.: Nutrition during adolescence, World Rev. Nutr. Diet. 33:1, 1979.
25. Sloane, B.A., Gibbons, C.C., and Hegsted, M.: Evaluation of zinc and copper nutritional status and effects upon growth of southern adolescent females, Am. J. clin. Nutr. 42:235, 1985.
26. Mahan, L.K., and Rosebrough, R.H.: Nutritional requirements and nutritional status assessment in adolescence. In Mahan, L.K., and Rees, J.M.: Nutrition in adolescence, St. Louis, 1984, The C.V. Mosby Co.
27. Clark, A.J., Mossholder, S., and Gates, R.: Folacin status in adolescent females, Am. J. Clin. Nutr. 46:302, 1987.

28. Daniel, W.A., Gaines, E.G., and Bennett, D.L.: Dietary intakes and plasma concentrations of folate in healthy adolescents, Am. J. Clin. Nutr. 28:363, 1975.

29. Huenemann, R.L., and others: A longitudinal study of gross body composition and body conformation and their association with food and activity in a teenage population: views of teenage subjects on body conformation, food and activity, Am. J. Clin. Nutr. 18:325, 1966.

30. Dwyer, J., and others: Adolescent attitudes toward weight and appearance, J. Nutr. Educ. 1(2):14, 1969.

31. Haugen, D.L.: The relationship of family meals to food habits and attitudes of youth in Minnesota, plan B, master's paper, Minneapolis, 1981, University of Minnesota.

32. Hinton, M.A., and others: Eating behavior and dietary intake of girls 12- to 14-years-old, J. Am. Diet. Assoc. 43:223, 1963.

33. Story, M.: Adolescent life-style and eating behavior. In Mahan, L.K., and Rees, J.M.: Nutrition in adolescence, St. Louis, 1984, The C.V. Mosby Co.

34. Santrock, J.W.: Adolescence, Dubuque, Iowa, 1981, Wm. C. Brown Group.

35. Ruben, A.M.: Television usage, attitudes, and viewing behaviors of children and adolescents, J. Commun. 21:355, 1977.

36. Kaufman, L.: Prime-time nutrition, J. Commun. 30:37, 1980.

37. Way, W.L.: Food-related behaviors on prime-time television, J. Nutr. Educ. 15:205, 1983.

38. Parham, E.S., Frigo, V.L., and Perkins, A.H.: Weight control as portrayed in popular magazines, J. Nutr. Educ. 14:153, 1982.

39. MacDonald, L.A., Wearring, G.A., and Moase, O.: Factors affecting the dietary quality of adolescent girls, J. Am. Diet. Assoc. 82:260, 1983.

40. Huenemann, R.L., and others: Food and eating practices of teenagers, J. Am. Diet. Assoc. 53:17, 1968.

41. Science and Education Administration: Nationwide Food Consumption Survey, 1977-1978, Preliminary Rep. No. 2, Food and nutrient intakes of individuals in 1 day in the U.S., Spring, 1977, Hyattsville, Md., 1980, U.S. Department of Agriculture.

42. Pao, E.M.: Eating patterns and food frequencies of children in the United States, Hyattsville, Md., 1980, U.S. Department of Agriculture, Human Nutrition, Science and Education Administration, Consumer Nutrition Center.

43. Thomas, J.A., and Call, D.L.: Eating between meals: a nutrition problem among teenagers? Nutr. Rev. 31:137, 1973.

44. McNutt, K.W., and McNutt, D.R.: Nutrition and food choices, Chicago, 1978, Science Research Associates, Inc.

45. Kintner, M., Boss, P.G., and Johnson, N.: The relationship between dysfunctional family environmentals and family member food intake, J. Marriage Fam. 43:633, 1981.

46. Bruch, H.: Eating disorders, New York, 1973, Basic Books, Inc., Publishers.

47. Minuchin, S., Rosman, B.L., and Baker, L.: Psychosomatic families: anorexia nervosa in context, Cambridge, Mass., 1978, Harvard University Press.

48. Rees, J.M.: Eating disorders. In Mahan, L.K., and Rees, J.M.: Nutrition in adolescence, St. Louis, 1984, The C.V. Mosby Co.

49. Gortmaker, S.L., and others: Increasing pediatric obesity in the United States, Am. J. Dis. Child. 141:535, 1987.

50. Abraham, S., and Nordsieck, M.: Relationship of excess weight in children and adults, Public Health Rep. 75:263, 1960.

51. Raymond, C.A.: Obesity many disorders; causes sought in genes, neurochemistry, psychology, J. A. M. A. 256:2301, 1986.

52. Keesey, R.E.: A set-point analysis of the regulation of body weight. In Stunkard, A.J., editor: Obesity, Philadelphia, 1980, W.B. Saunders Co.

53. Tobias, A.L., and Gordon, J.B.: Social consequences of obesity, J. Am. Diet. Assoc. 76:338, 1980.

54. Bullen, B.A., Reed, R.B., and Mayer, J.: Physical activity of obese and nonobese adolescent girls appraised by motion picture sampling. Am. J. Clin. Nutr. 14:211, 1964.

55. Stunkard, A.J., and Burt, V.: Obesity and the body image. II. Age at onset of disturbances in the body, Am. J. Psychiatry 123:1443, 1967.

56. Dietz, W.H.: Childhood and adolescent obesity. In Frankle, R.T. and Yang, editors: Obesity and weight control. The health professional's guide to understanding and treatment, Rockville, 1988, Aspen Publishers, Inc.

57. Coates, T.J., and Thoresen, C.E.: Treating obesity in children and adolescents: a review, Am. J. Public Health 68:143, 1978.

58. Brownell, K.D., Kelman, J.H., and Stunkard, A.J.: Treatment of obese children with and without their mothers: changes in weight and blood pressure, Pediatrics 71:515, 1983.

59. Seltzer, C.C., and Mayer, J.: An effective weight control program in a public school system, Am. J. Public Health 60:679, 1970.

60. Christakis, G., and others: Effect of a combined nutrition education and physical fitness program on the

weight status of obese high school boys, Fed. Proc. 25:15, 1966.

61. Crisp, A.H.: Anorexia nervosa: let me be, New York, 1980, Grune & Stratton, Inc.

62. Halmi, K.A., and others: Pretreatment evaluation in anorexia nervosa. In Vigersky, R.A., editor: Anorexia nervosa, New York, 1977, Raven Press.

63. Pugliese, M.T., and others: Fear of obesity: a cause of short stature and delayed puberty, N. Engl. J. Med. 309:513, 1983.

64. Bruch, H.: Perils of behavior modification in treatment of anorexia nervosa, J.A.M.A. 230:1419, 1974.

65. Rosman, B., and others: A family approach to anorexia nervosa: study, treatment, and outcome. In Vigersky, R.A., editor: Anorexia nervosa, New York, 1977, Raven Press.

66. Garfinkel, P.E., and Garner, D.M.: Anorexia nervosa: a multidimensional perspective, New York, 1982, Brunner/Mazel, Inc.

67. Drossman, D.A., Ontjes, D.A., and Heizer, W.D.: Anorexia nervosa, Gastroenterology 77:1115, 1979.

68. Hsu, L.K.G., Crisp, A.H., and Harding, B.: Outcome of anorexia nervosa, Lancet 1:61, 1979.

69. Hsu, L.K.G.: Outcome of anorexia nervosa, Arch. Gen. Psychiatry 37:1041, 1980.

70. Halmi, K.A., Falk, J.R., and Schwartz, E.: Binge eating and vomiting: a survey of a college population, Psychol. Med. 11:697, 1981.

71. Johnson, C.L., and others: Incidence and correlates of bulimic behavior in a female high school population, J. Youth Adolesc. 13:6, 1984.

72. Garner, D.M., Garfinkel, P.E., and O'Shaughnessy, M.: Clinical and psychometric comparison between bulimia in anorexia nervosa and bulimia in normal weight women. In: Understanding anorexia nervosa and bulimia, Report of the fourth Ross conference on medical research, Columbus, Ohio, 1983, Ross Laboratories.

73. Harris, R.T.: Bulimarexia and related serious eating disorders with medical complications, Ann. Intern. Med. 97:800, 1983.

74. White, W.C., and Boskind-White, M.: An experimental- behavioral approach to the treatment of bulimarexia, Psychother. Theory Res. Pract. 18:501, 1981.

75. Willard, S.G., Anding, R.G., and Winstead, D.K.: Nutritional counseling as an adjunct to psychotherapy in bulimia treatment, Psychosomatics 24:545, 1983.

76. Story, M.: Nutritional management and dietary treatment of bulimia, J. Am. Diet. Assoc. 86:517, 1986.

77. Fairburn, C.: A cognitive behavioral approach to the treatment of bulimia, Psychol. Med. 11:707, 1981.

78. National Center for Health Statistics: Weight by height and age for adults 18-74 years; United States. Vital and health statistics. Series 11, No. 208, Health Services and Mental Health Administration, Washington, D.C., 1979, U.S. Government Printing Office.

79. McAnarney, E.R.: Adolescent pregnancy and childbearing: new data, new challenges, Pediatrics, 75:973, 1985.

80. Committee on Adolescence, American Academy of Pediatrics: Statement on teenage pregancy, Pediatrics 63:795, 1979.

81. Zlatnik, F.J., and Burmeister, L.F.: Low "gynecologic age": an obstetric risk factor, Am. J. Obstet. Gynecol. 128:183, 1977.

82. Zuckerman, B., and others: Neonatal outcome: Is adolescent pregnancy a risk factor?, Pediatrics 71:489, 1983.

83. Garn, S.M., and others: Are pregnant teenagers still in rapid growth? Am. J. Dis. Child. 138:32, 1984.

84. Worthington-Roberts, B.S., and Rees, J.M.: Nutritional needs of the pregnant adolescent. In Worthington-Roberts, B.S., Vermeesch, J., and Williams, S.R., editors: Nutrition in Pregnancy and lactation, ed. 3, St. Louis, 1985, Times Mirror/Mosby Co.

85. Meserole, L.P., and others: Prenatal weight gain and postpartum weight loss patterns in adolescents, J. Adolesc. Health Care 5:21, 1984.

86. Endres, J., and others: Older pregnant women and adolescents: Nutrition data after enrollment in WIC, J. Am. Diet. Assoc. 87:1011, 1987.

87. Brown, R.T., and others: Iron status of adolescent female athletes, J. Adolesc. Health Care 6:349, 1985.

88. Bachman, J.G., Johnston, L.D., and O'Malley, P.M.: Smoking, drinking, and drug abuse among high school students: correlates and trends, 1975-1979, Am. J. Public Health 71:59, 1981.

89. Macdonald, D.I.: Patterns of alcohol and drug use among adolescents. Pediatr. Clin. North Am. 34:275, 1987.

90. Morrissey, E.R.: Alcohol-related problems in adolescents and women, Postgrad. Med. 64:111, 1978.

91. Roe, D.A.: Alcohol and the diet, Westport, Conn., 1979, Avi Publishing Co.

92. Farrow, J.A., Rees, J.M., and Worthington-Roberts, B.S.: Health, developmental and nutritional status of adolescent alcohol and marijuana abusers, Pediatrics 79:218, 1987.

93. Connolly, G.N., and others: The reemergence of smokeless tobacco, N. Engl. J. Med. 314:1020, 1986.

94. Committee on Drugs, American Academy of Pediatrics: Marijuana, Pediatrics 65:652, 1980.

95. Brown, J.: Diet and new drugs: eating habits of some drug users, Ecol. Food Nutr. 2:21, 1973.

96. Esterly, N.B., and Furey, N.L.: Acne: current concepts, Pediatrics 62:1044, 1978.

97. Michaëlsson, G., Juhlin, L., and Vahlquist, A.: Effect of oral zinc and vitamin A in acne, Arch. Dermatol. 113:31, 1977.

98. Robinson, N.M., and Robinson, H.B.: The mentally retarded child, ed. 2, St. Louis, 1976, McGraw-Hill Book Co.

99. Rees, J.M.: Nutritional counseling for adolescents. In Mahan, L.K., and Rees, J.M.: Nutrition in adolescence, St. Louis, 1984, The C.V. Mosby Co.

100. Frankle, R.T., and others: The door, a center of alternatives: the nutritionist in a free clinic for adolescents, J. Am. Diet. Assoc. 63:269, 1973.

101. Leverton, R.M.: The paradox of teenage nutrition, J. Am. Diet. Assoc. 53:13, 1968.

102. Mapes, M.C.: Gulp: an alternate method for reaching teens, J. Nutr. Educ. 9:12, 1977.

103. Alexson, J.M., and DelCampo, D.S.: Improving teenagers' nutrition knowledge through the mass media, J. Nutr. Educ. 10:30, 1978.

104. Wodarski, L.A., and others: Teaching nutrition by teams-games-tournaments, J. Nutr. Educ. 12:61, 1980.

9

Vegetarian Diets for Children

Cristine M. Trahms

OBJECTIVES

After studying this chapter, the student should:

1. Be aware of commonly reported health advantages to following a vegetarian food pattern.

2. Be aware of the effect of vegetarian and vegan food patterns on the nutritional status and growth of infants and children.

3. Know how to combine foods to provide adequate protein for children who follow vegetarian food patterns.

4. Know nutritional and growth parameters that should be monitored for children who follow vegetarian food patterns.

5. Know appropriate ways to counsel children and families who follow vegetarian food patterns.

Using plant foods as the primary source of nutrients in the food pattern is not a new concept, but is a fairly recent phenomenon in the United States.

In the past many religious groups have strongly advocated the importance of a meat-free food pattern, and this practice continues today. Traditionally, religious groups chose to be vegetarian for reasons of moral purity or food sanitation. The general populations of many countries have also long been vegetarian or near vegetarian, not necessarily by choice but because of limited food availability. The availability of food choices and the adequacy of the total food supply are often not considered when the adequacy of a vegetarian food pattern is discussed. The practice of eating meat does not inherently ensure good health, just as the practice of not eating meat does not ensure poor health. The interrelationships of nutrition, health, social mores, and food choices are very complex. The exclusion of one food source or food group does not necessarily swing the pendulum of health or nutritional adequacy in either the positive or the negative direction. Therefore when discussing vegetarianism—the concept of non–meat eating—one must consider other factors carefully.

Generally, a vegetarian is considered an individual who chooses to not eat meat, poultry, or fish, and a vegan (pure vegetarian) is an individual who chooses to not eat any animal products at all. Other definitions frequently used divide vegetarians into subsets based upon specific protein food choices. For example: a lacto-vegetarian is a person who drinks milk; a lacto-ovo-vegetarian is a person who chooses to use milk and eggs; and a pesco-vegetarian is a person who chooses to eat milk, eggs, and fish. However, individuals seldom describe themselves in these terms, and people do not base their food choices or lifestyles on tidy categories. Therefore many people who call themselves vegetarians may in fact eat meat as often as once a week or twice a month. On the other hand, people may choose extremely rigid food patterns that forbid them yeast and honey, or they may avoid the use of wool or leather because they are considered animal products. In this chapter a vegetarian is considered a person who has chosen to omit meat, poultry, and fish from his or her food intake pattern, and a vegan is considered a person who has chosen to eat only plant foods (i.e., no animal products). Individuals seldom make their personal food choices based on the accepted categories. It seems, then, most reasonable to work with individuals to evaluate foods as sources of nutrients rather than to force labels on individual food patterns. This method of evaluation also provides a reasonable basis for nutrition education.

HEALTH ADVANTAGES AND DISADVANTAGES

Recent work with population subgroups has indicated that there are health advantages to the vegetarian food pattern. Among the health advantages of a non-meat food pattern are positive decreases in cholesterol, triglycerides, and other blood lipid constituents.[1-3] Although there is disagreement on the specific dietary factors that support these changes, the vegetarian food pattern, both in long-term evaluations and in short-term cross-over studies, appears to exert a positive effect on blood lipids. A vegetarian food pattern also seems to reduce hypertension;[2, 4-6] and a decreased incidence of osteoporosis,[7] gallstones,[8] and diabetes[9] has been noted.

Much of this research has centered on adults in industrialized countries and specialized subgroups of the population that have made other life-style changes in addition to omitting meat from their food patterns. Life-style factors, such as abstinence from smoking and alcohol, great interest in exercise, or seclusion from the rest of society, must be considered as potential intervening or modifying variables for religious subgroups.

In the United States, a recent survey indicated that vegetarians come from relatively affluent and educated families, that the food patterns of more than half of those interviewed could be described as lacto-ovo-vegetarian, and that less than 10% adhered to a vegan food pattern.[10] Only 11% of those interviewed had parents who were also vegetarian, but most expected their own children to continue the vegetarian food pattern. About one fourth of the vegetarians were affiliated with traditional religious groups.

Much of the work that points out the disadvantages of a vegetarian food pattern has been conducted in third world countries, where the total amount of food and food choices available are very limited. Thus, many of these people would probably not choose to be vegetarians, but they have no alternative. Energy deficit and lack of food to provide specific nutrients must be considered when interpreting these reports. The negative impact of a vegetarian food pattern has also been reported in this country. Often young adults become overzealous in following specific teachings or omitting specific foodstuffs from their food patterns. One classic example of overzealousness is the Zen macrobiotic followers, who felt that tea and brown rice were the way to ultimate purity of body and soul. Even the leaders of the group warned against this extreme practice and encouraged a more moderate food intake pattern that included grains, legumes, fruits, and vegetables. The health disadvantages of the vegetarian food pattern have been documented primarily among those people who have chosen the vegan (pure vegetarian) food pattern. In general, the more restricted the pattern of food choices, the more likely that individual is to be at high nutritional risk. (The same can be said for popular weight-reduction formats.) Young children and pregnant women, who are generally considered to be at high nutritional risk, are thought to be particularly vulnerable to food intake patterns that limit the quantity or the kinds of food for consumption.

INDIVIDUALS WITH SPECIAL NEEDS

Pregnant Women

In the few sketchy reports on the outcome of the pregnancies of women who were vegans or vegetarians, there appear to be no detrimental effects to the mother or the offspring if the mother chooses a food pattern that provides the required nutrients in appropriate quantities to support the pregnancy. Hardinge and Stare[11] included several pregnant vegetarian women in one of their early nutritional status reports. The food intake patterns and calculated nutrient intakes were grouped with those of other adults, but they appeared adequate. The infants were reported to be of normal birth weight. Thomas, Ellis, and Diggory[12] reported on the health of vegans during pregnancy, comparing 14 vegans (28 pregnancies) and 18 control subjects (41 pregnancies). There were no differences in rates of stillbirths, toxemia, or anemia between the groups. There were also no differences in the birth weights of the infants. Only 3% of the women who were vegan took iron supplements during pregnancy. The vegan women also breast-fed their infants more frequently and for longer periods than did the control mothers. No data on weight gain during pregnancy were reported. Another report found no differences in birth weights between the vegetarian infants (both extensive and limited food group avoidances) and the control infants.[13]

Infants

It has been well documented that infants can indeed grow normally on food patterns comprised entirely of cereal proteins if the food patterns are carefully formulated. Knapp and others[14] rehabilitated 102 malnourished male infants 5 to 14 months of age and then offered nine different formulations that were isocaloric (100 kcal/kg) and contained 2 gm of protein/kg. The infants fed soybean, rice, cottonseed, cottonseed and rice, cottonseed and peanut, rice and soybean, soybean and peanut, or cow's milk formulas all demonstrated equivalent nitrogen retention. In crossover studies, the infants fed wheat plus lysine, rice and cottonseed, and peanut and rice formulas grew at rates equivalent to those of infants fed cow's milk. The infants fed only peanut formulas did not retain as much nitrogen as did the infants fed cow's milk, and the infants fed only rice formulas did not grow as well as did the infants fed cow's milk. It should also be noted that although the growth curves were equivalent, the infants fed cow's milk food patterns demonstrated smoother growth curves.

Preschool Children

Recent reports have indicated that deficits in height and weight may occur among young children on vegan diets in the United States. Young vegan children were significantly shorter ($p < 0.001$) and lighter ($p < 0.005$) than were age- and sex-matched vegetarian children and control children.[15] Dwyer and others[16] suggested an environmental influence on the size of young children.

When adjusted for midparental height, 61% of 119 preschool vegetarian children were less than the 20th percentile for height. In another report, 72 white children less than 5 years of age living at home were longitudinally measured using a standardized technique.[13] Thirty-four children had parents who consumed macrobiotic food patterns, 12 were members of yoga groups, 12 were Seventh-Day Adventists, and 14 had no group affiliation. Almost all (96%) of the children had been or were still being breast-fed. The vegetarian children younger than 2 years of age showed mean weight and length velocities that were lower than the Harvard norms, whereas those of the older vegetarian children were comparable with the Harvard norms. This pattern of growth was also reported for Dutch children.[17]

School-Age Children

Recently, the growth patterns of 142 vegetarian and 228 nonvegetarian schoolchildren were compared.[18] The two groups of children demonstrated differing growth patterns. It appeared that the more limiting the food choices, the more growth was affected. In general, length was more affected than weight although measurements were generally within normal limits. Evaluation of food intakes suggested that protein intakes for these children were adequate and energy intakes were less than the accepted recommendations. It would appear that, again, the availability of adequate nutrients to the individual child was a more significant factor than the beliefs of the parents and the concommitant prescribed food pattern. A summary of recent reported growth patterns of vegetarian children is shown in Table 9-1.

Nutrients of Concern

Young children consuming food patterns consisting only of plant foods seem to be at greater risk for nutritional inadequacies related to intakes of protein, calcium, total energy, essential fatty acids, riboflavin, iron, zinc, and vitamins B_{12} and D. Absorption of nutrients may also be a problem if the fiber content of

the infant's food pattern is high. Very high fiber intakes are believed to decrease intestinal transit time and bind iron, calcium, zinc, and other trace metals. These limitations in nutrient availability may be in part related to family food choice patterns and in part to the individual preferences of the child who may or may not eat the foods that are offered. An example of nutritional risk caused by limited food choices is the young child who was offered a grain beverage called kokoh consisting of rice, sesame seeds, and oats in a reasonable protein complement. However, the quantities offered to the child or that the child was willing to take did not provide adequate nutrients to support normal growth. In some cases, the deficiencies were severe and prolonged enough to cause death.[22] The young infant being exclusively breast-fed by a mother who has a marginal or definite vitamin B_{12} deficiency may have an increased risk of deficiency. Older children who consume diets severely restricted in animal foods may also be at risk if the choices of foods available to them are severely restricted and exclude all animal foods.

Young children in developing countries who are breast-fed but whose food patterns are not supplemented with additional foods may suffer adverse nutritional effects after 4 to 6 months of age, especially if they are weaned to a cereal gruel or other form of predominantly vegan food pattern. However, in these cases it must be remembered that other factors (e.g., poor sanitation and poor health care) may be important variables.

Reports of cases in the Unites States describe several cases of kwashiorkor among infants whose parents were vegetarian,[23] and poor weight gain in children fed cereal-base formulas.[24, 25] The infants were fed restricted quantities of kokoh and limited quantities of other foods. The children were rehabilitated on appropriate vegetarian or near vegetarian food patterns within a few months. In all of these reports, the number of children evaluated was

Table 9-1   Selected reported weight and height of vegetarian children

Report (Ref. No.)	No. of Subjects	Mean Age (Yr)	Growth Standard	Food Pattern	Size of Children
Brown, Bergen[19]	10	1–6	—	Zen macrobiotic (vegan)	Mean weight and height = 40%
Fulton et al.[20]	48	3.8	Hanes	"The Farm" Vegan	Mean height and weight less than mean of Hanes; height more affected; 83%had height less than 50th Percentile
Shull et al.[13]	72	< 5	Harvard	Vegetarian	Greater than 2 years of age subjects = control for weight and height; less than 2 years of age subjects = shorter, lighter than control
				Macrobiotic (vegan)	Slightly lower size attainment than vegan (not significant)
Dwyer et al.[21]	39	4	NCHS	Vegetarian	Height, weight within normal limits
Dwyer et al.[16]	119	2.33	Harvard	Vegetarian extensive vs. limited food group avoidances	Adjusted for mid-parent height, 61% = < 10th percentile, more pronounced with increased avoidances
van Staveren et al.[17]	92	1–3	Dutch Standards	Vegetarian macrobiotic (vegan)	Height and weight for age shorter and lighter; weight for length ok

small, and long-term observations on growth or nutrient intake were not made, but the questions these reports raise are disturbing.

Nutrient Intakes

Calculation of nutrient intakes of preschool children has shown that children whose food patterns excluded all animal products consumed significantly less total protein, fat, calcium, and riboflavin (p < 0.01) than did vegetarian children and control children.[26] Intakes of iron and calcium were also calculated at lower than acceptable levels. Ten children on Zen macrobiotic diets were described as being at the 40th percentile for height and weight.[19] Nutrient intakes were calculated as less than optimal, that is, less than 60% of the recommended dietary allowance for most nutrients except calcium and riboflavin, which were even lower.

Recently, the intakes of a small number of children (mean age of 4 years) consuming different types of vegetarian food patterns were evaluated. The findings suggested that these food patterns met the dietary goals for the United States for carbohydrate, fat, protein, sodium, and cholesterol. Some children had intakes limited in iron and in vitamins D and B$_{12}$.[21]

Recent reports indicate that infants and preschool children may also be at risk for vitamin D and B$_{12}$ deficiency if they are consuming food patterns restricted in animal products.

Vitamin D deficiency, rickets, and vitamin B$_{12}$ deficiency have been reported in breast-fed infants of vegan and vegetarian mothers. All of the infants had hypocalcemia and three fourths had *tetany* or convulsions.[27] Case reports cite growth failure and other clinical signs of vitamin B$_{12}$ deficiency in infants who were breast-fed by vegan women.[28, 29] Apparently, these infants required more vitamin D and B$_{12}$ than could be supplied by breast-milk of women with marginal vitamin D and B$_{12}$ stores. An increase in clinical identification of rickets has recently been reported in older infants[30] who demonstrated the classic symptoms: growth failure, listlessness, delayed motor development, and abnormal gait. Bone deformity was evident on further investigation. The children received little or no cow's milk or formula and no vitamin D supplements. Not all of the children were vegetarian or vegan. However, healing occurred with dietary changes in all cases. Of 52 children on macrobiotic food patterns 88% had vitamin D intakes of less than 100 IU/day[31] compared with vegetarian children, of whom only 18% had vitamin D intakes this low. Although five children had pathological findings related to bone mineralization, roentegenograms did not indicate rickets. Clinically, only three children demonstrated signs (bowed legs) that could possibly be attributed to vitamin D deficiency. The serum calcium and serum phosphorous levels of both the children on macrobiotic food patterns and the vegetarian children were within normal limits. Eight of the children on mac-

robiotic food patterns and two of the vegetarian children had elevated serum alkaline phosphatase levels. Calcium deficiency and osteomalacia in the presence of an adequate intake of protein and energy[32] further emphasize the need to evaluate all of the nutrient components of a food pattern.

The status of zinc nutriture in these children has not been evaluated to date. It would seem that zinc may be a limiting nutrient in some very restricted food patterns. A summary of reported nutrient intakes of vegetarian children is shown in Table 9-2.

Factors Influencing the Intakes of Young Children

The young child depends on caregivers to provide adequate foods as sources of nutrients. The adequacy of nutrient intake may also be affected by food preferences, which are demonstrated early in life. The older infant and toddler with rigid food preferences may be at risk for deficits of protein, energy, calcium, iron, zinc, vitamin D and vitamin B$_{12}$ despite adequate food availability.

The young child on a food intake pattern comprised totally or primarily of plant proteins may have problems obtaining an adequate intake of energy if the volume of food required to meet energy needs is large. Often a legume milk (commercially prepared or home prepared with a sufficient energy concentration) will provide an easily ingested volume of protein, energy, and other nutrients for the young child.

In addition to volume, texture may also influence the adequacy of the intake of the young child on a vegetarian food pattern. Many foods that contain adequate quantities of protein and are rich sources of nutrients must be texture modified for the young child; for instance, beans must be well cooked and mashed or pureed. Even rice must be mixed with liquid and mashed for the infant. The young child may not chew whole grain breads well, and consequently the nutrients may not

Table 9-2 Selected reported mean nutrient intakes of vegetarian children

Report (Ref. No.)	No. of Subjects	Mean Age (Yr)	Food Pattern	Energy (kcal)	Protein (gm)	Calcium (mg)	Iron (mg)	Vit D (µg)	Vit B12 (mcg)	Fiber (gm)
Brown, Bergen[19]	10	1–6	Zen macro-biotic (vegan)	1002–1267	34.4–41	359–402	0.1–11.9	—	—	—
Fulton et al.[20]	48	3–8	"The Farm" vegan, boys	1580–2141	52–62	323–426	18–25	—	10.8–19.2	—
			"The Farm" vegan, girls	1509–2249	49–65	296–340	14–16	—	10.9–15.8	—
Dwyer et al.[21]	39	4	Vegetarian	103/kg	3.3/kg	685	12–16	51–395 IU (1.3–9.9 µg)	0.6–4.4	—
van Staveren et al.[17]	92	1–3	Vegetarian	1020 (84–98/kg)	36 (2.8–3.5/kg)	783	7.1	0.5 µg	—	16
			Macrobiotic (vegan)	1010 (85–92/kg)	31 (2.2–3.3/kg)	345	10.8	0.3 µg	—	24.9
RDA, 1980*		1–3		1300	23	800	10–15	10 µg (400 IU)	2.0–3.0	—
		4–6		1700	30	800				

*Recommended Dietary Allowances, 9th ed., National Academy of Sciences, 1980.

be well absorbed. The same is true for nuts, seeds, dried fruits and some vegetables.

PROTEIN NEEDS OF YOUNG CHILDREN

Protein utilization is affected by a variety of factors, including quality and quantity of ingested protein, percent of calories as fat, total energy intake, biological variation of the individual, and growth and maintenance needs (e.g., age and nutritional state). Calculating protein utilization, and consequently protein needs, is a complex undertaking because many of the relationships are not clearly defined or are extremely difficult to measure.

Much work is being done to document protein utilization among young children and to evaluate the ability of vegetable protein food patterns to maintain growth and nitrogen balance for young children or to rehabilitate them from malnutrition or illness. The infectious process is a confounding variable that is difficult to quantitate but affects the utilization of nutrients.

Many combinations of grain and legume proteins have been evaluated in terms of maintenance of nutritional health or the rehabilitation of malnourished children in developing countries. Evaluation of a macaroni product containing 60% corn (maize), 30% defatted soy flour, and 10% wheat germ indicated nutritional recuperation in both the experimental and control groups of children.[33]

A CSM (68% corn, 28% defatted soy flour, 5% nonfat dry milk) infant food demonstrated that a small percentage of protein from animal foods enhances the value of a food product as a sole source of nutrients for young infants. This formulation promoted nitrogen retention similar to that of casein.[34]

A soybean protein textured food (soy protein isolate) with added egg albumin and wheat gluten has a protein quality of about 80% of that of milk. Children required 138 mg of nitrogen from the soy food as compared with 97 mg of nitrogen from milk to maintain

nitrogen equilibrium.[35] This food was readily accepted by the children.

Fat absorption in young children depends on levels of dietary protein intake.[36] Very low protein intakes even with adequate energy intakes are detrimental to maximum fat absorption and may ultimately increase total energy requirements. Children on diets containing 5% or more of total calories as protein (FAO/WHO recommendation) showed improvement of apparent fat absorption as protein intakes increased.

All this information on relative biological value or utilization of protein is interesting, but in this country few if any children must exist on a single food that, in turn, must supply all or the majority of nutrients. The young formula-fed infant is the exception. Formulations of infant food must be done very carefully to meet the rigorous nutrient requirements to support normal growth and development.

Choosing Protein Foods for Young Children

It is important that the protein sources offered to children be appropriately combined so that the pattern of amino acid intake will be adequate to support normal growth and development. Careful attention to combining plant proteins in the best proportion for optimal utilization is a must. Appetites of young children fluctuate widely on a day-to-day basis, making it important that all foods eaten provide nutrients rather than only energy.

In combining plant proteins, not only must foods that supplement the most limiting amino acids of each other be combined, but they should be combined in specific proportion for the most efficient utilization of protein. The ratio is specific for each combination. Examples of satisfactory combinations include the following: (1) 3/4 cup of dry rice with 1/4 cup of dry beans; (2) 3/4 cup of dry rice with 1 cup milk or 1/4 cup of milk powder and (3) 3 1/4 cup of wheat flour with 1/4 cup of soy grits and 1/2 cup of sesame seeds. Complementation of proteins is also a useful and practical way to enhance the value of foods readily accepted by young children.

One can easily accomplish this by adding a small amount of soy grits while oatmeal is being cooked or by adding wheat germ, soy flour, or dry milk to muffins, pancakes, cookies, and breads. The simple method called the Cornell Triple Rich Flour Formula developed at Cornell University complements the proteins of baked products. According to this formula, before any flour is put into the measuring cup the following should be measured into the bottom of the cup: 1 tbsp of soy flour, 1 tbsp of dry milk, and 1tsp of wheat germ. The cup is then filled with flour.

Preschool children are in the process of developing their individual food patterns and are not amenable to eating foods because they are good protein sources. It is often difficult to persuade them to eat foods in a precise proportional relationship or to eat a sufficient volume of legumes, grains, seeds, and nuts in forms that they can easily digest. Therefore it is difficult to provide sufficient quality and quantity of proteins and an adequate amount of calories to support adequate growth for young children without dairy foods or eggs in their food patterns.[26]

ENERGY NEEDS OF YOUNG VEGETARIAN CHILDREN

It is possible that the volume of food required to meet the energy needs of young children may interfere with adequate intakes. This is especially true for those children who are offered foods without texture modification. In most studies, the foods offered to children were texture modified into beverages with constant energy per unit of volume so that the children could easily ingest the required volume to meet energy needs. This research strategy may not be appropriate for the practical application of foods as sources of nutrients for this age group.

A model proposed by Payne[37] suggests that an adequate, safe protein/energy ratio in young children is close to 5%. Since most cereal grains seem to provide protein levels close to this, energy deficit rather than protein deficit may be the cause of protein/energy malnutrition in children in developing countries.

Energy intake should be adequate to promote growth in channel on acceptable growth charts. As for any child, parental size should be considered when evaluating the growth of children.

MEETING THE NUTRIENT NEEDS OF YOUNG VEGETARIAN CHILDREN

Protein and energy needs of young children must be stated as a dyad to provide guidelines for the relative adequacy of these dietary components. This dyad should include some factors for individual variation in energy, for the possibility that these needs may to some degree be independent of protein needs, and for the degree of adaptation of expenditure to suit intake or vice versa. Examples of recorded food intakes of vegan, vegetarian, and nonvegetarian children that show the variety of foods and general quantities needed to provide reasonable intakes of nutrients are given in Table 9-3.

Special attention needs to be paid to providing adequate sources of vitamins, minerals, and trace metals in the food patterns of young children. Fortified soy formulas are appropriate sources of all of the critical nutrients.

Although the information on zinc and the intakes of children is limited, it is known that zinc intakes are likely to be inadequate in a vegan food pattern because animal foods are primary sources of zinc. Phytate and fiber in cereals and vegetables are also known to bind zinc and decrease its availability. It has been suggested that foods highest in zinc and lowest in fiber, such as tofu (soy cheese) and hard cheeses be emphasized in the vegetarian food pattern to maintain an adequate intake of this nutrient.[38]

Table 9-3   Recorded 1-day intakes of young children

Food	Portion Size	Food	Portion Size
Child no. 1 (age 12 months) — **inadequate vegan intake**		**Child no. 3 (age 13 months)—** **vegetarian intake**	
Oatmeal, cooked	$\frac{1}{2}$ cup	Milk, whole	9 oz
Raisins	1 tsp	Cereal mixture	
Yellow squash, cooked	$\frac{1}{2}$ cup	Cornmeal, dry	$\frac{1}{4}$ cup
Apple	1 medium	Wheat germ	3 tbsp
Oatmeal, cooked	1 cup	Milk	$\frac{1}{4}$ cup
Yams, cooked	$\frac{1}{2}$ cup	Apple	1 tbsp
Pudding		Soybeans, cooked	1 cup
Apple cider	1 cup	Apricot, dried	2 halves
Arrowroot flour	1 tsp	Apple	$\frac{1}{2}$ medium
No supplements		Potato, baked	$\frac{1}{2}$ small
TOTAL ENERGY INTAKE	610 kcal	Tomato	1 small
TOTAL PROTEIN INTAKE	12 gm	Cheddar cheese, grated	$\frac{1}{4}$ cup
		Soy oil	2 tsp
Child no. 2 (age 14 months) — **better vegan intake**		Milk	9 oz
		Milk	9 oz
Kokoh (cereal mixture)	$1\frac{1}{4}$ cup	No supplements	
Rice	$\frac{1}{2}$ cup	TOTAL ENERGY INTAKE	1280 kcal
Sweet rice	$\frac{1}{4}$ cup	TOTAL PROTEIN INTAKE	66 gm
Whole oats	$\frac{1}{8}$ cup		
Sesame seeds	$\frac{1}{8}$ cup	**Child no. 4 (aged 12 months) —** **nonvegetarian intake**	
Wakame (sea weed)	$\frac{1}{2}$ tsp		
Squash	$\frac{1}{3}$ cup	Peach, canned	$\frac{1}{2}$
Whole wheat noodles	$\frac{1}{2}$ cup	Link sausage	2
Miso soup		Toast, white	$\frac{1}{2}$ slice
Miso (fermented soy)	1 tsp	Margarine	$\frac{1}{2}$ tsp
Scallions	1 tsp	Egg yolk	1
Onion	1 tsp	2% Milk	8 oz
Kokoh	$1\frac{1}{4}$ cup	2% Milk	8 oz
Nori (sea weed)	1 piece	Veal	50 gm
Cauliflower	$\frac{1}{4}$ cup	Cracker	1
Aduki beans, cooked	$\frac{1}{3}$ cup	Rice, cooked	$\frac{1}{2}$ cup
Watercress	1 sprig	Tomato	$\frac{1}{4}$ medium
Brown rice Kayu (1:5)	$1\frac{1}{4}$ cup	2% Milk	8 oz
Squash, cooked	$\frac{1}{4}$ cup	2% Milk	8 oz
Apple, baked	2 tbsp	Supplement: Poly-vi-sol	6 ml/day
Raisins	1 tsp	TOTAL ENERGY INTAKE	1020 kcal
No supplements		TOTAL PROTEIN INTAKE	58 gm
TOTAL ENERGY INTAKE	1140 kcal		
TOTAL PROTEIN INTAKE	35 gm		

Miso, wheat germ, legumes, nuts, and sprouts are also reasonable food sources of zinc.[39]

Vitamin B_{12} deficiency for the infant and young child can be avoided by ensuring adequate maternal stores during lactation and by providing sources for the young child. These sources may be fermented soy products (such as miso or tempeh), supplemented brewer's yeast, vitamin B_{12} tablets, dairy foods, or eggs.

Vitamin D needs may be met via exposure to sunlight, fortified milk or soy formula, vitamin D supplements, or cod liver oil.

Calcium is readily available from cow's milk or a soy formula. Dark leafy green vegetables and legumes are also reasonable sources. A calcium supplement may be needed if adequate food sources are not ingested.

Iron deficiency anemia is a common occurrence in childhood, regardless of food choice patterns. The most bioavailable sources of iron are muscle meats. The bioavailability of plant sources of iron is variable and less than that of heme sources.[40] However, nonheme iron bioavailability is improved if ascorbic acid-rich foods are consumed at the same meal. It is not known at what level high fiber, phytate and oxalate intakes interfere with iron absorption.

Many nutrient needs can be met by careful planning and by including foods that are equivalent sources of specific nutrients. Table 9-4 defines foods as sources of nutrients and the foods that can be exchanged to provide the equivalent nutrients. This scheme may be used not only by vegetarians but also by those who have specific food likes and dislikes or by those who for some other reason feel the need to restrict the variety of choices in their food intake patterns.

COUNSELING THE VEGETARIAN FAMILY

The word *vegetarian* has a specific nuance or value system attached to it for each person who has chosen to apply that label to himself or herself. The health care professional in the counseling role should carefully examine his or her own biases and, whether they are negative or positive, try to approach the family or household as open-mindedly as possible.

It seems reasonable that one should first ask the family to describe the foods regularly included and excluded in the family's food pattern and the individual's food pattern (see Chapter 2). A recent survey of women in Seattle indicated the importance of this approach.[41]

Table 9-4   Key nutrients to consider when choosing food patterns

If These Foods Are Excluded	Then These Nutrients Are Limited	Replace with These Foods
Meat, fish, poultry	Protein, iron, energy, zinc, folate, vitamin B_{12}, thiamine, essential fatty acids	Milk, dairy products, grains, legumes
Milk, dairy products	Protein, energy, calcium, vitamin B_{12}, vitamin D, riboflavin	Legumes, soy milk (fortified), dark green vegetables
Grains	Protein, iron, niacin, riboflavin, zinc, fiber	Legumes, dairy products
Legumes	Protein, iron, zinc, calcium, fiber	Grains, dairy products
Fruits	Vitamin A, vitamin C, fiber, folate	Vegetables
Vegetables	Vitamin A, vitamin C, fiber, folate	Fruits

Less than 50% of the persons who described themselves as vegetarians never ate meat, 30% ate meat once or twice per month, and nearly 10% ate meat as often as once per week.

Every food pattern that a person chooses has some positive aspects which should be defined and reinforced. Clinical experience indicates that a counseling and supportive role is much more effective than a directive or argumentative approach. People can, in fact, adequately meet their nutrient needs in a wide variety of ways, and the individual variability or standard deviation of needs is quite wide.

For the infant and young child linear growth and rate of weight gain can be used as indices of appropriate energy intake. The mother of an exclusively breast-fed infant should be questioned about the adequacy of here own intake and should be advised of all the usual guidelines regarding adequate fluid, protein, calcium, and energy to maintain health and support lactation.

Some provisions should be made to ensure that the breast-fed infant receives adequate supplies of iron, vitamin B_{12}, and vitamin D. Evidence[42] indicates that iron in breast-milk is well absorbed by the infant, so if the mother's diet provides adequate amounts of iron the needs of the infant should be met. Well-nourished lactating women who are following a vegetarian food pattern have adequate supplies of nutrients in their breast-milk.[43, 44] However, vitamin B_{12} may be a concern, especially if the mother's levels are low or if she has chosen a vegan food pattern. A supplement or additional food choices may be necessary to provide adequate quantities of this nutrient. Usually, if the need for the particular nutrient can be clearly documented, the parents are willing to reexamine their philosophical basis for making food choices, and a reasonable decision or compromise can be reached for the ultimate nutritional welfare of the child.

When breast-feeding is not feasible, the infant needs to receive adequate quantities of a properly prepared formula. This can be a commercial soy formula or a cow's milk formula, but it must provide adequate quantities of critical nutrients such as protein, calcium, iron, energy, and vitamins B_{12}, A, and D. It has been demonstrated that fortified soy formulas can promote normal growth and development in infants.[45] Less work has been done on evaluation of the nutrient properties of grain milks. Reports indicating poor growth in young children consuming grain milks were complicated by the inappropriate dilution and volume of milk offered to the children.[22, 24, 25]

Home-prepared infant formulas with a cow's milk or goat's milk base and supplemented with calcium, yeast, lactose, and other vitamin and mineral preparations are not advised. These types of formula are susceptible to errors in measurement and dilution; thus they put the infant at risk of excess of specific nutrients and potential renal solute problems.

Home-prepared soy milk supplemented with vitamin B_{12} can provide an appropriate base for the child who also consumes a wide variety of other foods. One family in our clinical experience prepared soy milk for the children. The soy milk was supplemented with crystalline vitamin B_{12}, and the hulls and pulp of the soy remaining after milk preparation were carefully used in mixed dishes and baked goods. Tofu was used frequently in mixed dishes. The children enjoyed all these foods and drank adequate quantities of the milk with enthusiasm, particularly if it was flavored with vanilla and served ice-cold.

Many adolescents and young adults who choose vegetarian or semivegetarian food patterns are concerned with their own health and the nutrition that is basic to it. Often their food choices are based, at least in part, on political and philosophical convictions. These people need information and supportive counseling to make sound health decisions, as well as the political or philosophical statement of their choice.

Young adolescents who are not yet emancipated from the nuclear family may use food selection as a means of establishing independence. In this situation parents must remain flexible, tolerant, and interested in the adolescent's convictions regarding food choices. When there is little understanding, the food pattern can quickly become another point of intense family conflict. It must be remembered that an unusual food pattern is not necessarily a harmful food pattern. The parents and the adolescent need guidance to discern the difference. Any direct criticism of food choices may be considered personal criticism, so counseling must be supportive. It should reinforce the positive aspects of the chosen food pattern and consider the energy and nutrient needs required for growth, development, and physical activity. Nonjudgmental discussion of alternatives and a mutual decision-making process among health care worker, adolescent, and parent can guide adolescents in making healthful and responsible food choices (Table 9-5).

In addition to the food guide (Table 9-6), the following point should be kept in mind when counseling a family that has chosen to become vegetarian: the goal of the health care professional is the same as when counsel-ing a nonvegetarian family, that is, to promote good health through reasonable food choices. Responsibilities would include the following:

1. To support the individual and the family in every positive aspect of the chosen food pattern
   a. By being nonjudgmental about the stated reasons for specific food choices
   b. By recognizing the wide variety of food choices that are appropriate to maintain good health
   c. By understanding the food taboos and food preferences and the reasons for them
2. To evaluate the food intake of a specific family member, identifying those nutrients that might be at risk of deficient intake because of food choices or food preparation methods
   a. By helping the family recognize the differing needs of infants, young children, adolescents, adults, pregnant women, and sedentary individuals
   b. By working with the individuals to identify food as sources of nutrients
3. To encourage the family members to pur-

Table 9-5 Combinations of food for vegetarian diets

Food	Ingredients
Oatmeal, cooked	$\frac{3}{4}$ cup of cooked oatmeal with 2 tsp of soy grits, $\frac{1}{3}$ cup of milk
Scalloped potatoes	$\frac{1}{2}$ cup of potatoes, $\frac{1}{2}$ cup of milk
Macaroni and cheese	$\frac{1}{2}$ cup of cooked macaroni, 3 tbsp of grated cheese
Rice pudding	$\frac{1}{2}$ cup of cooked rice, $\frac{1}{4}$ cup of milk
Peanut butter sandwich on whole wheat bread	$\frac{1}{2}$ tbsp of peanut butter, 1 slice of bread
Tortillas with beans	2 tortillas, $\frac{1}{4}$ cup of cooked beans
Whole wheat and soy muffin	2 tbsp of whole wheat flour, 1 tsp of soy flour, 1 tbsp of milk
Sesame and oatmeal cookies	1 tbsp of oatmeal, 1 tbsp of whole wheat flour, 1 $\frac{1}{2}$ tsp of sesame, $\frac{1}{2}$ tbsp of milk

Table 9-6 Vegetarian food guide

Food Group	Portion Size	Number of Portions		
		Pregnant	2 to 3 Years	4 to 6 Years
Breads, cereals, pasta	1 slice of bread $\frac{1}{3}$ cup of granola $\frac{3}{4}$ cup of cooked cereal 1 biscuit, muffin 1 tbsp of wheat germ $\frac{3}{4}$ cup of cooked rice	6	3	3
Protein foods				
Legumes, meat analogues	1 cup of cooked beans $\frac{1}{4}$ cup of peanut butter 6 oz of tofu	$\frac{3}{4}$	$\frac{1}{8}$	$\frac{1}{4}$
Nuts and seeds	3 tbsp	1	$\frac{1}{8}$	$\frac{1}{4}$
Dairy Products				
Milk	1 cup of milk, yogurt 1 oz of cheese 4 tbsp of cottage cheese	4	2-3	2-3
Eggs		$1\frac{1}{2}$	1	1
Fruits and vegetables	1 cup, raw $\frac{1}{2}$ cup, cooked $\frac{1}{2}$ cup of juice	5-6	2	3
Extra foods	No requirement (recommendation)			

Modified from Smith, E.B.: J. Nutr. Educ. 7:109, 1975.

chase foods that provide the most nutrients for the money

a. By encouraging the evaluation of foods for their nutrient content, packaging, and processing
b. By encouraging the use of simple foods, whole grains, fresh fruits, and vegetables
c. By encouraging the use of cooking methods that conserve nutrients

Summary

The more restrictive food choices become, the more difficult it is to plan a nutritionally adequate food pattern. Vegetarian food patterns that include prudently chosen plant foods and a reasonable amount of dairy foods are adequate to support normal growth and development for people of all ages, including young children and pregnant and lactating women. These recommendations are supported by a recent position paper from the American Dietetic Association,[46] as well as others.[47, 48] General recommendations to support an adequate nutritional intake for vegetarians and vegans include:

1. Use of a variety of fruits and vegetables
2. Use of whole grain breads and cereals
3. Limitation of foods that are high-energy, low-nutrient density
4. Provisions of adequate quantities of the limiting nutrients iron, calcium, folate, zinc,

and vitamin B_{12} either by appropriate food choices or fortified food supplements
5. Use of an appropriately supplemented cow's milk formula or soy formula for infants who are not breast-fed
6. Use of a suitable supplement or daily exposure to sunlight to provide adequate vitamin D.

Robertson, Flinders, and Ruppenthal[49] have compiled a helpful manual that includes nutrition information as well as recipes for those who choose nonmeat food patterns.

SUGGESTED LEARNING ACTIVITIES

1. Plan a menu for a 2-year-old vegetarian boy who weighs 10 kg. He is unwilling to consume beans of any kind. His mother is unwilling to offer more than 1 cup of milk or yogurt per day because "it causes phlegm."
2. Outline teaching objectives and a food pattern for a young woman with a 6-month-old infant who is at the 25th percentile for length and weight. The mother prefers to avoid all animal products. The infant is totally breast-fed. The mother plans to continue breast-feeding until the infant is 1 year of age.
3. Judy is a 4-year-old girl enrolled in the Head Start Program. She has been labeled "anemic" on the entrance physical examination. Her weight/stature is at the 10th percentile. Her mother is strongly opposed to all supplements. The family is vegan. Outline a plan for the family and for the classroom.
4. A mother of 2 young children (5 and 6 years of age) has recently become vegetarian and is adjusting her cooking habits and the family food pattern. Her children are picky eaters in both the variety and quantity of food they are willing to consume. She feels that they may have lost weight on the vegetarian food pattern. Suggest how she can provide appropriate intakes for her children.

REFERENCES

1. Masarei, J. R. L., and others: Vegetarian food patterns, lipids and cardiovascular risk, Aust. N. Z. J. Med. 14:400, 1984.
2. Adulla, M., and others: Nutrient intake and health status of lactovegetarians: Chemical analyses of diets using the duplicate portion sampling technique, Am. J. Clin. Nutr. 40:325, 1984.
3. Burr, M. L., and Sweetman, P. M.: Vegetarianism, dietary fiber, and mortality, Am. J. Clin, Nutr. 36:873, 1982.
4. Ophir, O., and others: Low blood pressure in vegetarians: the possible role of potassium, Am. J. Clin. Nutr. 37:755, 1983.
5. Margetts, B. M., and others: Vegetarian diet in mild hypertension: a randomised controlled trial, Br. Med. J. 293:1468, 1986.
6. Rouse, I. L. and others: Blood-pressure-lowering effect of a vegetarian diet: controlled trial in normotensive subjects, Lancet i:5, 1983.
7. Ellis, F. R., Scura, H., and Ellis, J. W.: Incidence of osteoporosis in vegetarians and omnivores, Am. J. Clin. Nutr. 25:555, 1972.
8. Pixley, F., and others: Effect of vegetarianism on development of gall stones in women, Br. Med. J. 291:11, 1985.
9. Snowdon, D. A., and Phillips, R. L.: Does a vegetarian diet reduce the occurrence of diabetes? A.J.P.H. 75:507, 1985.
10. Freeland-Graves, J. H., and others: A demographic and social profile of age- and sex-matched vegetarians and nonvegetarians, J. Am. Diet. Assoc. 86:907, 1986.
11. Hardinge, M. G., and Stare, F. J.: Nutritional studies of vegetarians. I. Nutritional, physical, and laboratory studies, J. Clin. Nutr. 2:73, 1954.
12. Thomas, J., Ellis, F. R. and Diggory, P. L. C.: The health of vegans during pregnancy, Proc. Nutr. Soc. 36:46A, 1976.
13. Shull, M. W., and others: Velocities of growth in vegetarian preschool children, Pediatrics 60:410, 1977.
14. Knapp, J., and others: Growth and nitrogen balance in infants fed cereal proteins, Am. J. Clin. Nutr. 26:586, 1973.
15. Trahms, C. M., and others: Restriction of growth and elevated protoporphyrin in children deprived of animal protein, Clin. Res. 25:179, 1977.
16. Dwyer, J. T., and others: Preschoolers on alternate lifestyle diets, J. Am. Diet. Assoc. 72:264, 1978.
17. van Staveren, W. A., and others: Food consumption and height/weight status of Dutch preschool children on alternative food patterns, J. Am. Diet. Assoc. 85:1579, 1985.

18. Dwyer, J. T., and others: Growth in "new" vegetarian preschool children using the Jenss-Bayley curve fitting technique. Am. J. Clin. Nutr. 37:815, 1983.

19. Brown, P. T., and Bergan, J. G.: The dietary status of "new" vegetarians, J. Am. Diet. Assoc. 67:455, 1975.

20. Fulton, J. R., and others: Preschool vegetarian children: dietary and anthropometric data, J. Am. Diet. Assoc. 76:360, 1980.

21. Dwyer, J. T., and others: Nutritional status of vegetarian children, Am. J. Clin. Nutr. 35:204, 1982.

22. Shinwell, E. D., and Gorodisches, R.: Totally vegetarian diets and infant nutrition, Pediatrics 70:582, 1982.

23. Chase, H. P., and others: Kwashiorkor in the United States, Pediatrics 66:972, 1980.

24. Robson, J. R. K., and others: Zen macrobiotic dietary problems in infancy, Pediatrics 53:326, 1974.

25. Roberts, I. F., and others: Malnutrition in infants receiving cult diets: a form of child abuse, Br. Med J. 1:296, 1979.

26. Trahms, C. M., and Feeney, M. C.: Evaluation of diet and growth of vegans, vegetarian, and nonvegetarian preschool children, Fed. Proc. 34:675, 1975.

27. Hellebostad, M., and others: Vitamin D deficiency rickets and vitamin B_{12} deficiency in vegetarian children, Acta Paediatr. Scand. 74:191, 1985.

28. Higginbottom, M. C., and others: A syndrome of methylmalonic aciduria, homocystinuria, megaloblastic anemia and neurologic abnormalities in a vitamin B_{12} deficient breast fed infant of a strict vegetarian. N. Engl. J. Med. 299:317, 1978.

29. Lampklin, B. C., and Saunders, E. F.: Nutritional vitamin B_{12} deficiency in an infant, J. Pediatr. 75:1053, 1969.

30. Rudolf, M., and others: Unsuspected nutritional rickets, Pediatrics 66:72, 1980.

31. Dwyer, J. T., and others: Risk of nutritional rickets among vegetarian children, Am. J. Dis, Child. 133:134, 1979.

32. Marie, P. J., and others: Histological osteomalacia due to dietary calcium deficiency in children, N. Engl. J. Med. 307:584, 1982.

33. Beghin, I., and others: Assessment of biological value of a new corn-soy-wheat noodle through recuperation of Brazilian malnourished children. Am. J. Clin. Nutr. 26:246, 1973.

34. Graham, G. G., and others: Dietary protein quality in infants and children. IX. Instant sweetened corn-soy-milk blend, Am. J. Clin. Nutr. 26:491, 1973.

35. Bressani, R., and others: Protein quality of a soybean protein textured food in experimental animals and children, J. Nutr. 93:349, 1967.

36. MacLean, W. C., and others: Effect of the level of dietary protein intake on fat absorption in children, Pediatr. Res. 11:774, 1977.

37. Payne, P. R.: Safe protein-calorie ratios in food patterns: the relative importance of protein and energy intake as casual factors in malnutrition, Am. J. Clin. Nutr. 28:281, 1975.

38. Freeland-Graves, J. H., and others: Zinc and copper content of foods used in vegetarian food patterns, J. Am. Diet. Assoc. 77:648, 1980.

39. Truesdell, D. D., and others: Nutrients in vegetarian foods, J. Am. Diet. Assoc. 84:28, 1984.

40. Lynch, S. R., and others: Iron absorption from legumes in humans, Am. J. Clin. Nutr. 40:42, 1984.

41. Johnston, P. K.: Infant feeding among Seventh-Day Adventists, unpublished master's thesis, Seattle, 1979, University of Washington.

42. Saarinen, U. M., and Siimes, M. A.: Iron absorption from breast milk, cow's milk, and iron supplemented formula, Pediatr. Res. 13:143, 1979.

43. Finley, D. A., and others: Inorganic constituents of breast milk from vegetarian and nonvegetarian women: Relationships with each other and with organic constituents, J. Nutr. 115:772, 1985.

44. Finley, D. A., and others: Breast milk composition: fat content and fatty acid composition in vegetarians and nonvegetarians, Am. J. Clin. Nutr. 41:787, 1985.

45. Fomon, S. J., and others: Requirements for protein and essential amino acids in early infancy: studies with soy-isolate formula, Acta Paediatr. Scand. 62:33, 1973.

46. American Dietetic Association: Position paper on vegetarian approach to eating, J. Am. Diet. Assoc. 77:61, 1980.

47. Truesdell, D. D., and Acosta, P. B.: Feeding the vegan infant and child, J. Am. Diet. Assoc. 85:837, 1985.

48. Dwyer, J.: Health implications of vegetarian diets, Comp. Ther. 9:23, 1983.

49. Robertson, L., Flinders, C., and Ruppenthal, B.: The new Laurel's kitchen; Berkeley, 1986, Ten Speed Press.

10

Nutritional Considerations for Children in Sports

Bonnie Worthington-Roberts

OBJECTIVES

After completing this chapter, the student should:

1. Explain energy metabolism in the child participating in vigorous activity.
2. Summarize current thinking about the degree to which athletes need to increase protein intake.
3. Discuss the importance of iron for the performing athlete.
4. Define *sports anemia*.
5. Summarize data that suggest that athletic amenorrhea may be harmful.
6. Explain the consequences of dehydration as related to athletic performance.
7. Describe why glycogen loading might work.
8. Recommend an appropriate pregame meal.
9. Outline sensible weight management strategies for athletes.

Introduction

Interest in sports and physical fitness has increased dramatically among children and adolescents. No longer is athletic competition and training restricted to boys in varsity team sports. Much enthusiasm has developed among women, and individual sports have gained in popularity among girls and boys of all ages.

This interest in athletic performance is beneficial to the health of our youth, provided that the intensity of involvement is not excessive and when sensible health maintenance practices are encouraged.

Health maintenance for growing athletes is multifaceted, including attention to diet and nutrition. Primary objectives include the following:

1. Relaxed, supportive, loving home environment
2. Sufficient (but not excessive) training or athletic practice
3. Sufficient sleep
4. Adequate food and fluid
5. Appropriate medical attention for disease prevention and injury management
6. Support and encouragement in the face of error or defeat

The area of diet is unfortunately filled with superstition and myth about "optimum practices." Special diets or foods are sometimes advocated, and the use of supplements is frequently recommended. These diets and supplements often have no scientific proof to support their use; however, the enthusiasm of the trainer may be more than adequate to motivate compliance. Very few studies have been undertaken on nutritional needs of *growing* athletes. Most published research has dealt with adolescents who agreed to be studied while training for specific sports. Data on normal, moderately active children may also be considered in determining nutritional recommendations for athletes (see Chapter 2).

CALORIES

Sports activities differ widely in the amount of energy required to support them (Table 10-1). In general, however, a child in sports requires a greater caloric intake than does the sedentary youngster. The average 10-year-old boy may expend between 2000 and 2800 kcal/-day, whereas the majority of boys this age who are running great distances or exerting themselves in other physical activities may expend an additional 300 to 700 kcal/day. The caloric needs of preadolescent girls are similar to those of boys for moderate and heavy exercise. In adolescence, however, when boys become relatively larger, their total daily needs in all circumstances become greater. By adulthood, women expend approximately 10% fewer calo-

ries than men, assuming physical conditioning and training regimens are comparable. Extensive training decreases energy expenditure in both males and females; the trained individual burns about 7% less energy than the nontrained person to complete any specified task. The size of the individual, the level of training, and the type of sports activity engaged in are major factors determining total daily caloric needs (Figure 10-1).

Since very young children are now participating in athletic events, which in some cases are quite demanding, Torún, Chew, and Mendoza[1] measured 47 preschool children (17 to 45 months of age) under basal metabolic conditions and while participating in various exercises. In all situations, preschool children required more kilocalories per unit of body weight than did adults (Table 10-2). Freedson and others[2] examined 6- and 7-year-old children and reported similar observations. In addition, however, these workers found that males expended 11% to 16% more energy than females in completing treadmill running tests at slow, medium, and fast speeds. Although there are no satisfactory guidelines for calculating energy costs of activities for children, Torún, Chew, and Mendoza[1] propose the following strategy for estimating the energy expenditure of preschool children in time-motion studies: (1) use the energy costs of activities that have been measured in children whenever available, and (2) use 1.2, 2, and 2.5 times the child's basal metabolism for sedentary, light, and moderately heavy activities, respectively; or use the values determined in adults per unit of body weight multiplied by 2 for sedentary activities and 1.2 for all other activities.

Besides being used for basal metabolism and physical activity, calories are required to support normal growth. Growing athletes therefore demand somewhat more calories per kilogram of body weight than those athletes who are mature. During adolescence

Table 10-1   Approximate energy cost of various exercises and sports as estimated for adults

Sport or Exercise	Total Calories Expended/Minute of Activity	Sport or Exercise	Total Calories Expended/Minute of Activity
Climbing	10.7-13.2	Rowing—cont'd	
Cycling		97 strokes/minute	11.2
5.5 mph	4.5	Running	
9.4 mph	7.0	Short distance	13.3-16.6
13.1 mph	11.1	Cross-country	10.6
Dancing	3.3-7.7	Tennis	7.1
Domestic work		Skating, fast	11.5
Bed making	3.5	Skiing	
Dusting	2.5	Moderate speed	10.8-15.9
Ironing	1.7	Uphill, maximum speed	18.6
Cleaning floors	3.5	Squash	10.2
Football	8.9	Swimming	
Golf	5.0	Breaststroke	11.0
Gymnastics		Backstroke	11.5
Balancing	2.5	Crawl	14.0
Abdominal exercises	3.0	Walking	
Trunk bending	3.5	2 mph	2.5
Arms swinging, hopping	6.5	3 mph	3.5
Rowing		5 mph	5.5
51 strokes/minute	4.1	Watching television	1.5
87 strokes/minute	7.0	Wrestling	14.2

Modified from Nutrition for athletes: a handbook for coaches, Washington, D.C., 1971, American Alliance for Health, Education and Recreation.

(especially for boys), when the growth rate is extremely rapid, the caloric needs may be very great.

The most frequently encountered nutritional problem among athletes is failure to consume sufficient food energy. This may be related to an over-committed lifestyle, a disorganized or poverty-stricken background, or an overaggressive effort to limit body fatness. When athletes ingest too few calories they lack sufficient energy to perform optimally in sports events, and in some cases their growth may be impaired.

In general, the athlete's greatly increased caloric expenditure automatically increases the appetite, with the result that he or she ingests more food. Although it is unlikely that an athlete in heavy physical training will gain too much weight, caloric intake greater than the daily expenditure is not recommended, as it results in unnecessary fat deposition with subsequent increased work load to the heart. The increased caloric requirements are best met by increasing food intake across the board, without significantly altering the proportions of the micronutrients or macronutrients of the diet. There are no known "special" food sources that supply extra reserves of energy that are not provided by other foods with the same nutrients.

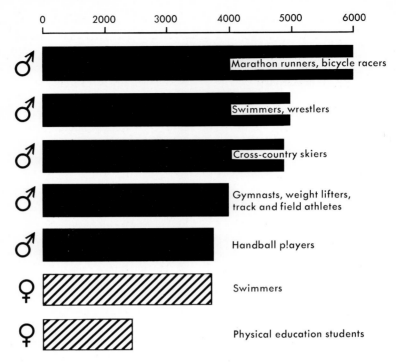

Figure 10-1   Typical daily calorie expenditure of athletes training for various sports. (Data from Saltin, B.: Fluid electrolyte and energy losses and their replenishment in prolonged exercise; and from Rogozkin, V.A.: Some aspects of athlete's nutrition. In Parizkova, J., and Rogozkin, V.A., editors: Nutrition, physical fitness, and health, Baltimore, 1978, University Park Press.)

Table 10-2   Comparison of energy expenditures of preschool children with those of adult men and women (cal/kg/min)*

Activity	Children	Adult Men	Adult Women
Basal metabolism	38	18	17
Lying down, awake	44	20	21
Sitting quietly, playing, or sedentary work	47	22	22
Walking leisurely on level ground	71	64	53
Walking uphill and downhill	87	83	77
Walking rapidly at a grade	98	85	—
Leisure ride on tricycle or bicycle	75	58	58
Climbing stairs	94	—	—

Data from Torun, B., Chew, F., and Mendoza, R.D.: Nutr. Res. 3:401, 1983.
*Note: This is cal/kg/min, not kcal/kg/min.

The reportedly low daily energy intake of some weight-conscious athletes is rather startling.[3-6] In a four-year study at Syracuse University,[3] 10 men's and 6 women's athletic teams were observed. Male gymnasts averaged 2080 kcal/day and male wrestlers consumed 925 to 1821 kcal/day, depending on whether intake was measured before a match for which the athlete restricted his food intake. Female dancers averaged 1909 kcal/day. Other researchers reported that female marathon runners consumed 1400 kcal/day in one case[4] and 1990 kcal/day in another.[5] Similar low levels of energy intake have been documented in ballet dancers, figure skaters, gymnasts, and others.

Brownell, Steen, and Milmore[7] speculate that food efficiency at burning increases as weight falls below the level at which the person regulates normally and that energy efficiency increases to the greatest degree in sports where low body weight is a factor, irrespective of the metabolic selection factors which draw individuals to certain sports. The extent to which low daily calorie intakes, such as those reported above, affect the growth and health of boys and girls remains to be determined (although the negative consequences of amenorrhea are becoming apparent). It is also unclear what longterm effects such restrictive eating patterns may have on calorie requirements in those months and years following active athletic competition. Suffice to say, rigorous calorie limitation during periods of growth carries the potential of short-term or permanent effects on health. Overly aggressive efforts at minimizing body fatness are therefore not to be encouraged.

Energy Sources

The immediate source of energy for muscle work is adenosine triphosphate (ATP), which is formed in muscles largely by metabolism of carbohydrates and fats. It can be metabolized rapidly to meet the needs of sudden episodes of activity in intensive short-term exercise. Since ATP is metabolized without the use of oxygen,

the reaction is classified as *anaerobic*. This type of reaction is important during strenuous exercise, when the heart and lungs cannot deliver oxygen quickly to the muscles. If energy is needed for more than brief spurts, the high-energy compound in muscles, called phosphocreatine (PC), can almost instantaneously provide the energy required to regenerate ATP. Within a matter of minutes of vigorous exercise, however, the small stores of ATP-PC are used up, and then the body must turn to another source of energy to regenerate the ATP-PC system.[8]

Glycogen is the second energy source for muscles. It is stored in limited amounts in muscle cells and can be metabolized within the muscle cells to restore ATP. This activity is carried out primarily in the absence of oxygen; thus it is also classified as anaerobic. The level of glycogen storage in skeletal muscles is modified to some degree by dietary composition. It is possible to load muscles with unusually high levels of glycogen by adherence to a specially designed nutrition program used in conjunction with proper conditioning. The principles of glycogen loading and the available data on its effectiveness and safety are discussed on pp. 248-249.

As prolonged exercise gradually depletes the stores of ATP-PC and muscle glycogen, the body increasingly resorts to another source of energy. This last type of fuel comes from the aerobic metabolism of carbohydrates (glucose) and fats (Figure 10-2). In most children, a considerable amount of stored fat is available, but its slow rate of metabolism makes it a less efficient source of quick energy. For reasons that are not presently clear, fat does not seem to be available to maintain performance at very high intensities of muscle work (i.e., 60% to 70% VO_2max*). Neither the supply of free

---

*VO_2max is a term used to express the percentage of maximum oxygen consumption of a working individual; work physiologists use this term to express the severity of a specific type of work or exercise.

Figure 10-2   **A,** Variation in energy over time. **B,** Changes in the respiratory quotient (*RQ*) or oxygen and carbon dioxide, indicating a shift in the utilization of carbohydrates and fats by the working muscles.

fatty acids exogenous to active muscle nor the endogenously available muscle triglyceride can fully replace the essential role of carbohydrates. It is true, however, that the highly conditioned competitor works long hours in conditioning activities to improve oxygen-burning capacity. With intensive training, athletes can significantly increase their efficiency in using fatty acids and **ketones** as energy sources. This is particularly important for endurance events in which glycogen usage may be partially spared as fat is burned. In sports activities requiring much endurance, glucose metabolism makes a minor contribution to total energy needs.

Figure 10-3 summarizes the predominant energy systems required in the more common physical activities. The relative contributions of the anaerobic and aerobic systems to the overall energy requirement differ markedly with the time and intensity of the specific activity to be performed. With an intense burst of energy, like a tennis serve, the energy is provided anaerobically and supplied almost exclusively by the stored high-energy phosphates, ATP and PC. As the duration of the activity increases, energy from lactic acid plays a much more important

role. As the intensity of the activity diminishes somewhat and the duration extends to between $1\frac{1}{2}$ and 4 minutes, dependence on energy from the phosphate stores decreases while energy release from aerobic reactions becomes more important. After 4 minutes of continuous exercise, an activity becomes more dependent on aerobic energy. In a cross-country ski race or a marathon, the body is powered almost exclusively by the energy from aerobic reactions.

Carbohydrate is widely recognized as the most readily available source of energy.[9] The simple sugars from digested carbohydrate are absorbed from the small intestine and are taken by means of the bloodstream to the liver; here fructose and galactose are largely converted to glucose, which reenters the bloodstream for transport to body tissues, particularly brain and skeletal muscle. A fairly small amount of circulating glucose is converted to glycogen for storage in liver and muscle. The importance of glycogen is substantial when athletic involvement extends over long periods. Carbohydrate administration during competitive efforts may prevent the premature depletion of liver glycogen stores and

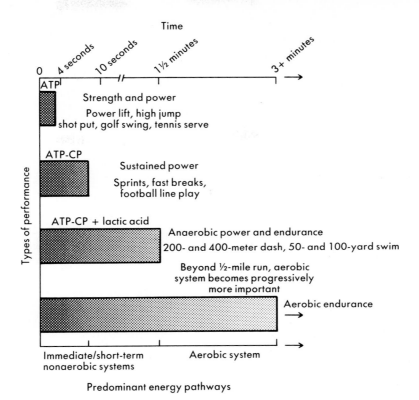

Figure 10-3   Classification of activities based on duration of performance and the predominant energy pathways.

improve endurance performance.[10] With provision of a high-carbohydrate diet, long-distance cyclists have ridden farther,[11] long-distance cross-country skiers have raced faster,[12] long-distance canoeists have paddled faster,[13] and soccer players have scored more goals in the latter parts of games.[14] Availability of carbohydrate is a major limiting factor, and its ingestion during performance or in conjunction with prior exercise recovery plays an important role in the total well-being of the athlete.

PROTEIN

For many years, it has been generally believed that physical activity does not significantly increase the need for dietary protein.

Recent data suggest, however, that protein metabolism *may* change somewhat during endurance exercise or rigorous weight training. The earlier view that skeletal muscle functions as a fairly inert protein reservoir is no longer tenable. Evans and others[15,16] reported a substantial decrease in the rate of protein synthesis and an increase in gluconeogenesis during exercise. They estimated that protein can provide up to 5.5% of the total caloric cost of exercise. Additional research is required to evaluate the accuracy of this estimation.[17]

The continual flux of amino acids between muscular tissue and nonmuscular tissue, particularly the liver and kidney, supports the view that proteins play a role in the generation of energy. During periods of stress, glucocorticoids are released from the adrenal cortex to cause amino acid mobilization from muscle. The amino acids that originate from muscle can be used by the liver as gluconeogenic precursors. The amino acids that originate from muscle can be used by the liver as gluconeogenic precursors. The elevated flux of amino acids to the liver originates from the skeletal muscle in two ways. The circulating glucocorticoids can accelerate muscle protein breakdown to augment hepatic gluconeogenesis.

In addition to their role in gluconeogenesis, amino acids contribute to whole body energy metabolism. During rest, and to a greater degree during exercise, there is significant interorgan flux that results in the redistribution of amino acids from one tissue to another. Alanine makes up only about 11% of the free amino acids in skeletal muscle, yet during exercise, alanine far exceeds all other amino acids in the net release from muscle. This means that alanine synthesis increases tremendously during exercise. Pyruvic acid, derived either from glucose or from other amino acids, is converted to alanine using nitrogen donated by the branched chain amino acids. Alanine is thus able to serve an important carrier function for the transport of amino groups, in a nontoxic form, from skeletal muscle to liver. Although serum alanine from skeletal muscles has been found to increase during exercise, branched chain amino acids are selectively taken up by exercising muscles. Alanine from the skeletal muscles eventually reaches the liver where it is reconverted to glucose by means of gluconeogenesis. Presumably, the alanine nitrogen, which originally was derived from the branched chain amino acid molecule, is transferred to the urea cycle in the liver, where it is eventually excreted.

The alpha-ketoacid, which results from the glucose-alanine cycle during exercise, can be converted irreversibly to acetyl-coA, which ultimately provides high-energy fuel to meet metabolic demands. The oxidative potential of this cycle led recent investigations toward a more extensive account of the relationships between branched chain amino acids and muscle amino acids and their role in exercise. The prediction that a greater than tenfold increase in oxygen consumption is common in working muscle supports the theory that branched chain amino acid oxidation occurs in working muscle.

Of the three branched chain amino acids, only leucine can be completely degraded in muscle to carbon dioxide, after transamination and decarboxylation. Therefore, only leucine can supply a considerable fraction of the muscle's energy during exercise. Dohm, Hecker, and Brown[18] found that a substantial amount of energy can come from leucine oxidation in exercising rats. They found that when humans exercise leucine oxidation rates increase by 240%; leucine flux decreases by 21%. This means that protein synthesis decreased significantly. Therefore the elevated efflux of hepatic amino acids can be made available to muscle as an energy source without an increase in muscle protein breakdown.

So protein may provide up to 5.5% of the total caloric cost of exercise. Unlike carbohydrates and fats, leucine is a nonrenewable source of energy in that it is an essential amino acid. Evans and others[19] have estimated that 853 mg of leucine is oxidized during a 2-hour ride on a cycle ergometer at 55% of VO_2max. This represents almost 90% of the current estimated leucine requirement. Because essential amino acid requirements have been determined only for resting humans, a reevaluation of minimum daily requirements should be considered for physically active humans.

In addition to using amino acids for energy (to a limited extent), the athlete who is training or competing may demand greater amino acid retention when muscles are being developed and blood volume is increasing. Increases in lean body mass, enzymatic protein, *myo-*

globin, and hemoglobin are typical effects of training that may temporarily require greater protein utilization. Athletes who develop proteinuria, hemoglobinuria, or myoglobinuria as a result of prolonged intense exercise may also require higher levels of protein until these conditions subside. Overall, the increased need for protein is easily accommodated through common food selections.

Sweating usually does not significantly increase the need for protein in the athlete. Sweating as a result of vigorous physical activity does increase nitrogen loss, and this may amount to 600 mg after 2 hours of strenuous exercise by the mature man. If this activity lasts for 4 hours in 1 day, the nitrogen lost through sweat would be about 1.2 gm; replacing this loss through dietary sources would require and extra 7.5 gm of protein, an amount obtained in three or four bites of meat.

The performing athlete, like everyone else, must replace nitrogen losses incurred each day. The child and adolescent must go one step further and provide sufficient nitrogen (from dietary protein) for physical growth. Precise data are unavailable on protein requirements of either the mature adult who is developing his muscle mass or the growing child or adolescent who is engaged in a muscle development program. Obviously their needs are measurably greater than those of comparable persons not engaged in rigorous physical conditioning.

Table 10-3 provides a liberal estimate of protein requirements for the rapidly growing, tall, adolescent male athlete. To begin with, the 70-kg adult male loses approximately 4 gm of nitrogen/day through the urine, feces, and skin; this level of nitrogen is equivalent to approximately 25 gm of protein. Obviously, there is individual variation that could conceivably (according to available data) increase the protein needs of some adults by about 30%. This estimation increases protein needs from 25 to 32.5 gm/day. Allowing for 4 hours of strenuous exercise with consequent sweat losses of

nitrogen, an additional 7.5 gm of protein is required, or a total of 40 gm of protein/day for the 70-kg male. If muscle mass is being markedly increased, an extra 7 to 8 gm of protein might be added to the requirements, but only during the phase of active muscle building. If one liberally estimates an extra 10 gm of protein/day for the rapidly growing adolescent boy, the total daily protein requirement should be approximately 55 to 60 gm. Protein needs may be greater for those young males who are

Table 10-3   Liberal estimate of daily protein need for the large, rapidly growing male athlete with a developing muscle mass

Basis for Need	Protein (gm)
Replacement of nitrogen lost through urine, feces, skin, and other sites (for 70-kg male)	24.5
Provision of 30% extra protein for individual variation (for 70-kg male)	7.5
Replacement of nitrogen lost through sweat during 4 hours of strenuous exercise (for 70-kg male)	7.5
Coverage of increased protein need of growing muscle mass (for 70-kg male)	7.5
Coverage for extra protein associated with rapid growth in adolescence (liberal estimate)	10.0
Extra protein allotment for the exceptionally large male (liberal estimate)	10.0
Provision of extra protein to cover that burned during rigorous endurance events or weight training	12.0
TOTAL	79.0

Data obtained in part from Durnin, J.V.G.A.: Protein requirements and physical activity. In Parizkova, J., and Rogozkin, V.A., editors: Nutrition, physical fitness, and health, Baltimore, 1978, University Park Press; and Evans, W.J., and others: Protein metabolism and endurance exercise, Phys. Sports Med. **11**:53, 1983.

exceptionally large or engaged in endurance sports or demanding weight training (Figure 10-4). Even if the needs were to reach 80 gm/day, this amount is readily obtained through ingestion of ordinary foods (Table 10-4).

The majority of athletes tend to consume more protein than the estimated requirement. It is known, for example, that most common diets provide 10% to 15% of calories from protein. It follows, then, that with high-calorie diets substantial amounts of protein may be readily obtained (Table 10-5). Athletes emphasizing high-protein foods may consume even higher levels of protein each day.

An obvious question is whether excessive protein consumption improves in any measurable way the short- or long-term performance of athletes. One investigation assessed the effect

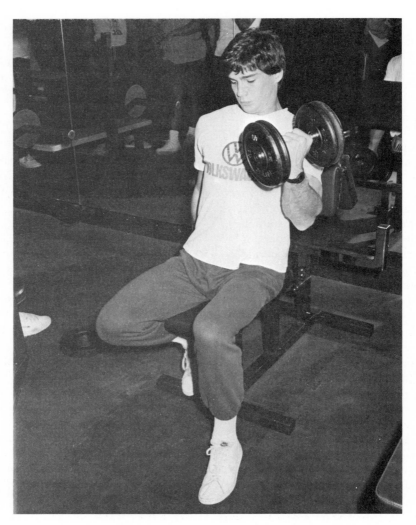

Figure 10-4   Dumbbells provide an excellent means for strength development.

Table 10-4 Protein content of representative American foods

Food	Portion Size	Protein (mg)
Milk	1 cup	8
Hamburger patty, broiled	3 oz	23
Egg	1	7
Yogurt	1 cup	8
Steak	3 oz	20
Cheddar cheese	1 oz	7
Chili con carne	1 cup	19
Chicken drumstick	1	12
Tuna	3 oz	24
Peanut butter	1 tbsp	4
Whole wheat bread	1 slice	3
Spaghetti (noodles only)	1 cup	5
Minestrone soup	1 cup	5

Table 10-5 Representative levels of protein intake associated with varying levels of calorie intake

Calorie Intake	Calories Derived from Protein		Protein Intake (gm)	
	10%	15%	10%	15%
2000	200	300	50	75
2500	250	375	65	94
3000	300	450	75	113
3500	350	525	88	132
4000	400	600	100	150
4500	450	675	113	169
5000	500	750	125	187
6000	600	900	150	225
7000	700	1050	175	263

of protein supplements on 32 male competitors during their basic training in Marine Officer Candidate School.[20] Sixteen of the men were given a protein supplement. Physical performance was evaluated in all subjects before, during, and after the program. Both the supplemented and nonsupplemented groups significantly improved their physical performance scores from program onset to program termination, but no significant difference was observed between the groups.

Most growing athletes consume more protein than can be effectively used for maintenance or growth. Consequently, a portion of each day's protein supply is used for energy or is stored as fat with the nitrogen waste being excreted in the urine. Although this high protein intake is generally not hazardous, it is usually expensive and it promotes loss of appetite and sometimes diarrhea. Production of excessive nitrogen waste always increases fluid requirements, so that efficient urinary excretion

of this waste is achieved. For the athlete at risk for dehydration, this latter observation clearly suggests some cause for concern.

VITAMINS

Much misinformation and exaggeration exist regarding the relationship between vitamins and exercise. Popular fitness magazines, coaches' newsletters, and the training practices of sports superstars convey the message that supplemental vitamins are needed to boost energy, maximize performance, and help alleviate the stress of competition. Advocates of supplementation have exaggerated the needs for all 13 recognized vitamins and have even created new "vitamins," such as vitamin B_{15} or pangamic acid.

The connection between exercise and vitamins has been examined from two points of view (Figure 10-5).[21] For many years, nutritionists have been interested in the effects of exercise on vitamin requirements while exercise physiologists have been concerned with the effects of vitamin supplementation on athletic performance. There is some evidence that

Figure 10-5   Vitamin-exercise interactions.

exercise may increase the need for certain vitamins such as C[22] and riboflavin[23-25] in individuais with marginal vitamin stores. Other recent work suggests that exercise may acutely affect metabolism of certain vitamins such as vitamin B_6.[26] There is no conclusive evidence to suggest that supplementation improves performance in individuals with adequate nutrition. In a series of over 250 experiments conducted during the 1940s, Keys and Henschel[27] examined the effect of megadose vitamin supplementation on fatigue and ability to work. Metabolic tests and biochemical evaluation of blood samples detected no effect of any single vitamin or combination of vitamins on physiological and biochemical functions. These researchers concluded that "supercharging" with vitamins did not affect performance. During the 1960s and 1970s, there was another surge of interest in vitamins with emphasis on vitamin C,[28, 29] vitamin E,[30, 31] and niacin.[32-34] Although the findings were somewhat controversial, researchers concluded that vitamin supplementation did not improve performance in individuals with adequate nutrition.[35]

Several studies have examined the value of vitamin E supplements for athletes.[30, 31, 36] Sharman[30] studied two groups of adolescent swimmers who were provided daily with either 400 mg of α-tocopherol acetate or placebos in addition to their normal diets. The swimmers were studied for 6 weeks, and all were involved in daily swimming workouts and supportive exercises. Before and after supplementation program, anthropometric measurements were recorded, and cardiorespiratory efficiency and motor fitness were evaluated to test performance. Although training was found to significantly improve the performance of swimmers in both experimental groups, vitamin E did not produce any obvious benefits.

In a later study by Lawrence and others,[36] two groups of well-trained competitive swimmers were observed. The first group was given 90 IU of α-tocopherol acetate/day for 6 months, whereas the second group was given placebos. A swimming endurance test was given before the start of the supplementation and after 1, 2, 5, and 6 months. No difference in swimming endurance was observed between the two groups during the 6 months. A comparable study on a younger, less trained group of competitive swimmers again revealed that vitamin E supplementation did not affect swimming endurance.

The effect of vitamin C supplementation has also been studied by several investigators. Bailey and others[37] observed 40 young males, 20 of whom were classified as trained and the remainder, as untrained. Performance on various treadmill tests was recorded before and after a 5-day ingestion of 2 gm of ascorbic acid/day or placebos. The purpose of the study was to determine if vitamin C had any effect on oxygen uptake and ventilatory adjustment in trained and untrained subjects before, during, and after exercise. The results provided no indication that ascorbic acid supplementation improved performance in any measurable way.

Since 1980, several experiments have studied the impact of vitamins on exercise. It is difficult to interpret the results of many of these studies because of inadequacies in research design. Lack of control or placebo groups, inadequate measures of exercise performance, and incomplete nutritional information are common problems. Several groups, however, paid careful attention to both vitamin intake and exercise performance.

The effects of thiamin restriction were examined in 18 young men who participated in a double-blind study.[38] For 5 weeks the subjects followed a low thiamin diet with either a 5 mg thiamin supplement or a placebo. The control and supplemented subjects showed marked variation in thiamin status as measured by urinary and blood levels, with values in the low group indicative of deficiency. Even still, there was no difference between the groups in minutes to exhaustion or watts generated during a progressive cycle ergometer test.

Buzina and others[22] examined the relationship between vitamin C and physical work capacity in adolescent boys. These young people from rural Yugoslavia showed biochemical evidence of vitamin B_6 and riboflavin deficiency as well as low plasma vitamin C. All of the boys therefore received vitamin B_6 and riboflavin supplementation; half received 70 mg of vitamin C daily. Aerobic capacity increased in the vitamin C group and did not change in the control group. Since the subjects did not have impaired iron status, the authors concluded that the effect of vitamin C was not related to its role in the improvement of iron absorption.

In a series of studies conducted at Oregon State University, the impact of exercise on vitamin B_6 requirements was evaluated. Exercise appeared to increase the level of pyridoxal phosphate in the bloodstream;[39] an explanation for this finding was never found. However, based on urinary excretion of vitamin B_6 metabolites, there was no evidence that exercise adversely affected vitamin B_6 status.

Cornell University was the site for a number of studies related to exercise and riboflavin requirements in young women.[23-25] During these studies, women were fed carefully controlled amounts of riboflavin during periods of nonexercise and during periods of supervised exercise. Thus both diet and exercise were carefully controlled. In all three studies, the riboflavin requirement appeared to increase with training in women who had low biochemical riboflavin status. Supplemental riboflavin did not improve the ability to train.

From the results of these studies, it is possible to conclude that exercise may affect requirements for vitamin C and riboflavin. There was no detectable effect of low thiamin intake on performance. Exercise effects on vitamin B_6 metabolism appeared to be related to the acute substrate demands of the working muscle. Vitamin supplementation improved the ability to train only in the vitamin-C depleted subjects of Buzina and others.[22] There was no measurable effect of supplemental thiamin, riboflavin, or vitamin B_6.

What recommendations should be made to athletes regarding vitamin supplementation? Because of the close relationship between calorie and vitamin intake, the major group at risk are those athletes who limit their caloric intake and thus, their vitamin intakes. These athletes include those groups concerned about the cosmetics of extra weight, such as gymnasts, dancers, figure skaters and divers, and those who are required to "make weight," such as wrestlers, boxers, jockeys, and light-weight football or crew participants. In those athletes, a basic multivitamin-mineral pill might be appropriate in order to ensure adequate intake.

MINERALS

The most significant effect of exercise on mineral nutrition is the loss of electrolytes through sweat. In general, sweat contains approximately 20 to 30 mEq (460 to 690 mg) of sodium/liter, so when sweating is excessive, losses up to 350 mEq (8050 mg) may occur each day in the acclimated adult male. This amount may be greater in the nonacclimated individual, and in either case it is great enough to disturb fluid and electrolyte homeostasis.

Observations of children during strenuous running show that children under 12 years of age sweat less but stay cooler.[40] Apparently, younger children have a better ratio of surface area to weight than do older children and adults, and thus they are able to dissipate heat more effectively without as great a fluid loss. Young children therefore exhibit less risk of dehydration and electrolyte imbalance than adolescents and adults. This situation does not mean, however, that attention to fluid replacement should be overlooked in this population.

Salt can be replaced on a regular basis by salting foods to a satisfying taste. Use of salt tablets is generally unnecessary, and sometimes they may even cause gastrointestinal disturbances resulting from fluid movement into the gut. If water loss exceeds 5 to 10 pounds in a given contest or workout, some consideration might be given to specific salt replacement. Adding salt to the normal diet may adequately cover needs, but use of *dilute* salt-containing fluids may also be considered. Commercially available electrolyte drinks are pleasantly flavored and may be diluted since most are more concentrated than they need to be for greatest effectiveness and comfort. Since thirst alone may not prompt sufficient water intakes during intense competition or extreme heat, regularly scheduled periods for fluid replacement should be part of any athletic training program.

Attention to potassium and magnesium replacement may be more important than consideration of sodium needs. The amount of these minerals lost through sweat is negligible when environmental temperature is mild and exercise level is moderate. Under conditions of moderate to extreme heat, however, potassium losses may be considerable if exercise is heavy and prolonged. Liu, Borowski, and Rose[41] recently described a patient with bouts of carpopedal spasm after exercise. The patient played six hours of tennis daily, swam and sunbathed. She was found to have hypomagnesemia. After receiving magnesium supplements, her symptoms abated and her serum magnesium normalized. Lane and others[42] and Lane and Cerda[43] assessed potassium and sodium imbalance in volunteer runners performing in a hot climate with high humidity. Estimated losses of potassium tended to exceed the daily level of intake recommended for healthy Americans, especially in persons who were poorly acclimated. Costill, Cote, and Fink[44] reported somewhat different findings in eight men examined during two 4-day exercise-dietary regimens. Whether the men consumed a control or a low-potassium diet, no significant diminishment in total body potassium content was observed. Similarly, Dressendorfer and others[45] studied the plasma mineral levels in 12 male marathon runners during a 20-day road race. The runners consumed an unrestricted, isocaloric diet that averaged 4800 kcal/day (range 4100-5600). All subjects maintained normal plasma mineral levels without using mineral supplements during the 312-mile road race. These latter reports suggest that there is usually no need for trained athletes to take salt pills, special electrolyte solutions, or mineral supplements. It seems reasonable, however, to emphasize to sports enthusiasts the value of high-potassium foods

(Table 10-6). Electrolyte beverages may also be provided if they are *palatable, hypotonic,* and *balanced* in their content of glucose, chloride, sodium, and potassium.

Iron is another mineral of major importance for maintenance of optimal condition in the athlete.[46] Aerobic metabolism involves the utilization of oxygen, which must be conveyed to body tissues via hemoglobin in red blood cells (RBCs). Since aerobic metabolism plays a major role in athletic undertakings (especially endurance sports), maintenance of normal hemoglobin levels is essential. Iron is required for hemoglobin synthesis but is also involved in oxygen utilization within muscles. Here, iron-containing myoglobin helps to transport oxygen across the cell to mitochondria where much of the ATP is produced for muscle

Table 10-6 Potassium content of common foods

Food	Portion Size	Potassium (mg)
Banana	1 small	370
Orange	1 small	200
Grapefruit	$\frac{1}{2}$ medium	135
Potato	1 $2\frac{1}{4}$" diameter	407
Tomato	1 small	244
Carrot	1 large	341
Celery	1 small inner stalk	68
Beef steak	$\frac{1}{4}$ lb	325
Chicken breast	$3\frac{1}{2}$ oz (uncooked)	350
Salmon	$3\frac{1}{2}$ oz (uncooked)	399
Bread, white	1 slice	20
Bread, whole wheat	1 slice	63
Milk, whole	$\frac{1}{2}$ cup	176
Cheese, American	1 oz	23

contraction. In the mitochondria, other iron-containing substances (cytochromes, enzymes) are required for aerobic metabolic processes involved in energy production. Thus iron status may be important to performance through effects at either circulatory or metabolic levels.

Enough iron must be consumed each day to replace that which is lost and to provide the normal accumulation of iron in growing children. Usual daily losses in some athletes may exceed those of non-athletes, especially if perspiration is excessive.[47] There is also evidence of enhanced RBC breakdown with some types of training (mainly running).[48] Since much of the iron from RBC breakdown is recycled, however, it is unclear how significant this phenomenon of RBC destruction might be.

Iron losses have recently been calculated for eight young female runners[49]; daily losses were about 2.7 mg, a level considerably above the estimated 1.5 mg/day losses typical of menstruating women. Male distance runners have also been reported to demonstrate elevated daily iron losses; these individuals may use iron twice as fast as the normal adult male.[50] Causes of faster iron turnover may be related to increased RBC destruction and/or increased loss of iron in sweat. Increased gastrointestinal blood loss associated with prolonged strenuous exercise has also been observed.[51–56] Large iron losses from various sources could ultimately affect iron status and nutritional iron requirements.

Several studies have reported evidence of iron depletion and iron deficiency in highly trained athletes. Among Olympic athletes, 5% of female and 2% of the male athletes had iron deficiency anemia.[57] Several recent studies have reported evidence of poor iron stores in both female and male athletes,[50, 58] yet this problem is substantially more common in women due to their normal high iron losses through menstruation.[59,60,62] Interestingly, iron absorption may be better in endurance athletes than in non-athletes.[50, 53] Even if this is true, risk of iron depletion is substantial in most populations of athletes.

Research on iron deficiency in animals and humans indicates that inadequate iron intake results in loss of strength and endurance, easy fatigability, shortening of attention span, loss of visual perception, and compromised learning ability.[46] The iron-deficient athlete therefore should be identified and provided with both iron supplements and dietary counseling on food sources of iron. Female athletes using the intrauterine device are especially good candidates for iron supplements, because excessive menstrual blood loss often occurs when the device is used. Most sensibly, however, prevention of iron deficiency is a better approach than treatment of the problem once established; thus general dietary guidelines for athletes should emphasize iron-rich foods of both animal and vegetable origin. When the self-selected diet appears inadequate to fulfill daily needs for iron, a low-level supplement may then be worthwhile in the maintenance of satisfactory long-term iron status.

Studies on the use of iron supplements with athletes have produced mixed results. In general, those studies which used small amounts of iron (50 mg iron or less per day) in the supplement found little improvement in hemoglobin and iron status,[64–66] while those which used larger amounts of iron in the supplement (100 mg iron or more per day) reported beneficial effects.[49, 61, 67, 68] In general, in the studies that reported beneficial effects the populations examined had a high proportion of iron deficient subjects. If an athlete is iron deficient, then an iron supplement is quite likely to be beneficial and should be used.

It should be noted, however, that a phenomenon exists, called *sports anemia, runner's anemia*, or *pseudoanemia*.[69,70] This condition has been reported in some athletes, especially those involved in long-distance running or swimming or those who are subjected to recurrent trauma (e.g., football play-

ers and boxers).[63] Suggested causes of sports anemia include inadequate absorption of iron, blood loss, expansion of blood volume, inadequate dietary protein intake, and intravascular hemolysis caused by onset of heavy training and trauma, resulting in hemoglobinuria. However, few of these causes have been studied in depth in athletes.

One definition of sports anemia is the presence of clinical anemia (hemoglobin levels below 12 gm/100 ml in females, 14 gm/100 ml in males) in an athlete who is usually experiencing a decline in athletic performance. Such a definition, however, may not be entirely satisfactory, because in recent years the generalization regarding the optimal hemoglobin concentration has been challenged in several studies. Although some investigators believe that optimal hemoglobin concentration for athletes may be at the upper end of the normal range, others support the concept that sports anemia is a normal physiological adaptation that should provoke no concern.

In support of the concept that sports anemia is normal, Yoshimura[71] believes the evidence from Japan indicates that sports anemia is caused by increased destruction of RBCs, which is a result of an increase in fragility. He cites evidence suggested that the spleen releases a hemolyzing factor during exercise. He also quotes studies indicating that the destruction of RBCs allows the protein from the hemoglobin to be used to "promote growth or hypertrophy of muscles and regeneration of new and strong RBCs."

A scheme of adaptation that is easier to study relates oxygen transport to hematocrit and blood viscosity.[69] As the hematocrit (or hemoglobin level) increases, the oxygen-carrying ability of the blood improves. The optimum hematocrit for carrying oxygen would be 100%, but the viscosity of the blood increases with an increasing hematocrit. As the blood becomes thicker, it becomes more difficult to pump. Therefore the hematocrit should be at a level that combines an optimum oxygen-carrying capacity and viscosity. Crowell and Smith[72] determined that a hematocrit of 40% is optimal for oxygen transport. This roughly corresponds to a hemoglobin concentration in the range of 13 to 14 gm/100 ml. Guyton, Jones, and Coleman[73] suggest that the "borderline anemia state" is optimal for oxygen transport and that the factors governing RBC production are fine-tuned to meet the daily stresses athletes impose on their bodies. If this hypothesis is correct, the guidelines for the diagnosis of sports anemia are those outlined in Table 10-7.

Support for the belief that sports anemia may indeed be physiological is provided by Dressendorfer, Wade, and Amsterdam,[74] who observed marathon runners during a 20-day road race. RBC count, blood hemoglobin concentration, and related hematological factors were recorded in 12 young men during a 312-mile run. The RBC and hemoglobin levels decreased significantly (Figure 10-6), and the runners became marginally anemic during the race. Running speeds, however, were not adversely affected, and no abnormal clinical signs (other than rare instances of hematuria) were noted. The investigators suggest that a sudden increase in long-distance running mileage above the regular training level may cause sports anemia, a functional pseudoanemia that, in mild cases, does not impair endurance performance.

In a similar study, Frederickson, Puhl, and Runyan[75] examined indices of iron status in female high school cross-country runners during and after the competitive season. The runners experienced sports anemia in that their hemoglobin concentrations and packed RBC volumes declined significantly during the first week of training (Figure 10-7). Between weeks 1 and 8 of the season, the runner's hemoglobin concentrations and packed RBC volumes gradually returned to preseason values; the serum iron and percent transferrin saturation showed steady but nonsignificant declines (Figure 10-7). By the end of the detraining period, all the iron indices had returned to initial values (except total iron-binding capacity). The authors suggest that in young women the *recovery from* sports anemia may impose a demand on body iron reserves and that it would be prudent to assess iron status as well as hematological indices in such women before and during aerobic training.

Others have found that mild anemia is not harmful to performance. Early studies in Norway on students found no relationship between hemoglobin concentration and maximal oxygen uptake after correcting for body size of students with mild anemia or low normal hemoglobin levels. Other researchers have found no difference in ventilation or heart rate in subjects with hemoglobin values between 8 and 15 gm/100 ml.

But more severe anemia is clearly associated with retarded oxygen delivery to tissues.

Table 10-7 Guidelines for the diagnosis of sports anemia

Hemoglobin Concentration in Men and Women

	Normal range	Approximate population mean
Men	14-18 gm/100 ml	16 gm/100 ml
Women	12-16 gm/100 ml	14 gm/100 ml

Suggested Criteria for Sports Anemia and Suboptimal Hemoglobin Concentration

	Sports anemia	Suboptimal hemoglobin concentration
Men	< 14 gm/100 ml	< 16 gm/100 ml
Women	< 12 gm/100 ml	< 14 gm/100 ml

Modified from Pate, R.R.: Phys. Sports Med. **11**:115, 1983.

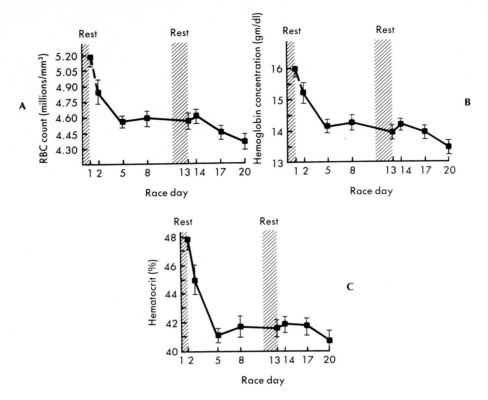

Figure 10-6 Red blood cell concentration (**A**), hemoglobin concentration (**B**) and hematocrit reading (**C**) during 312-mile race held over 20 days. Values are means (± S.E.M.) (*vertical bars*) for 12 marathon runners. (Modified from Dressendorfer, R.H., Wade, C.E., and Amsterdam, E.A.: Development of pseudoanemia in marathon runners during a 20-day road race, J.A.M.A **246**:1215, 1981)

Several studies in rats and humans support this belief. Anemia subjects have been found to demonstrate increased anaerobic metabolism during exercise, prolonged recovery times after performing standardized work loads on a bicycle ergometer, decreased maximum aerobic power, and elevated peak exercise heart rates and lactate levels following exercise.

Diagnosis of sports anemia is based on the history of athletic participation and the exclusion of other forms of anemia. A complete blood cell count is recommended along with an RBC count. (The RBC count is usually normal in athletes with sports anemia.) Serum iron levels and iron-binding capacity should be obtained to rule out iron efficiency as a cause. After the less common causes of anemia such as folic acid deficiency, vitamin B_{12} deficiency, thalassemia, and chronic disease have been eliminated, it is possible to determine the haptoglobin level immediately before and after a workout. A drop in the haptoglobin level implies that hemolysis has occurred and supports mechanical destruction of RBCs as a con-

Figure 10-7 Mean hemoglobin concentration and packed cell volume of runners and comparison subjects. Vertical lines indicate ± S.E.M. (Modified from Frederickson, L.A., Puhl, J.L., and Runyan, W.S.: Effects of training on indices of iron status of young female cross-country runners, Med. Sci. Sports Exerc. **15**:271, 1983.)

tributor to the anemia, although one cannot be sure it is the only cause.[69]

After being diagnosed as having sports anemia, many athletes ask about the usefulness of supplemental iron, even when they have been told that their iron level is normal. There is little evidence that additional iron in a non-deficient person will lead to increased RBC production. If all other causes of anemia have been eliminated and sports anemia is diagnosed, no treatment is believed to be necessary.

It should be remembered, however, that true iron deficiency may be identified in athletes

and when treated may lead to improvement in their performance. High-risk individuals should be monitored for change in iron status and provided appropriate dietary or supplementation guidelines when deemed appropriate. The incidence of iron deficiency in an otherwise healthy group of athletes is significant. Since iron deficiency is known to be the most common specific nutrient deficiency among Americans, attention to its presence should not be ignored.

Iron "conservation" is occasionally noted in the female competitor of menstrual age.[76-84] Menarche reportedly is delayed in young women who are actively involved in physically demanding athletics (Figure 10-8).[85] Secondary amenorrhea is known to result from rigorous exercise, as well as excessive weight loss leading to the establishment of a low percentage of body fat. Although many young athletes with amenorrhea have low body weights, no obvious association between fatness and menstrual regularity has been observed among athletes.[86] Theoretically, amenorrhea may ultimately improve the iron status of the competitor. It is uncertain, however, whether ongoing suppression of the normal female menstrual pattern provides any lasting harm to the health and reproductive performance of such women.

The major concern derived from recent observations is that ongoing amenorrhea in mature women may simulate menopause as far as the bony skeleton is concerned.[87-91] Cann,[87] for example, observed 25 amenorrheic patients 19 to 49 years of age and found that all demonstrated significant bone loss, as measured by a quantitative computed tomographic technique for assessing vertebral mineral content. The total group of 25 women had a mean of 28% less bone mass than 45 age-matched control subjects. Not all the women with amenorrhea developed the condition as a result of athletic participation, but bone loss in women with

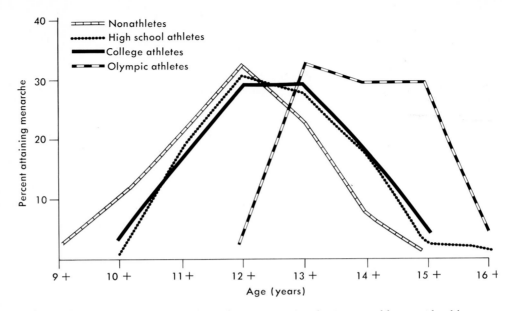

Figure 10-8   Relative distributions of ages at menarche in nonathletes and athletes at different competitive levels. The athletes attained menarche significantly later than did the nonathletes, and the Olympic athletes attained menarche significantly later than did the high school and college athletes. (From Malina, R.M., and others: Age at menarche and selected menstrual characteristics in athletes at different competitive levels and in different sports, Med. Sci. Sports 10:218, 1978).

amenorrhea for whatever cause was similar. The lingering question that is still unanswered is "Are some female athletes in danger of developing early osteoporosis?" There is also concern over the effects of prolonged hypoestrogenism on the genitourinary and vascular systems.

One alarming consequence of suboptimal bone density in amenorrheic athletes is the apparent increased risk of fracture. This possibility is supported by several recent reports of female ballet dancers and competitive runners.[92, 93] Warren and others[92] conducted a survey of 75 dancers in four professional ballet companies. The incidence of fractures in this group was 61%; it rose with increasing age of menarche. Sixty-nine percent of the fractures were stress fractures (mostly in the metatarsals)

and their occurrence had an even stronger correlation with increased age at menarche. The incidence of secondary amenorrhea was twice as high among the dancers with stress fractures and its duration was longer. In seven of ten dancers in whom endocrine studies were performed, the amenorrheic intervals were marked by prolonged hypoestrogenism. These data suggest that a delay in menarche and prolonged intervals of amenorrhea that reflect prolonged hypoestrogenism may predispose ballet dancers to stress fractures.

In another study, researchers performed a three-phase retrospective study to evaluate the effect of menstrual status upon musculoskeletal injuries in women athletes.[93] Data were gathered on the menstrual and running histories of women participants in a regional 10 km footrace. Sixty-one percent of the subjects reported an interruption of at least three months in their running program; the most common cause of interruption was injury. Those who interrupted their running were more likely to have irregular or absent menses and less likely to have been using oral contraceptives than the group of continuous runners. Subsequently, this same research team obtained information on the relationship between bone injury and menstrual status in 207 collegiate women athletes. It was found that x-ray–documented fractures occurred in 9% of the athletes with regular menses and in 24% of women athletes with irregular or absent menses. Similar data were later collected from a large group of serious recreational runners. These authors conclude that premenopausal women who have absent or irregular menses are at increased risk for musculoskeletal injury while engaged in vigorous exercise programs.

An obvious question to ask from these observations is to what degree, if any, is the amenorrhea-induced reduction in bone density reversible. This issue was addressed recently by Drinkwater and others[94] who evaluated a group of female athletes 15.5 months after an initial assessment of bone density and endocrine profile. Bone density was evaluated in (1) athletes who regained menses, (2) athletes who remained amenorrheic, and (3) athletes with regular cycles. Changes in vertebral bone mineral density were significant for the amenorrheic women who resumed menstruation (+ 6.3%) but not for the cyclic women (−0.3%); two athletes who remained amenorrheic during this period continued to lose bone (−3.4%) (Figure 10-9). These researchers conclude that resumption of menses was the primary factor for the significant increase in the vertebral bone density of the formerly amenorrheic athletes.

If amenorrhea in young women leads to bone loss or other adverse consequences, there is a need to carefully examine the contributing factors. There is a consensus that active women need not significantly change their lifestyles and eliminate exercise. That alone might provide additional stress that would contribute to menstrual irregularity. As more information is accumulated, it should be reported in such a way that it ultimately will enhance the health care provided to women. It is definitely premature, at best, to recommend that women abandon exercise programs that offer positive contributions to self-image and stress management and probably assist in the prevention of osteoporosis.

WATER

Attention to daily water requirements is of major importance to athletes of all calibers. Water is needed as the supporting medium in which all body reactions occur. In addition, it is extremely important in body temperature regulation, for excessive heat generated by exercise must be dissipated. This is done most effectively through the evaporation of sweat. This mechanism fails to function effectively, however, if the water supply is inadequate to meet the needs of the sweat glands.

A well-conditioned athlete who exercises in high temperatures will voluntarily drink more fluid. Some conscientious attention to water needs must be maintained, however, because a water deficit of approximately 3% of total body water is associated with a deterioration in performance in both males and females (Table 10-8). Individuals in prime physical condition can function effectively until body water equal to 4% to 5% of body weight is lost; at this point, athletic performance clearly deteriorates. The conscientious athlete never allows such a deficit to develop.

It should be noted, however, that although children can acclimatize to exercise in the heat, the rate of their acclimatization is slower than that of adults. Therefore the child needs more exposure to the new climate to sufficiently

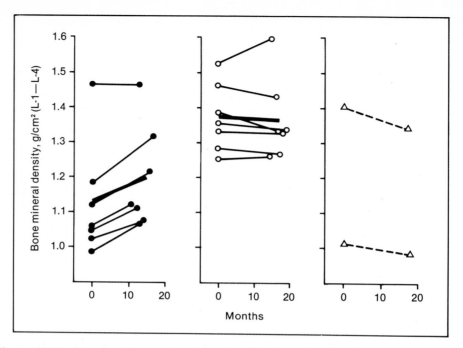

Figure 10-9   Changes in bone mineral density of lumbar spine (L-1 through L-4) with time between test 1 and test 2 for athletes who regained menses (**left**), athletes who remained cyclic (**center**), and athletes who remained amenorrheic (**right**). Broad lines represent mean values. (From Drinkwater, B.L., and others: Bone mineral density after resumption of menses in amenorrheic athletes. J. Am. Med Assoc. **256**:380, 1986.)

acclimatize. Whatever the circumstance, children frequently do not instinctively drink enough fluids to replenish fluid lost during prolonged exercise and may become gravely dehydrated. A major consequence of dehydration is an excessive increase in body temperature during exercise. For a given level of dehydration, children are subject to a greater increase in core temperature during exercise than are adults. The dehydrated child is more prone to heat-related illness than the fully hydrated one.[95]

According to the American Academy of Pediatrics,[95] children with the following conditions are at a potentially greater risk of heat stress: obesity, febrile state, cystic fibrosis, gastrointestinal infection, diabetes insipidus, diabetes mellitus, chronic heart failure, caloric malnutrition, anorexia nervosa, sweating insufficiency syndrome, and mental deficiency. The parent, the coach, and the clinician should be especially careful about monitoring children with these conditions who choose to participate in rigorous physical activities.

Negative fluid balance is commonly noted in competitive wrestlers attempting to make weight. Aggressive efforts to lose pounds quickly may involve spitting and induced sweating. Vaccaro, Zauner, and Cade[96] assessed dehydration and rehydration in college wrestlers before competition. Body weight, hematocrit, and plasma protein concentration were determined at the normal state, at weight

Table 10-8   Food restriction and fluid deprivation and dehydration produce the following:

1. Decreased muscular strength
2. Decreased work performance
3. Decreased plasma and blood volumes
4. Decreased cardiac function
5. Decreased oxygen consumption
6. Impaired thermoregulatory processes
7. Decreased kidney blood flow
8. Depletion of liver glycogen stones

certification, and just before competition. Results of analysis confirmed that wrestlers cannot regain in 5 hours all the fluid lost in the process of making weight. Thus they enter most wrestling matches in a relative state of dehydration.

Dehydration is known to produce undesirable changes in several physiological processes; these changes ultimately compromise physical performance and health (Table 10-8). The American Medical Association's guidelines for weight management in young wrestlers should be the foundation for practice of coaches and trainers (box, below).

American Medical Association's Guidelines for Weight Management in Young Wrestlers

1. 7% to 10% body fat is desirable for the wrestler.
2. The wrestler should participate in a 6-week intensive training and conditioning program with no regard for his weight.
3. Weight at the end of this period is to be his minimum effective weight for competition and certification
4. Any effort to maintain a weight below this would be a hardship on the body.

CASE STUDY: Dehydration and Pulmonary Embolism in a High School Wrestler*

A 16-year-old high school wrestler had flu-like syndrome with fever, nausea, weakness, and myalgia 2 days before a match. He lost 3.5 kg to make weight for the match and fell to an opponent he had easily defeated earlier. He was dyspneic for 30 minutes after his fall. He lost 2.5 kg by sweating and fluid restriction before another match 4 days later. He became exhausted in the second period and was pinned; cyanosis was noted and oxygen administered. The next day his physician heard a heart murmur and hospitalized the boy. Most clinical indices appeared to be normal at admission. A third heart sound was heard, and an ECG showed tachycardia with right axis deviation. A systolic murmur was heard 12 hours later, and premature ventricular beats appeared; left scapular pain was reported. Hypotension and cyanosis with severe chest pain were evident the following day. A total cardiopulmonary bypass was performed; large amounts of embolic material of varying ages were removed from both pulmonary arteries. There is presumptive evidence that dehydration before a match helped to increase blood viscosity and venous stasis, which, combined with lower extremity trauma, led to asymptomatic deep vein thrombosis and massive pulmonary embolism.

One common consequence of dehydration is the development of muscle cramps. Muscle cramps are painful, involuntary contractions of muscles caused by dehydration, electrolyte imbalance, or ischemia (an inadequate supply of blood to the muscle). These conditions are produced by exposure to severe hot or cold temperatures, overexercise, injury, or anything that irritates the muscles and causes pain. Pain impulses travel to the spinal cord, which responds by sending back impulses that cause reflex muscle contractions. These contractions create more pain, causing the vicious cycle to continue.

Heat cramps are the most familiar type of muscle cramps. They occur in people who

*Data from Croyle, P.H., Place, R.A., and Hilgenberg, A.D.: J.A.M.A. **241:**827, 1979.

sweat profusely and become dehydrated. Four to six pounds of water can be lost in an hour by some athletes performing in even moderate climates. Water is the best fluid replacement and should be consumed at the rate of 8 oz per 20 minutes of activity. Chronic dehydration can occur over several days of activity in the heat. This is avoided by checking weight regularly and conscientiously replacing lost fluid. This may require that the athlete consume fluid beyond the point of satisfying his thirst.

Under unusual circumstances, overhydration can occur. This was recently made clear by two ultramarathon runners who were hospitalized with hyponatremic encephalopathy (brain abnormalities related to low blood sodium concentration) after completing 80 and 100 km (50 and 62 miles), respectively, of an ultramarathon race in Chicago.[97] The two runners consumed such large quantities of free water during the race that apparent water intoxication developed, since sodium losses in perspiration were not satisfactorily replaced. Symptoms included disorientation, confusion, restlessness, and elevated blood pressure, heart rate, and body temperature. Treatment with intravenous saline allows for satisfactory recovery.

Ultraendurance athletes should be made aware that their salt needs are different from those of the sedentary public. Race directors and their medical personnel should know that ultraendurance athletes should never receive hypotonic intravenous fluids after extended exercise. These athletes should be encouraged to develop, train, and race with a palatable salt replacement plan.

FIBER

Fiber is now recognized as a valuable component of the diet in human beings. Even though the human gastrointestinal tract is incapable of effective digestion and absorption of this material, it promotes normal motility and regulates the rate and character of digestive and absorptive processes. But because fiber does remain in the gut along with fluid, which it may retain, it may add to body weight at a time when the athlete would prefer to be lighter weight. In addition, it may be broken down, to some degree, by bacteria in the large bowel. This may produce gas, which may disturb the feeling of optimal readiness for precise athletic competition. On occasion therefore it may behoove the competitor to moderate consumption of fiber before weigh-in or actual competition.

ALCOHOL

Some adolescent athletes have the mistaken notion that moderate alcohol consumption improves their performance.[98] In fact, ethanol cannot be used as an energy source for exercise; it does not influence maximal oxygen consumption during exercise nor does it affect anaerobic energy expenditure through sources such as ATP and PC. In addition, alcohol is a depressant to the central nervous system: it accentuates fatigue by increasing the production of lactate; it slows the reaction time; it interferes with reflexes; and it destroys coordination. Overall, the effect of alcohol on physical performance appears to be negative on all counts; decreased performance has been reported thus far in tests of dynamic balance, visual tracking, arm steadiness, body sway, and various other psychomotor tasks. However, as one high school alcoholic noted:[98] the sensation promoted by alcohol is deceptively positive, that

> I would drink before going to school, and I'd get to physical education class rarin' to go. But the coordination wasn't there. I *felt* I could perform better, but it was all in my head. In reality, I really performed worse.

"HEALTH FOODS" AND THE VEGETARIAN DIET

A wide variety of foods are presently available to consumers in the United States. Most of these foods provide valuable nutrients along with the ever-present calories; some provide more nutrients per 100 calories than others. Ingestion of an array of basic foods may allow for establishment and maintenance of health. No foods carry magical properties that make them especially effective in promoting optimal physical performance.

It is generally wise to be leery of advertisements that tout the value of a new "health food." Often such products are quite expensive and provide nothing more than can normally be obtained from a balanced diet. The typical athlete usually consumes a sizable number of calories each day. The majority of such individuals obtain their required nutritional support through food sources in the daily menu.

The vegetarian diet can support good health, providing that basic pitfalls are avoided (see Chapter 9). Satisfactory nonmeat sources of iron, calcium, vitamin B_{12}, zinc, protein, and calories must be selected. Combining vegetable proteins so that they complement each other is especially important for the strict vegetarian athlete. Since most vegetables provide calories in a more dilute form than do animal materials, the athlete must be careful about meeting calorie needs so that both growth and the energy level for athletic competition are maintained.

NUTRITIONAL PREPARATION FOR ATHLETIC PERFORMANCE

Short-Term Events

Before a short-term athletic contest a general well-balanced diet should be consumed. Immediately before the competition, muscular work should be limited, so that muscle sources of energy will be plentiful. Between several scheduled short-term events, time should be allowed to replenish these energy sources (e.g., ATP, PC, and glycogen) and clear the by-products of anaerobic metabolism (e.g., lactic acid). An adequate supply of carbohydrate and water should be available throughout the day. Fruit juices are popular with many athletes, but some prefer complete liquid meals or other eas-

ily digested foods. To avoid a heavy, sluggish feeling, athletes should restrict their intake of high-fiber foods, such as the following:

1. Whole grains (e.g., cereals, breads, and other derivatives)
2. Dried peas and beans
3. Nuts and seeds
4. Fruits, especially raw with skins
5. Vegetables, especially raw with skins, stems, and seeds.
6. Bran

Avoidance of high-fat foods, which demand long-term digestion, will also support a feeling of readiness. The following is a list of representative high-fat foods:

1. Butter and margarine
2. Cream, sour cream, ice cream, mayonnaise, gravy, and salad dressings
3. Meats, especially fried or fatty
4. Creamed dishes
5. Most cheeses and cheese dishes
6. Pastry
7. Bacon and sausage
8. Chocolate

Gas-forming foods should be minimized in the diet if gas formation is disturbing or distracting to the athlete. Gas-forming foods include the following:

1. Melons
2. Sulfur-containing vegetables such as cabbage, cauliflower, radishes, brussels sprouts, turnips, onions, rutabagas, green peppers, dried peas and beans, lentils, apples, corn, and avocados
3. Others (different for each person)

Long-Term Events

Preparation for lengthy competitive activities involves attention to the same basic nutrition principles encountered in other circumstances. In addition, sensible eating practices on the day of the event should be followed. On the morning of the competition high-bulk foods and fatty foods should be avoided, and choices should be made from available carbohydrate sources. In preparation for a lengthy afternoon competition, a light lunch that is low in residue and fatty foods should be taken at least $2\frac{1}{2}$ hours before the starting time. Foods that are satisfying to the individual should be selected.

When choosing high-carbohydrate foods for consumption on competition day, athletes should avoid those that are too concentrated in form. Such foods include honey, glucose syrups, and high-sugar/high-electrolyte beverages. Such concentrated solutions, when present in the gut, may provoke the movement of water from body tissues into the gut lumen to balance the osmotic condition; this may cause abdominal discomfort and diarrhea, which may aggravate poor gastric function already present in the nervous athlete. Diluted, sweetened fruit juices or fruit-flavored drinks are tolerated better than are more concentrated products.

Caffeine-containing beverages (e.g., cola drinks) are of questionable merit because of their initial ability to act as stimulants followed by a tendency to produce depression in young athletes. Individuals who are particularly sensitive to caffeine may develop adverse central nervous system and cardiovascular effects as well as ringing in the ears, insomnia, gastric irritation, and diuresis. The diuretic effect of caffeine may not only increase risk of dehydration, but it may also bring on the urge to urinate at a critical point during the athletic competition. Whether or not caffeine consumption improves endurance is a subject of debate since both positive and negative results have been reported.[99,100] Since the International Olympic Committee has ruled that using caffeine as a "stimulant" is unacceptable, it should not be considered an issue for children in sports.

Some athletes in recent years have used the glycogen-loading diet to maximize muscle glycogen stores for moderate to long-term activities.[101] Since the readily available anaerobic energy sources in muscle cells are exhausted within 5 minutes of heavy physical activity and since enough oxygen cannot be supplied to muscle to meet energy needs through metabolism alone, a substantial store of glycogen is very useful. Glycogen stores support an increase in anaerobic energy production just when it is needed. An example of the value of extra muscle glycogen is provided in Figure 10-10. The work times of men on bicycle ergometers markedly increased as muscle glycogen stores were augmented.

Glycogen stores can be greatly increased by adherence to a high-carbohydrate regimen during the week preceding competition. For some athletes a high-carbohydrate diet has proved successful for improving performance when moderate to long-term energy support is demanded. The glycogen-loading diet was developed as a follow-up to data originally collected by Swedish physiologists. These workers conducted studies of muscle glycogen content during the course of a week of controlled dietary intake (Figure 10-11). It was found that on a normal diet, the average concentration of glycogen in muscle tissue was approximately 1.75 gm/100 gm of muscle. When the diet was reversed to include large amounts of carbohydrate, the level increased to 3.5 gm/100 gm muscle. The same studies demonstrated that if the specific muscle was exercised strenuously to specifically deplete it of glycogen while on a low-carbohydrate diet, the subsequent institution of a high-carbohydrate diet caused the glycogen to rise to 4.7 gm/100 gm in the exercised muscle. This Swedish work thus demonstrated that glycogen stores could be practically tripled through diet modification in conjunction with a program to first deplete then replete muscle glycogen content.

Figure 10-10 Relationship between initial muscle glycogen content in quadriceps femoris and work time in six subjects on bicycle ergometers with the same relative load three times each with 3-day intervals. Diets before exercise: (**1**) mixed (*open circle*), (**2**) carbohydrate free (*closed circle*), and (**3**) carbohydrate rich (*triangle*). (Redrawn from Bergstrom, J., and Hultman, E.: Nutrition for maximal sports performance, J.A.M.A. **221**:999, 1972.)

The glycogen-loading diet as it traditionally is prescribed involves 6 days of attention to dietary manipulation, as illustrated in Figure 10-12. If the event is to be held on Saturday, the athlete starts on the preceding Sunday evening or early Monday morning by consuming a diet that is rich in protein and fat, with carbohydrate representing only approximately 10% of the daily calories. After several days of this depletion phase, most athletes find that they tire easily and perform suboptimally during practice sessions. On the third day, the high-protein, high-fat regimen is replaced by a high-carbohydrate diet. Carbohydrate-rich foods are emphasized in this period, but protein and fat may still be consumed at reasonably normal levels. Some athletes have used flavored beverages that are rich in glucose to supply part of the carbohydrate needs.

Adherence to the glycogen-loading diet requires dedication on the part of the athlete, particularly during the first phase, when carbohydrate intake is rigorously restricted. During this time, the specified diet is significantly different from that usually consumed. The fatigued feeling that often develops during this period may prove frustrating and discouraging to the athlete in training. Consequently,

Figure 10-11   Effect of dietary composition on muscle glycogen content of endurance athletes. *CHO*, Carbohydrate. (From Bergstrom, J., and Hultman, E.: Nutrition for maximal sports performance, J.A.M.A. **221**:999, 1972. Copyright 1972, American Medical Association.)

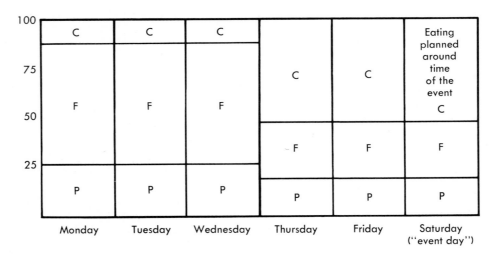

Figure 10-12   Diagrammatic representation of daily dietary composition of an athlete following the strict glycogen-loading routine. *C*, Carbohydrate; *F*, fat; *P*, Protein. (In some cases, Wednesday's routine may be like Thursday's and Friday's if a shorter depletion period is specified.)

it is wise to use the glycogen-loading regimen with considerable discretion; it probably should not be undertaken for every competition during the season, but should be reserved for those few occasions when special preparation is clearly in order. In fact, it is impossible to attain extremely high muscle glycogen storage at more frequent intervals than a few weeks, even if the program is carefully followed. At other times, the athlete may prefer to emphasize the high-carbohydrate aspect of the diet for 3 to 4 days preceding competition. This is obviously much easier to accomplish, because the several days of fatigue associated with the high-fat, high-protein depletion phase may then be avoided. In fact, more recent research has shown that levels of glycogen storage close to that achieved with the full depletion/loading regimen can be reached with just a high-carbohydrate diet and rest.[102]

Just how safe the glycogen-loading diet is remains to be confirmed through continued observation. Glycogen retains water, and both substances may be deposited in muscle to such an extent that the athlete may feel heavy and stiff. The weight increase caused by water retention may reduce the ability of the athlete to take up oxygen maximally. Based on individual case studies, fears have been raised that glycogen loading may cause cardiac arrhythmias, raise serum triglyceride levels, and destroy muscle fibers by the excessive glycogen storage. Little definitive proof has been found to support these fears. Recently, however, an Oregon State University researcher reported observation of cardiac arrhythmias during the depletion of the carbohydrate-loading regimen four health male runners.[103] This scientist suggests that the diet causes the skeletal muscles to rob from the heart muscle, using the glycogen the heart should be using. He suggests that marathon runners should skip the glycogen-depletion phase if carbohydrate loading is attempted.

The onset of exhaustion is thought to reflect depletion of glycogen stored in the muscles and liver. The terms *bonking* and *hitting the wall* are used (box, below). When muscle glycogen is depleted, muscle contraction fails. When liver glycogen is depleted, the blood glucose level falls, causing exercise-induced hypoglycemia, which impairs the functioning of the nervous system, muscular tissue, and RBCs.

When the skeletal muscle is depleted of glycogen, glycogen synthetase activity increases (Figure 10-13). This enzyme stimulates the synthesis of glycogen, a process that begins soon after rigorous activity ceases. The time required for glycogen repletion depends on the intensity of the exercise that was undertaken and the amount of carbohydrate that is consumed in the diet. Even when carbohydrates provide 90% of the calories, after exhaustive exercises 46 to 48 hours are required to restore muscle glycogen to preexercise levels. Restoration rates appear to vary; some athletes are not able to restore muscle glycogen on a high-carbohydrate diet, even after a 5-day rest.

During repeated days of endurance training, Costill noted a small restoration of muscle glycogen when subjects are fed a mixed diet containing 250 gm of carbohydrate per day. Figure 10-14 illustrates the steady decline in muscle glycogen content with successive days

---

**Definitions of Terms
Describing Glycogen Depletion**

Bonking—running out of liver glycogen, which causes hypoglycemia, dizziness, shakiness, and confusion. An athlete can recover from a bonk by eating immediately.

Hitting the wall—running out of muscle glycogen with the development of fatigue. The athlete usually cannot come back or continue, even if he or she eats some carbohydrate.

Figure 10-13 Changes in muscle glycogen concentration and in muscle glycogen synthetase activity during and after a marathon run.

Figure 10-14 Muscle glycogen content during 3 days of heavy training with diets whose caloric compositions were 40% carbohydrate (low *CHO*) and 70% carbohydrate (high *CHO*) (Modified from Costill, D., and Miller, J.M.: Nutrition for endurance sports: carbohydrate and fluid balance. Int. J. Sports Med. 1:2, 1980)

of training that these subjects show. A diet rich in carbohydrates (550-600 gm/day), on the other hand, effectively restores muscle glycogen in the 22 hours between training sessions.

The high carbohydrate diet of greater than 500 gm/day often requires that people continue eating after satiation.[9] When athletes are allowed to eat ad libitum, they often underestimate their caloric needs and consume too little carbohydrate to fully restore muscle glycogen. It appears that individuals who perform prolonged, intense exercise on repeated days must consume a diet rich in carbohydrate to minimize the cumulative effects of glycogen depletion and chronic fatigue.

The source of carbohydrate used for repletion appears to make some difference. Costill and others[104] compared diets containing simple sugars with those containing complex carbohydrates. They found no differential effects after 24 hours; after 48 hours, however, the muscle glycogen levels were higher after eating starches than after eating simple sugars (Figure 10-15). The researchers suggested that the different responses in insulin and glucose could explain their results. Although insulin levels after a starch meal are lower, they remain elevated over baseline levels longer when compared with an equivalent glucose meal.[104]

Pregame Meal

Many superstitions exist in our society about which foods to consume before competition. In reality, there is no magic formula for every person. Since individuals differ with regard to food preferences, psychological crutches, and digestive response to stress, a variety of food items and eating schedules may support good

Figure 10-15   The effects of wheat products (bread and pasta) and sugar on replacement of skeletal muscle glycogen levels. One day after a depleting exercise there was no difference in glycogen levels; however, 48 hours after exercise the complex carbohydrate diet caused a significantly higher glycogen level. (Redrawn from Costill, D.L. and others: The role of dietary carbohydrates in muscle glycogen resynthesis after strenuous running. Am. J. Clin. Nutr. **34**:184, 1981.)

preparation. Still, the following recommendations for sensible pregame food apply to all athletes:

1. The diet should include familiar foods that the athlete believes "will make him win."
2. Energy intake should be sufficient to prevent hunger and faintness during the period of competition.
3. The foods chosen should be relatively easy to digest, so that the stomach and upper gut are empty at the time of competition.
4. Fluid intake should be sufficient to maintain an optimal level of hydration throughout the day.
5. Gas-forming foods should be selected with discretion and should be avoided if they pose problems for the athlete.
6. Meals should not be skipped entirely, because the overall performance capacity of the athlete may ultimately suffer.

At times the liquid pregame meal may be chosen as a sound alternative to other available options. Commercial products such as Sustagen, Sustacal, and Ensure provide a palatable high-carbohydrate, high-calorie, high-fluid pregame diet. These products typically provide sufficient amounts of fat and protein to promote satiation and palatibility, but the fluid character of the meal allows for its easy passage through the stomach and small intestine. Aside from these characteristics, a liquid diet has no particular advantage that warrants its serious consideration as a diet of choice. If the team or athlete accepts such a preparation and believes that it optimizes performance, it may be justifiably selected as a sound, nutritious pregame diet.

A common practice of part-time athletes is consuming "quick-energy foods" (candy, honey, and concentrated sugar drinks) 20 to 30 minutes before a sports event. This may actually impair their performance. Eating such concentrated sugars increases plasma insulin, which in turn inhibits the utilization of free fatty acids by the muscle. Another objection to quick energy foods is that the osmotic effect of concentrated sugars may cause retention of fluids in the gastrointestinal tract. The athletes may experience nausea, stomach cramps, and, during endurance events, dehydration.

A dilute sugar solution (2% or less), which can be safely consumed periodically during an endurance sport, helps to restore fluids lost and to maintain blood sugar levels. Once an athlete begins to exercise, periodic ingestion of dilute glucose solutions does not significantly increase plasma insulin concentration. One study has shown that drinking a solution containing glucose polymers alone or with fructose every 25 minutes during a 55-mile bicycle ride resulted in a better finishing time and reduced fatigue in highly conditioned cyclists.[105] Another observation of stationary cyclists showed that blood glucose and carbohydrate metabolism were significantly higher throughout the trials when a carbohydrate-containing solution was ingested than when water was ingested (Figure 10-16).

One final comment about pregame preparation relates to the controversial practice of soda loading. The theory behind this practice is that sodium bicarbonate will raise the pH level of the muscle, and thus rid the muscle more quickly of hydrogen ions; the buildup of these ions is known to bring on muscle fatigue. The study providing the most support for this practice was conducted by Wilkes, Gledhill, and Smyth in 1983.[106] Six trained middle-distance runners were studied after ingestion of sodium bicarbonate ($NaHCO_3$) or a placebo such as calcium carbonate ($CaCO_3$) to determine the effect of an acute metabolic alkalosis on the time it took to run an 800-meter race. In the alkalotic state subjects ran faster (2.9 seconds), and the corresponding postexercise values for blood lactate concentration and extracellular hydrogen ion (H^+) levels were higher than in the control conditions, suggesting an increased anaerobic energy contribution. These results support

Figure 10-16   Blood glucose and the rate *CHO* oxidation during 4 hours of cycling at 50% of VO_2max with (*CHO*) and without (control) sugar feedings. (Redrawn from Costill, D.L., Carbohydrate nutrition before, during, and after exercise. Fed. Proc. 44:364, 1985.)

the speculation that the increase in extracellular buffering following $NaCHO_3$ ingestion facilitated H^+ efflux from the cells of working muscle, thereby delaying the decrease in intracellular pH and postponing fatigue. It was concluded that the ingestion of $NaHCO_3$ (300 mg/ kg/-body weight) by middle-distance runners before an 800-meter race had an ergogenic effect.

Since this report was published, several others groups have attempted to evaluate the merits of soda loading[107]; negative findings were reported. According to the 1983 researchers, however, these negative results should be expected since the practice is helpful only in anaerobic situations with durations up to 4 minutes. Whether or not soda loading works remains to be confirmed by future research. In the meantime, its efficacy should be irrelevant

to performing athletes, since it is contrary to the ethics of competition.

WEIGHT MANAGEMENT

Adjustment of body weight is sometimes necessary to prepare an athlete to perform optimally in certain sports. Neither weight loss nor weight gain is easily achieved, and both adjustments require appropriate early planning so that goals may be reached within a *reasonable* period. Weight that is lost or gained represents mainly fat and muscle; ideally, weight that is lost should consist mostly of fat, whereas weight that is gained should consist predominantly of muscle and its associated fluid. Major changes of this sort do not occur overnight, especially in the absence of physical activity. Planning well in advance of the scheduled competition is an absolute must; and any sound program in weight management must emphasize rigorous physical training, not just diet, to satisfactorily meet and maintain weight gain or weight loss goals. Last-minute attention to weight modification may compromise both the health and performance of the athlete.

Three components are vital to the success of any organized weight management program. First, sufficient time should be allowed; in most cases, a maximum rate of gain of 0.5 to 1 kg of muscle mass/week should be anticipated. Weight loss at a rate of 1 kg/week is usually the desired rate; never should this rate exceed 2 kg/week. Second, all special diets or food plans for weight management should fulfill all nutritional needs, including those for protein, vitamins, and minerals. Thus vitamin, mineral, and protein supplements are not necessary; although occasionally iron supplements may be justifiably recommended for women of reproductive age. Third, weight management programs are ideally supervised by individuals other than the head coach. This duty is best delegated to a team nutritionist, physician, trainer, or assistant coach.

During the season of scheduled competitions, some sports (e.g., wrestling) require that pre-event body weight be recorded. Athletes can safely minimize weight at the time by avoiding salty foods, which promote excessive water retention, and by reducing intakes of dietary fiber, which may linger in the gut lumen and provide unneeded weight. Water intake should not be compromised during this period, and efforts to promote dehydration as a means of making weight (e.g., vomiting, spitting, exercising in plastic suits, sauna bathing, and using diuretics and cathartics) should never be undertaken.

Some young athletes go to incredible extremes to lose body weight or maintain it at a low level.[108-114] This is especially evident in the individual whose basal metabolic rate is low to moderate and whose typical level of body fat is well above 10% of total body weight. To maintain a body composition of 5% fat requires considerable training and dietary self-control for the majority of athletes, male or female. Since females normally support a much higher body fat content, however, the effort required in training and diet is often tremendous. Unfortunately, some athletes place so much emphasis on achievement of minimum body fatness that starvation diets and demanding training schedules are undertaken. Such practices may adversely affect endurance, physical growth, and psychological stability.

Excessive weight loss and food aversion similar to that seen in anorexia nervosa are problems among some seriously committed young athletes. This pathological aversion to food and fatness differs from anorexia nervosa in that male and female athletes appear to be at equal risk, the affected athlete is usually recognized relatively early, and the emotional stresses leading to the weight loss are not usually deep-seated or chronic, but are short-term concerns that respond well to counseling. According to Dr. N. Smith,[115] "the athlete at greatest risk of abusive weight loss is typically a serious student and outstanding athlete with unrealistic goals who fears failure to meet the high expectations of coaches, parents, and friends."

Most successful athletes do not function optimally at very low levels of body fatness. Many recent studies have examined the physical and physiological characteristics of various types of elite athletes. Several of these studies have focused on children and thus provide some reference for the concerned parent, coach, or health care provider. Thorland and others[116] examined boys and girls (15.2 to 18.6 years of age) who were participating in the Junior Olympics (Table 10-9); their percentage of body fat ranged between 7.3% and 13.9% for the boys and between 12.5% and 22% for the girls. Mayers and Gutin[117] looked at elite

Table 10-9   Percentage body fat in a group of Junior Olympians by event

Event Category	Percent Body Fat (Males)	Percent Body Fat (Females)
Middle-distance runs	7.3	12.5
Mile walk	9.9	15.1
Sprints and hurdles	8.4	13.4
Throws	13.9	22.0
Jumps and vaults	8.5	12.9
Gymnastics and diving	8.4	14.8
Wrestling	9.7	—

Data from Throland, W.G., and others: Med. Sci. Sports Exerc. **13**:332, 1981.

prepubertal male cross-country runners; their percentage of body fat ranged from 14% to 18.6%. Sady and others[118] recorded the body composition and physical dimensions of 9- to 12-year-old experienced wrestlers; their mean percentage of body fat was 13.3%, a level nearly 30% higher than that found in more mature wrestlers and almost twice that recommended by the American College of Sports Medicine (7%).

Some athletes desirous of improving performance attempt to increase body weight. This practice is most common in the United States among young men playing football. To gain weight, a person must ingest sufficient calories and protein to support tissue deposition. A variety of diets have been tried by athletes seeking to gain weight, but simple ingestion of larger portions of basic foods may provide what is needed. Alternatively, nutritious high-calorie snacks may be added to the diet. Diets that are rich in saturated fats and cholesterol should be avoided. Vitamin and protein supplements serve no useful purpose in the overall plan.

Increases in body weight ideally result from creation of lean body mass instead of fat. Increasing muscle mass can only result from muscle work. An intake of approximately 2500 extra calories is needed to acquire 0.5 kg of muscle tissue. The addition of 750 to 1000 kcal/day to a regular diet will provide the energy needs for gaining 0.5 to 1 kg/week as well as for the increased energy output of the muscle-training program. Specific details of a muscle development program should be geared to the age and condition of the athlete. Progress should be assessed at regular intervals by measuring fatfold thickness and body weight, reviewing dietary practices and problems, and judging psychological and emotional status. Excessive deposition of body fat may indicate that the muscle-training program requires modification.

ERGOGENIC AIDS

A variety of products and programs are marketed for the athlete, often with claims that performance will be markedly enhanced if the product or program is adopted (Table 10-10). Very little evidence exists to support the use of these agents and in some cases adverse side effects are cause for concern.

Vitamin B_{15} (pangamic acid) is widely used by amateur and professional athletes because they believe it lowers blood lactic acid, stabilizes blood sugar during exercise, and reduces the effects of fatigue. This substance is actually not a vitamin at all but a mixture of calcium gluconate and Dimethylglycine. Russian stud-

Table 10-10   Characteristics of selected ergogenic agents

I. Bee Pollen

A. Composition

Bee pollen is a mixture of bee saliva, plant nectar, and pollen (the male germ cells of flowering plants). Traditionally, the pollen is brushed off the back legs and pollen basket of worker bees forced to enter the hive through a portal partially obstructed by a wire mesh. But with the increasing popularity of pollen as a health food, this means of pollen collection has proved inadequate to meet demand. Instead, tons of bee pollen are now being produced after direct collection from hives.

The pollen material is sold either as loose powder, compressed into tablets of 400-500 mg with or without other nutritional supplements, or as capsules.

Manufacturers' data suggest that after removal of the water, the protein varies from 10%-36% with an average of 20%; the essential amino acid content is reasonably high. Simple sugars, such as those in honey, make up 10%-15% of the content, and in addition to small quantities of fats, pollen contains significant amounts of minerals, such as potassium, magnesium, phosphorus, calcium, copper, and iron. Some vitamins are also present including thiamine, riboflavin, niacin, pantothenic acid, ascorbic acid, biotin, and carotenes.

B. Problems Claimed to be Helped by Product

A vast body of literature, especially in the lay press, has extolled the curative properties of pollen in diseases ranging from colitis, premature aging, and renal disease to skin blemishing and weight loss. A flier from a local health food store claims that "pollen has a dramatic effect upon mental perception in athletic performance. In documented clinical trials, IQs of children have been doubled and resistance to stress has been increased significantly in both animals and humans. Experiments by French doctors suggest that pollen contains both antibiotic and growth factors."

C. Proven Assets of Product

Scientific literature on the composition and healthful properties of bee pollen is almost nil, and evidence defining health benefits is entirely anecdotal.

D. Adverse Side Effects of Use (Especially in Large Amounts)

A recent report describes three patients who experienced systemic reactions after ingesting bee pollen. Another patient was reportedly treated after suffering an anaphylactic reaction from ingestion of bee pollen for remedy of his allergic rhinitis. In most of the cases, the specific allergen causing the problem derived from a plant pollen contaminating the bee pollen.

Since bee pollen contains nucleic acids, high intakes are not recommended for those individuals predisposed to gout or who have signs of renal disease.

E. Other Comments

Taken as a supplement, it appears that bee pollen might provide a satisfactory nutritional contribution to the diet of an individual who cared to pay the price for the product.

II. Brewer's Yeast

A. Composition

Brewer's yeast is the nonfermentative, nonextracted yeast of the botanical classification *Saccharomyces* and is derived as a by-product from the brewing of beer and ale. It is generally sold in dry form since the fresh form spoils readily.

Table 10-10   Characteristics of selected ergogenic agents — *cont'd*

A suitable daily portion of the dried yeast is 1-2 tbsp (15-30ml) and may be mixed in vegetable drinks (e.g. tomato juice), cooked cereals, flavored instant breakfast drinks, gravies, meat loaf, and various sauces.

If there is a choice of product, one that is "debittered" should be selected. Tablets are also available for those who prefer a more convenient and palatable form of the product.

B. Problems Claimed to be Helped by Product

Brewer's yeast is promoted as a natural potent source of protein, vitamins, minerals, and nucleic acids: consequently, athletes have used it as an energy food.

Claims for its usefulness in diabetes are related to its content of GTF-chromium. In fact, one investigation showed that a group of elderly subjects provided with brewer's yeast (rich in available chromium) significantly improved in glucose tolerance and serum cholesterol levels compared with torula yeast (low in chromium).

C. Proven Assets of Product

Brewer's yeast is used primarily as a rich supplemental source of B vitamins, although it is also a good source of fair quality protein, with a minimum of 35% crude protein. When irradiated with ultraviolet light, it provides vitamin D.

It is rich in chromium and selenium, minerals that are limited in the diets of some Americans. Chromium is present in an organic form (glucose tolerance factor) that is much more beneficial to the body than the inorganic form of the mineral.

D. Adverse Side Effects of Use (Especially in Large Amounts)

Since brewer's yeast is rich in nucleic acids, individuals susceptible to gout should be cautious in their use of the product.

Systemic saccharomyces yeast infections have resulted from daily oral ingestion of viable organisms in brewer's yeast. As a supplement, it is important to make sure the yeast is dead.

III. Ginseng

A. Composition

Ginseng is the root of the ginseng plant and is sold in capsules, extract, instant powder, paste, tea (sometimes made with leaves), and whole root.

Ginseng's growing popularity is attributed to pharmacologically active agents that exert stimulant action. Ginseng contains peptides, steroids, and many unidentified substances that appear responsible for its stimulant effect. Nevertheless, some commercial ginseng products are devoid of these active agents. Others may be "spiked" with synthetic products and drugs. In addition, most of the ginseng sold in the United States may be derived from a North American plant related to the original *Panax schinseng* plant. Though little work has been done, evidence suggest that extracts from the original plant may not have the same pharmacological effects as extracts from related plants.

B. Problems Claimed to be Helped by Product

Ginseng is claimed to be a general tonic for digestive troubles, impotence, and overall lack of vitality.

C. Proven Assets of Product

Report of effectiveness are largely anecdotal. The amounts consumed (1 tsp or 5 gm) are too small to contribute much in the way of nutrients. Recently, however, extracts from ginseng root powder were shown to have cholesterol-lowering effects in birds. This effect has been attributed to saponins (ginsenosides) in ginseng.

Continued.

Table 10-10   Characteristics of selected ergogenic agents — *cont'd*

D. Adverse Side Effects of Use (Especially in Large Amounts)

In China, doses of ginseng up to 50 gm have been tested, and 2-3 gm is considered the amount needed to elicit behavioral stimulation. However, recently, what has become known as the Ginseng Abuse Syndrome has been associated with use of the herb. With doses as low as 3 gm, hypertension and neurological symptoms such as insomnia, nervousness, feelings of depersonalization, confusion, and depression have been reported. Also, skin eruptions, edema, and diarrhea are seen. Abrupt withdrawal of ginseng may lead to hypotensive crises.

Ginseng has been reported to produce a physiological estrogen-like effect on the vaginal mucosa, mastalgia with diffuse mammary nodularity in postmenopausal women, and, experimentally, stimulation of corticotropin secretion and altered RNA hepatic metabolism. After a bilateral oophorectomy, one research team observed a notable vaginal effect in a patient ingesting an unstated amount of Romanian ginseng only 2 weeks per month. A 72-year-old woman experienced vaginal bleeding and a moderate estrogen effect after ingesting one tablet daily of a Swiss-Austrian geriatric formula containing 200 mg ginseng of an unspecified source.

IV. Protein supplements

A. Composition

Protein supplements are available as liquids, powders, and tablets. They contain either all the essential amino acids to make a "high quality" protein or only specific amino acids.

B. Problems Claimed to be Helped by Product

Products are often promoted to improve physical performance, assist in weight reduction, or build skeletal muscles.

C. Proven Assets of Product

Most Americans consume far more protein than they can use; excess protein can be converted to fat that the body eventually can burn. No evidence exists that athletes or physically active people require protein in excess of levels normally required by adolescents or that extra protein improves physical performance.

D. Adverse Side Effects of Use (Especially in Large Amounts)

Excess protein can lead to ketosis, dehydration, tendency for gout, and increased urinary excretion of calcium.

V. Royal jelly

A. Composition

Royal jelly is a milky white substance produced by worker bees to nourish the queen bee. Queen bees differ from worker bees; they are about twice the size, they live up to 8 years (about 40 times longer than worker bees), and they lay about 2000 eggs per day (female worker bees are infertile).

While the egg of the queen starts out like all the others, the royal jelly fed to this bee is the basis for the difference that develops during the growth state.

Royal jelly is sold in capsule form as a nutritional supplement, but it is also an ingredient in certain expensive cosmetics.

B. Problems Claimed to be Helped by Product

The implication of promoters of royal jelly is that it will do as much for humans as it does for queen bees—it will increase size, longevity, and fertility. Although it is a rich source of certain B vitamins (like pantothenic acid), it has not been shown to possess any recognizable preventive, therapeutic, or rejuvenating characteristics.

Table 10-10   Characteristics of selected ergogenic agents — *cont'd*

C. Proven Assets of Product
None known.

D. Adverse Side Effects of Use (Especially in Large Amounts)
None reported.

VI. Wheat germ
A. Composition
Wheat germ is the embryo of the sprouting part of the wheat seed. It constitutes only 2.5% of the kernel and is the source of wheat germ meal and wheat germ oil.

Wheat germ meal is low in fiber, high in fat and vitamin E, and fairly rich in protein (minimum 25% crude protein). Defatted wheat germ is the product that remains after removal of part of the oil from the meal; it contains at least 30% crude protein, but is much lower in vitamin E than regular wheat germ meal.

The defatting process is desirable, however, in that the fat decomposes readily and markedly reduces the shelf-life of the product. The label indicates whether the germ is defatted.

Wheat germ is a good source of calories, essential fatty acids, protein, minerals, vitamin E, and the B vitamins.

B. Problems Claimed to be Helped by Product
Wheat germ and its oil are on the list of popular ergogenic foods. A well-known athletic trainer with good academic credentials published experiments that led him to propose the benefit of wheat germ in improving physical performance. His findings received considerable attention. However, other researchers have been unable to reproduce his work or show evidence that wheat germ or its oil improves physical performance. This same athletic trainer also claimed to have isolated from wheat germ a compound, octacosanol, that provides energy and builds endurance. Recently, octacosanol has become available as a single supplement. It is a solid white alcohol extracted from wheat germ, but again the criticisms raised against wheat germ also apply to its components.

C. Proven Assets of Product
Wheat germ meal is used chiefly as a livestock feed, although some of it is now used as a human nutritional supplement. Wheat germ oil is used primarily as a rich vitamin E supplement for humans and animals. It can be added to many kinds of foods, such as bread, cookies, cereals, and milkshakes.

D. Adverse Side Effects of Use (Especially in Large Amounts)
None reported.

---

ies suggest that use of this substance promotes increased oxygen efficiency, but these investigations were not properly controlled. Several American studies support the claims of reduced lactic acid and increased performance, but others show no measurable effects. It may be that further studies are justified, but presently it is illegal to sell vitamin B_{15} as a dietary supplement or a drug.

Since the Italian soccer team won the World Cup in 1982, claiming their carnitine supplements gave them the winning edge, carnitine has been a popular product in health food establishments. Enthusiasts claim this amino acid derivative strengthens athletes for the long haul, bolsters ailing hearts, and abets dieting. This all sounds plausible, since L-carnitine is responsible for moving fatty acids into mitochondria to be burned for fuel. Endurance depends on fat metabolism, hence the high hopes for high performance. But there are no data on human need for carnitine; we get carnitine from food (meat and dairy products, mostly) and we manufacture our own supply in the liver and kidneys. Vegetarians, who get very little dietary carnitine, apparently make up the difference with little trouble.

Most of the carnitine available for purchase is in the DL form. Several reports suggest that D-carnitine may inhibit the action of the L-isomer,[119-121] thus possibly creating a carnitine-deficiency state. Deficiency of an enzyme that uses carnitine, carnitine palmityl transferase, produces symptoms of muscle cramps, myoglobinuria, and muscle weakness in humans. Symptoms become progressively worse during prolonged exercise, after consumption of high fat diets, with fasting, and during cold weather.

The case of a 35-year-old male distance runner demonstrates an adverse reaction to supplemental DL-carnitine. This experienced runner ate 500 mg of DL-carnitine each night for two nights before a half-marathon race. He noticed a slight tingling sensation after ingestion of carnitine although no problems were encountered in the race. During the following weeks, urine samples after training runs ranged from pink to brown in color; he had never had an previous episodes of blood or myoglobin in the urine. In addition, he had extreme weakness of the quadriceps muscles. Urine discoloration and weakness were worse on cold, windy days. After one month of reduced activity, the runner had to cease training altogether for a period of four to five weeks. Training was then resumed with no further ill effects.[122]

Bee pollen continues to be very big business. Sales by one company in Sweden totaled more than $2.5 million in 1984. That company manufactured more than 140 million pollen tablets from a harvest of 20 tons of pollen. Lay literature claims that bee pollen improves athletic and sexual performance; prevents infection, allergy, and cancer; prolongs life; and improves digestion. Despite these claims, only one medical study about the effects of bee pollen on athletic performance has been published.[123] Results from that study indicated that bee pollen does not improve athletic performance.

Concern remains about the continued popularity of anabolic steroids, even among young boys and women.[124] Users generally assume that these agents increase strength, lean muscle mass, and athletic performance. Data on the effects of androgenic anabolic steroids on physical performance are generally negative both in humans[125] and in animals.[126, 127] Moreover, steroid treatment has been shown to be followed by a reduction of endogenous testosterone production; side effects include liver disorders, growth disorders, cardiovascular disease, reproductive abnormalities, and possibly other problems, like hypertension. The Black Market in steroids is estimated at $100 million a year, according to the FDA. Since 1985, federal investigations have resulted in indictments, convictions, and the seizure of $7 million in illegal steroids. In one of those convictions, a California man was found guilty on 21 counts of dispensing human and animal steroids without prescriptions. On December 5, 1986, he was sentenced to six years in prison and was ordered to pay more than $210,000 in fines and penalties.[128]

Of course arresting the dealers is only half the battle to stop the illegal market. As long as there are buyers, there will be new dealers to take the places of the ones who were caught. To really stop the problem, athletes must be convinced that the dangers are not worth whatever extra edge the steroids might give them. Recently, the FDA sent brochures with warnings about steroids to high schools throughout the United States. In addition, the agency is sending those schools 100,000 posters of professional wrestler Jesse Ventura telling athletes "Don't Pump Trouble. . .Stay Away From Steroids."

Summary

Common sense clearly should prevail in assessing the nutritional needs of the growing athlete. Sufficient calories must be consumed to support growth and activity. Fluid and electrolytes lost during practice or competition must be replaced to avoid the consequences of dehydration and electrolyte imbalance. Protein, vitamin, or mineral supplements are generally unnecessary, but occasionally an iron supplement may serve to correct iron deficiency or maintain iron balance in adolescent boys and girls. Weight management efforts should be approached sensibly, without efforts to achieve minimal weight through promotion of fluid loss. Eating before competition should be scheduled to avoid retention of undigested food material in the gut at the time of the event. Foods that are easy to digest should be selected with avoidance of unnecessary fat, fiber, and gas-forming fruits and vegetables. No special diet is recognized as clearly the ticket to success. However, if ingestion of a certain food provides a psychological edge, selection of it must be considered potentially advantageous.

SUGGESTED LEARNING ACTIVITIES

1. Define typical calorie requirements for adolescents participating in various sports
2. Calculate approximate protein requirements for a growing 70-kg adolescent and a mature 80-kg adolescent.
3. What athletes should be monitored closely for iron deficiency?
4. Define the adverse effects of secondary amenorrhea.
5. Explain the consequences of dehydration both in general and in regard to athletic performance.
6. Identify sports in which glycogen loading may prove advantageous.
7. Outline major features of a good pregame meal.
8. Summarize reasonable weight loss and weight goals for male and female athletes. Identify healthful levels of body fatness for both groups.

REFERENCES

1. Torún, B., Chew, F., and Mendoza, R.D: Energy costs of activities of preschool children, Nutr. Res. 3:401, 1983.
2. Freedson, P.S., and others: Energy expenditure in prepubescent children: influence of sex and age, Am. J. Clin. Nutr. 34:1827, 1981.
3. Short, S.H., and Short, W.R.: Four-year study of university athletes' dietary intake, J. Am. Diet. Assoc. 82:632, 1983.
4. Marcus, R., and others: Menstrual function and bone mass in elite women distance runners, Ann. Intn. Med. 102:158, 1985.
5. Nelson, M.E., and others: Diet and bone status in amenorrheic runners, Am. J. Clin. Nutr. 43:910, 1986.
6. Cohen, J.L., and others: A nutritional and hematologic assessment of elite ballet dancers, Phys. Sports Med. 13:43, 1985.
7. Brownell, K.D., Steen, B.N. and Milmore, J.H.: Weight regulation practices in athletes: analysis of metabolic and health effects, Med. Sci. Sports Exerc. 19:546, 1987.
8. Gollnick, P.D.: Metabolism of substrates: energy substrate metabolism during exercise and as modified by training, Fed. Proc. 44:353, 1985.
9. Costill, D.L.: Carbohydrate nutrition before, during and after exercise, Fed. Proc. 44:364, 1985.
10. Ryan, A.: Round table—balancing heat stress, fluids and electrolytes, Phys. Sports Med. 3:43, 1975.
11. Brooke, J.D., Davies, G.J., and Green, L.F.: The effects of normal and glucose syrup work diets on the performance of racing cyclists, J. Sports Med. Phys. Fitness 15:257, 1975.
12. Karlsson, J., and Saltin, B.: Diet, muscle glycogen and endurance performance, J. Appl. Physiol. 31:203, 1971.
13. Green, L.F., and Bagley, R.: Ingestion of glucose syrup drink during long distance canoeing, Br. J. Sports Med. 6:125, 1972.

14. Muckle, D.S.: Glucose syrup ingestion and team performance in soccer, Br. J. Sports Med. 7:340, 1973.

15. Evans, W.J., and others: Protein metabolism and endurance exercise, Phys. Sports Med. 11:53, 1983.

16. Dohm, G.L., and others: Protein metabolism during endurance exercise, Fed. Proc. 44:348, 1985.

17. Lemon, P.W.R.: Protein and exercise: update 1987, Med. Sci. Sports Exerc. 19:S179, 1987.

18. Dohm, G.L., Hecker, A.L., and Brown, W.E.: Adaptation of protein metabolism to endurance training: increased amino acid oxidation in response to training, Biochem. J. 164:705, 1977.

19. Evans, W.J., and others: Changes in whole body leucine dynamics during submaximal exercise, Med. Sci. Sports Exerc. 13:89, 1981.

20. Rasch, P., and others: Protein dietary supplementation and physical performance, Med. Sci. Sports Exerc. 1:195, 1969.

21. Belko, A.Z.: Vitamins and exercise—an update, Med. Sci. Sports Exerc. 19:S191, 1987.

22. Buzina, K., and others: Vitamin C status and physical working capacity in adolescents, Int. Z. Vitam. Nutr. Res. 54:55, 1984.

23. Belko, A.Z., and others: Effects of exercise on riboflavin requirements of young women. Am. J. Clin. Nutr. 37:509, 1983.

24. Belko, A.Z., and others: Effects of aerobic exercise and weight loss on riboflavin requirements of moderately obese, marginally deficient young women. Am. J. Clin. Nutr. 40:553, 1984.

25. Belko, A.Z., and others: Effect of exercise on riboflavin requirements: biological validation in weight reducing women. Am. J. Clin. Nutr. 41:270, 1985.

26. Leklem, J.E. Physical activity and vitamin B_6 metabolism in men and women: interrelationships with fuel needs. In Leklem, J.E., and Reynolds, R.D., editors: Vitamin B6: Its Role in Health and Disease, New York, 1984, Alan R. Liss, Inc.

27. Keys, A., and Henschel, A.F.: Vitamin supplementation of U.S. Army rations in relation to fatigue and the ability to do muscular work, J. Nutr. 23:259, 1942.

28. Gey, G.O., Cooper, K.H., and Bottenberg, R.A.: Effect of ascorbic acid on endurance performance and athletic injury, J.A.M.A. 211:105, 1970.

29. Hoogerwerf, A., and Hoitink, W.J.H.: The influence of vitamin C administration on the mechanical efficiency of the human organism, Int. Z. Angew. Physiol. Einschl. Arbeitsphysiol. 20:164, 1963.

30. Sharman, I.: The effects of vitamin E and training of physiological function and athletic performance in adolescent swimmers, Br. J. Nutr. 26:265, 1971.

31. Watt, T., and others: Vitamin E and oxygen consumption, Lancet 2:354, 1974.

32. Bergstrom, J.E., and others: The effect of nicotinic acid on physical working capacity and on metabolism of muscle glycogen in man, J. Appl. Physiol., 26:170, 1969.

33. Carlson, L.A., and Oro, L.: Effect of nicotinic acid on plasma free fatty acids, Acta Med. Scand. 172:641, 1962.

34. Jenkins, D.J.A.: Effects of nicotinic acid on carbohydrate and fat metabolism during exercise, Lancet 2:1307, 1965.

35. Wilmore, J.H. and Freund, B.J.: Nutritional enhancement of athletic performance, Nutr. Abstr. Rev. 54:1, 1984.

36. Lawrence, J.D., and others: Effects of tocopherol acetate on the swimming endurance of trained swimmers, Am. J. Clin. Nutr. 28:205, 1975.

37. Bailey, D.A., and others: Effect of vitamin C supplementation upon the physiological response to exercise in trained and untrained subject, Int. J. Vitam. Nutr. Res. 40:435, 1970.

38. Wood, B.A., and others: A study of partial thiamin restriction in human volunteers, Am. J. Clin. Nutr. 33:848, 1980.

39. Leklem, J.E. and Schultz, T.: Increased plasma pyridoxal 5'-phosphate and vitamin B_6 in male adolescents after a 4500 meter run, Am. J. Clin. Nutr. 38:541, 1983.

40. Barnes, L.: Preadolescent training: how young is too young? Phys. Sports Med. 7:114, 1979.

41. Liu, L., Borowski, G., and Rose, L.I.: Hypomagnesemia in a tennis player, Phys. Sports Med. 11:79, 1983.

42. Lane, H.W., and others: Effect of physical activity on human potassium metabolism in a hot and humid climate, Am. J. Clin. Nutr. 31:838, 1978.

43. Lane, H.W., and Cerda, J.J.: Potassium requirements and exercise, J. Am. Diet. Assoc. 73:64, 1978.

44. Costill, D.L., Cote, R., and Fink, W.J.: Dietary potassium and heavy exercise: effects of muscle water and electrolytes, Am. J. Clin. Nutr. 36:266, 1982.

45. Dressendorfer, R.H., and others: Plasma mineral levels in marathon runners during a 20-day road race, Phys. Sports Med. 10:113, 1982.

46. Haymes, E.M.: Nutritional concerns: need for iron, Med. Sci. Sports Exerc. 19:S197, 1987.

47. Paulev, P.E., Jordal, R., and Pederson, N.S.: Dermal excretion of iron in intensely training athletes, Clin. Chim. Acta 127:19, 1983.

48. Puhl, J. The Elite Athlete. New York, 1985, Spectrum Publications, Inc.

49. Nickerson, J.H., and others: Decreased iron stores in high school female runners, Am. J. Dis. Child, 139:1115, 1985.

50. Ehn, L., Carlmark, B., and Hoglund, S.: Iron status in athletes involved in intense activity, Med. Sci. Sports Exerc. 12:61, 1979.

51. Schoch, D.R., and others: Gastrointestinal bleeding in an adolescent runner, J. Pediatr. 111:302, 1987.

52. Carlson, D.L., and Mawdsley, R.H.: Sports anemia: a review of the literature, Am. J. Sports Med. 14:109, 1986.

53. Clement, D.B., and Sawchuk, L.L.: Iron status and sports performance, Sports Med. 1:65, 1986.

54. MacMahon, L.F., and others: Occult gastrointestinal blood loss in marathon runners, Ann. Int. Med. 100:846, 1984.

55. Stewart, J.G., and others: Gastrointestinal blood loss and anemia in runners, Ann. Int. Med. 200:843, 1984.

56. Fisher, R.L., and others: Gastrointestinal bleeding in competitive runners, Dig. Dis. Sci. 31:1226, 1986.

57. DeWijn, J.F., and others: Haemoglobin, packed cell volume, serum iron, and iron binding capacity of selected athletes during training, J. Sports Med. 11:42, 1971.

58. Wishnitzer, R., Vorst, E., and Berrebi, A.: Bone marrow iron depression in competitive distance runners. Int. J. Sports Med. 4:24, 1983.

59. Dufaux, B., and others: Serum ferritin, transferrin, haptoglobin and iron in middle- and long-distance runners, elite rowers and professional racing cyclists, Int. J. Sports Med. 2:43, 1981.

60. Clement, D.B., and Asmundson, R.C.: Nutritional intake and hematological parameters in endurance runners, Phys. Sports Med. 10:37, 1982.

61. Plowman, S.A., and McSwegin, H.T.: The effects of iron supplementation on female cross-country runners, J. Sports Med. 21:407, 1981.

62. Lampe, J.W., Slavin, J.L., and Apple, F.S.: Poor iron status of women runners training for a marathon, Int. J. Sports Med. 7:111, 1986.

63. Selby, G.B., and Eichner, E.R.: Endurance swimming, intravascular hemolysis, anemia and iron depletion, Am. J. Med. 81:791, 1986.

64. Cooter, G.R., and Mowbray, K.: Effects of iron supplementation and activity on serum iron depletion and hemoglobin levels in female athletes. Res. Q. 49:114, 1978.

65. Haymes, E.M., Puhl, J.L., and Temples, T.E.: Training for cross-country skiing and iron status, Med. Sci. Sports Exerc. 18:162, 1986.

66. Pate, R.R., Maguire, M., and Van Wyk, J.: Dietary iron supplementation in women athletes, Phys. Sports Med. 7:81, 1979.

67. Nickerson, H.J., and Tripp, A.D.: Iron deficiency in adolescent cross-country runners. Phys. Sports Med. 11:60, 1983.

68. Schoene, R.B., and others: Iron repletion decreases maximal exercise lactate concentrations in female athletes with minimal iron deficiency anemia, J. Lab. Clin. Med. 102:843, 1983.

69. Williamson, M.R.: Anemia in runners and other athletes, Phys. Sports Med. 9:73, 1981.

70. Pate, R.R.: Sports anemia: a review of the current research literature, Phys. Sports Med. 11:115, 1983.

71. Yoshimura, H.: Anemia during physical training (sports anemia), Nutr. Res. 28:251, 1970.

72. Crowell, J.W., and Smith, E.E.: Determinant of the optimal hematocrit, J. Appl. Physiol. 22:501, 1967.

73. Guyton, A.C., Jones, C.E., and Coleman, T.G.: Circulatory physiology: cardiac output and its regulation, Philadelphia, 1973, W.B. Saunders Co.

74. Dressendorfer, R.H., Wade, C.E., and Amsterdam, E.A.: Development of pseudoanemia in marathon runners during a 20-day road race, J.A.M.A. 246:1215, 1981.

75. Frederickson, L.A., Puhl, J.L., and Runyan, W.S.: Effects of training on indices of iron status of young female cross-country runners, Med. Sci. Sports Exerc. 15:271, 1983.

76. Wentz, A.C.: Body weight and amenorrhea, Obstet. Gynecol. 65:482, 1980.

77. Baker, E.R.: Menstrual dysfunction and hormonal status in athletic women: a review, Fertil. Steril. 36:691, 1981.

78. Calabrese, L.H., and others: Menstrual abnormalities, nutritional patterns, and body composition in female classical ballet dancers, Phys. Sports Med. 11:86, 1983.

79. Speroff, L., and Redwine, D.B.: Exercise and menstrual function, Phys. Sports Med. 8:42, 1980.

80. Schwartz, B., and others: Exercise-associated amenorrhea: a distinct entity? Am. J. Obstet. Gynecol. 141:662, 1981.

81. Lutter, J.M., and Cushman, S.: Menstrual patterns in female runners, Phys. Sports Med. 10:60, 1982.

82. Caldwell, F.: Menstrual irregularity in athletes: the unanswered question, Phys. Sports Med. 10:142, 1982.

83. Vandenbroucke, J.P., van Laar, A., and Valkenburg, H.A.: Synergy between thinness and intensive sports activity in delaying menarche, Br. Med. J. 284:1907, 1982.

84. Frisch, R.E., and others: Delayed menarche and amenorrhea of college athletes in relation to age at onset of training, J.A.M.A. 246:1559, 1981.

85. Glass, A.R., Deuster, P.A., and Kyle, S.B.: Amenorrhea in Olympic marathon runners, Fertil. Steril. 48:740, 1987.

86. Sanborn, C.F., Albrecht, B.H., and Wagner, W.W.: Athletic amenorrhea: lack of association with body fat, Med. Sci. Sports Exerc. 19:207, 1987.
87. Nelson, M.E., and others: Diet and bone status in amenorrheic runners, Am. J. Clin. Nutr. 43:910, 1986.
88. Drinkwater, B.L., and others: Bone mineral content of amenorrheic and eumenorrheic athletes, N. Engl. J. Med. 311:277, 1984.
89. Cann, C.E., and others: Decreased spinal mineral content in amenorrheic women, J.A.M.A. 251:626, 1984.
90. Marcus, R., and others: Menstrual function and boned mass in elite women distance runners, Ann. Intern. Med. 102:158, 1985.
91. Lindberg, J.S., and others: Exercise-induced amenorrhea and bone density, Ann. Int. Med. 101:647, 1984.
92. Warren, M.P., and others: Scoliosis and fractures in young ballet dancers, New Engl. J. Med. 314:1348, 1986.
93. Lloyd, T., and others: Women athletes with menstrual irregularity have increased musculoskeletal injuries, Med. Sci. Sports Exerc. 18:374, 1986.
94. Drinkwater, B.L., and others: Bone mineral density after resumption of menses in amenorrheic athletes, J.A.M.A. 256:380, 1986.
95. American Academy of Pediatrics: Clinical heat stress and the exercising child, Phys. Sports Med. 11:155, 1983.
96. Vaccaro, P., Zauner, C.W., and Cade, J.R.: Changes in body weight, hematocrit and plasma protein concentration due to dehydration and rehydration in wrestlers, J. Sports Med. Phys. Fitness 16:45, 1976.
97. Frizzel, R.T., and others: Hyponatremia and ultramarathon running, J.A.M.A., 255:772, 1986.
98. Astrand, P.: Diet and athletic performance, Fed. Proc. 26:1772, 1967.
99. Lombardo, J.A.: Stimulants and athletic performance. I. amphetamines and caffeine, Phys. Sports Med. 14:128, 1986.
100. Eichner, E.R.: The caffeine controversy: endurance and cholesterol. Phys. Sports Med. 14:124, 1986.
101. Moore, M.: Carbohydrate loading: eating through the wall, Phys. Sports Med. 9:97, 1981.
102. Costill, D.L.: Carbohydrate-loading without depletion, Runner's World, August, 1978.
103. Leklem, J.: Personal communication.
104. Costill, D.L., and others: Carbohydrate feeding during prolonged strenuous exercise can delay fatigue, J. Appl. Physiol. 55:230, 1983.
105. Edwards, T.L., Santeusanio, D.M., and Wheeler, K.B.: Field test of the effects of carbohydrate solutions on endurance performance, selected blood serum chemistry, perceived exertion and fatigue in world class cyclists, Med. Sci. Sports Exerc. 16:190, 1984.
106. Wilkes, D., Gledhill, N., and Smyht, R.: Effect of acute induced metabolic alkalosis on 800-m racing time, Med. Sci. Sports Exerc. 15:277, 1983.
107. Groves, D. Studies: bicarbonate has no benefits, Phys. Sports Med. 15:51, 1987.
108. Peterson, M.S.: Nutritional concerns for the dancer, Phys. Sports Med. 10:137, 1982.
109. Cohen, J.L., and others: Exercise, body weight and professional ballet dancers, Phys. Sports Med. 10:92, 1982.
110. Niinimaa, V.: Figure skating: what do we know about it? Phys. Sports Med. 10:51, 1982.
111. Croyle, P.H., Place, R.A., and Hilgenberg, A.D.: Massive pulmonary embolism in a high school wrestler, J.A.M.A. 241:827, 1979.
112. Dummer, G.M., and others: Pathogenic weight control behaviors of young competitive swimmers, Phys. Sports Med. 15:75, 1987.
113. Borgen, J.S., and Corbin, C.B.: Eating disorders among female athletes, Phys. Sports Med. 15:89, 1987.
114. Rosen, L.W., and others: Pathogenic weight control behavior in female athletes, Phys. Sports Med. 14:79, 1986.
115. Smith, N.J.: Excessive weight loss and food aversion in athletes simulating anorexia nervosa, Pediatrics 66:139, 1980.
116. Thorland, W.G., and others: Body composition and somatotype characteristics of Junior Olympics athletes, Med. Sci. Sports Exerc. 13:332, 1981.
117. Mayers, N., and Gutin, B.: Physiological characteristics of elite prepubertal cross-country runners, Med. Sci. Sports Exerc. 11: 172, 1979.
118. Sady, S.P., and others: The body composition physical dimensions of 9- and 12-year-old experienced wrestlers, Med. Sci. Sports Exerc. 14:244, 1982.
119. Blum, K., Seifter, E., and Seifter, J.: The pharmacology of D- and L-carnitine and D- and L-acetylcarnitine: comparison with choline and acetylcholine, J. Pharmacol Exp. Ther. 178:331, 1971.
120. Bazzato, G., and others: Myasthenia-like syndrome after DL- but not L-carnitine, Lancet 1:1209, 1981.
121. Paulson, D.J., and Shug, A.L.: Tissue specific depletion of L-carnitine in rat heart and skeletal muscle by D-carnitine, Life Sci. 28:2931, 1981.
122. Keith, R.E.: Symptoms of carnitinelike deficiency in a trained runner taking DL-carnitine supplements, J. A. M. A. 255:1137, 1986.

123. Steben, R.E., and Bourdreaux, P.: The effects of pollen and protein extracts on selected blood factors and performance of athletes, J. Sports Med. Phys. Fitness 18:221, 1978.
124. Miller, R.W.: Athletes and steroids: playing a deadly game, FDA Consumer 21(11):17, 1987.
125. Ballarin, E., and others: Unmodified performance in runners following anabolic steroid administration, Int. J. Sports Med. 7:302, 1986.
126. Kuhn, F.E., and Max, S.R.: Testosterone and muscle hypertrophy in female rats, J. Appl. Physiol. 59:24, 1985.
127. Max, S.R., and Rance, N.E.: No effect of sex steroids on compensatory muscle hypertrophy, J. Appl. Physiol. 56:1589, 1984.
128. Stehlin, D.: For athletes and dealers, Black Market steroids are risky business, FDA Consumer 21(10):24, 1987.

11

Special Concerns of Dietary Intake During Infancy and Childhood

Peggy L. Pipes

OBJECTIVES

After studying this chapter, the student should:

1. Be aware of common concerns of food and nutrient intake during infancy and childhood.

2. Be aware of proposed nutritional approaches to the prevention of chronic disease.

3. Recognize factors that must be considered in controlling children's weight.

4. Be aware of approaches to the diagnosis and control of food allergies in infancy and childhood.

5. Recognize the diversity of opinions regarding the need to modify the fat and salt in children's diets to prevent cardiovascular disease.

6. Understand nutrition and food intake approaches to the prevention of dental caries.

Common concerns related to food and nutrient intake during infancy and childhood include excessive energy intakes, food allergies, dental caries, and lactose malabsorption. Diets of children who modify their food intakes to control these conditions often need to be monitored for adequacy of nutrient intakes. In addition, many conflicting opinions have been expressed about the need to modify children's diets to prevent chronic disease in later life. Whether a diet low in fat and cholesterol and

high in polyunsaturated fatty acids supports adequate growth and development remains an unanswered question. Some experts feel children should consume a limited salt intake; others feel this is unnecessary. These special concerns are discussed in this chapter.

OBESITY

Obesity is a frequent concern in clinics that serve adolescents. The lack of success in achieving sustained weight reduction of obese ado-

268

lescents has focused on identifying children at risk and motivating families to alter life-styles, environmental factors, and psychosocial factors that contribute to the development of this condition.

Obesity is a major health hazard predisposing affected adults to a greater risk of hypertension, cardiovascular disease, diabetes, gallbladder disease, and degenerative joint disorders than persons of normal weight. In addition to these health risks, obese individuals are often subjects to sociocultural prejudices. For example, obese adolescents face discrimination at college entrance, and obese adults are discriminated against in job placement and advancement. Obese adolescents often exhibit psychosocial difficulties. They frequently have distorted body images and low **self-esteem** and may become socially isolated. They have been described as leading a "Cinderella-like" existence.[1]

Incidence

Obesity in childhood is a growing problem, having increased by 54% among 6- to 11-year-old children and 39% among 12- to 17-year-old children in the past 15 to 20 years. Estimates indicate that 30% of males and 25% of females 6- to 10-years-old and 18% of males and 25% of females 12- to 17-years-old are obese. [2] Limited data exist on obesity in preschoolers. One study in Manhattan suggested an incidence of greater than 13%.[3]

Prognosis of Obesity

Many obese children become obese adolescents and adults. It has been estimated that 40% of children obese at 7 years of age and 70% of obese adolescents are obese as adults.[4] Retrospective investigations have shown that approximately 30% of the obese adults had a history of juvenile obesity.[5] Data from the United States Health Examination Study showed that three fourths of those classified as obese between 6 and 11 years of age were classified as obese 3 to 4 years later.[6] Ear-

ly-onset obesity is more severe and resistant to treatment than is obesity acquired later in life.[7]

Definition

Obesity is defined as an excessive deposition of adipose tissue. It differs from overweight, which implies only weight in excess of average for height. Overweight can result from increased lean body mass, adipose tissue, or both. Forbes[8] has suggested that there may be two types of obesity in childhood and adolescence: one type characterized by increased lean body mass in addition to fat, a tendency for tallness, advanced bone age, and a history of overweight since infancy; and another type with no increase in lean body mass, normal bone age and height, and weight gain in the midchildhood or late childhood years.

Weight greater than 20% of normal for height is one criterion that has been used to define obesity. Such standards, although they show trends for populations, are not applicable to individual children. The use of weight standards tends to underestimate fatness in children less than 6 or 7 years of age and frequently overestimates adiposity in adolescents.[9] Diagnosis of grossly obese children is easily made by visual inspection. Differentiating between less severely obese children and those who are overweight because of increased muscle mass requires measurements that give indications of body composition. Identification of children who are overfat and are settled into patterns of growth indicative of future obesity also requires that measurements of body composition be included in health examinations, just as other measurements of growth are obtained. As described in Chapter 1, standards for tricep fatfold measurements with calipers have been published for all age groups. Use of these measurements to define greater than normal increases in adipose tissue of infants and children as they grow older helps identify children for whom preventive measures should be applied.

Etiological Factors

Studies of rats and other animals have definitively shown that, in animals, genes carrying obese traits are transmitted to offspring.

Definition of human genetic obesities has been more difficult because of the mixed racial heritage of most individuals and the many environmental factors known to contribute to obesity that cannot be controlled in studies. The high incidence of obesity among parents of obese children and the fact that early-onset obesity appears to be almost intractable leads one to believe that hereditary factors are important. Studies have shown that 60% to 70% of obese adolescents have one or both obese parents,[9] and 40% of obese adolescents have obese siblings. Other studies have found that less than 10% of children of average-weight parents are obese.[10] A study of Danish adoptees found that an individual's relative weight strongly correlated with the body masses of his or her biological parents. There was no relation between the body masses of the individuals studied and their adoptive parents.[11]

Seltzer and Mayer[12] studied weight patterns of different body types. Using Sheldon's somatotypes they described obese adolescent females as more endomorphic and less ectomorphic than nonobese adolescent females. Inherited body type may predispose children to obesity.

Inactivity is another cause of obesity.[13] Obese adolescents and school-age children are less active than are those of normal weight. Most become obese by ingesting calorie intakes equivalent to or less than their peers. Activity patterns are acquired in childhood. Children learn to enjoy those activities in which their families and peers engage. Parents who enjoy hiking, swimming, and sports often teach their children to engage in and enjoy these physical activities. Parents who spend their hours at home urging their children to be still so that they can watch television or read reinforce inactivity and sedentary living.

Television viewing also contributes to obesity. Dietz found a dose-response effect: the more television viewed, the greater the risk of obesity. In addition to the inactivity while watching TV, children are reported to eat more and to eat more of the foods advertised on TV during the programs.[14]

Several researchers have reported increased birth weights of obese children compared with children of normal weight.[15,16] Others have found no differences in birth weights of the two groups of children. In their study, Fisch, Bilek, and Ulstrom[17] found that infants who were extremely obese at birth tended toward normal weight at 4 and 7 years of age but that an unusually high percentage retained their stocky physiques. The children who were very obese at 4 and 7 years of age tended to have had stocky physiques at birth. By 7 years of age, however, they were joined in their obese and overweight status by several children who had normal physiques at birth.

There has been speculation in the past that formula-feeding and the early introduction of semisolid foods might be one cause of excessive intakes of energy and obesity in infancy and that obese infants very often become obese adults. However, a number of studies have shown that breast-feeding, bottle-feeding, and the age of introduction of semisolid foods do not cause obesity in infancy or later childhood.[18,19,20] Obesity in infancy has not been found to be predictive of obesity in later life.[1] Fomon found measures of fatness at 8 years of age no greater in children who had been bottle-fed compared to those who had been breast-fed.[20] A longitudinal study of children found that obese infants at 6 months and at one year of age become progressively thinner as they grow older. Weight gain in infancy was not found to be predictive of obesity at 9 years of age.[21]

Obesity during the preschool and school-age years does increase the risk of obesity in later life. A channeling tendency that increases with age has been noted.[22]

Interestingly, retrospective studies of obese adolescents have shown that a large percentage of them had feeding problems in infancy, and some had even been hospitalized for failure to gain weight. Seven of ten mothers of obese adolescents studied by Hammar and others[1] reported seeking advice about feeding their children during infancy at least six times. Seven of the ten obese adolescents had had allergic reactions to food in late infancy and early childhood. Massengale[23] found that 28% to 30% of 92 obese adolescents had histories of feeding problems in the first year of life. Two children had had pyloric stenosis, and eight had been hospitalized for poor weight gain or dehydration.

Psychosocial factors and parent-child interactions are important factors that contribute to obesity in childhood. The obese child is often an only child or the youngest child and frequently the result of an unwanted pregnancy. These children are often given food and material objects instead of love and the opportunity to have experiences that lead to the development of coping skills.[24] Anxious and insecure parents frequently overfeed children as expressions of their concern and love. They usually measure their success as parents by the amount of food their children eat and by how much weight they gain.

Psychological trauma has been observed to be another factor associated with the onset of obesity. Bruch[25] noted that fear of hospitalization was associated with the onset of obesity in some children. Kahn[26] found a history of separation from their mothers in 32% of 72 obese children under 12 years of age. Fourteen of the children had experienced rapid weight gains that began shortly after the separations.

Differences have been noted in the incidence of obesity among children from the lower and higher socioeconomic groups. Garn, Clark, and Guire[27] reported, from analysis of data compiled during the Ten-State Nutrition Survey of 1968-1970 and the Preschool Nutrition Survey conducted by Owens and associates, that after the first few years of life and into adolescence the children of the poorest groups were leaner and the children of the affluent group were fatter. The higher the socioeconomic status, the greater the amount of adipose tissue. Females were fatter than males at all ages at comparable income levels. White children had more adiposity than blacks. In adults the relationship between fatness continued in males but reversed for females. Low-income female adults were fatter than those who had greater economic resources.

Garn, Hopkins, and Ryan[28] reevaluated the socioeconomic influences on adiposity with data from the Tecumseh, Michigan, Community Health Survey. Again they found low-income preadolescent males and females to be leaner than their higher income peers during the first examination. When the same individuals were reevaluated 18 years later, the low-income children had become fatter than their high-income peers.

Prevention

Regardless of its cause, obesity results when energy intakes exceed energy needs for growth, maintenance, and activity. Its manifestation is usually the result of small excesses of calorie intakes over expenditure for a period of weeks, months, or years. By monitoring rates of growth and deposition of adipose tissue, children can be identified who are accumulating more fat than would be anticipated, and measures to increase activity or decrease caloric intakes can be effected.

Adolescents often make their own decisions about what and when they eat. Counseling must be directed to the teenagers themselves. Parents control the food available to younger children, create the environment that influences their acceptance of food, and can influence energy expenditure by the opportunities they create for physical activity for their children. It may be important to explore first with parents their reason for encouraging children to consume amounts of food that result in rapid weight gain. Some parents may not recognize that their expectations for the quanity of food they encourage their children to consume are excessive and that the chubby child is not necessarily the healthy child.

Parents may need help in developing appropriate parenting skills. They may need to learn how to respond to hunger and other needs of their infants or how to interact with their children. They may need help in identifying ways to help their children develop initiative and to cultivate friends and outlets in the community.[24]

The activity pattern of both the child and the family should be explored; it may be important to help parents find ways of increasing their child's level of activity. Parents who live in apartments often reinforce sedentary activities to reduce the noise level and complaints from neighbors. Those who live in one-family dwellings may have limited space for activities for children. City park departments, preschools, and schools frequently have programs that offer opportunities to increase children's activities.

The range of appropriate energy intakes at any given age is large. Overweight children and children with familial trends to obesity may need fewer calories than their peers. Griffith and Payne[29] found that normal weight 4- to 5-year-old children of obese parents expended 1174 kcal/day as compared with 1508 kcal/day expended by children of the same size and age of normal weight parents. Children of normal weight parents expended twice as much energy in physical activity as did those of obese parents. Families of children with a familial tendency to obesity may need help in identifying the kinds and amount of food that provide an energy intake that support normal growth and weight gain.

Nutrition counseling should be family oriented and based on normal nutrition, emphasizing foods that provide a balance of nutrients as well as appropriate calorie intakes.

Families need to realize that efforts are directed at reduction in rates of weight gain and are not intended to effect weight loss. They must recognize that the food available and the models set for their child determine the child's response to efforts to control weight gain. Family meals may need to be modified to include fewer fried foods, less gravy, and fewer rich desserts. Parents and siblings may have to modify their own eating practices to set appropriate examples. Teachers, baby-sitters, and day-care workers should be alerted to and included in programs designed to control weight. Food experiences at school may need to be modified to exclude corn dripping with butter and chocolate cupcakes so frequently provided for special occasions. Low-calorie snacks such as raw fruits and vegetables can be provided instead of cookies, candy, and hot dogs. The use of food as reinforcers can be modified. Comparative energy values of snack foods are shown in Table 11-1.

Parents and children will need help in planning for parties and special occasions. Some children delete 50 kcal/day from their planned diet and have a calorie savings account that permits them to participate in the refreshments. Some prefer to have very special food. For example, one child has a "very special glass of water and gingersnap" for his preschool snack.

Care should be taken in approaches to prevention of obesity, because the preventive methods can have harmful results. For example, Pugliese and others[31] describe fourteen normal children with growth failure and delayed maturation due to an inadequate intake because of fear of obesity.

If the child is grossly obese, a very slow rate of weight reduction may be attempted; however, linear growth should be frequently monitored. My clinical experience has indicated that in grossly obese preschool and school-age handicapped children, a weight reduction of 2 pounds per month did not affect linear growth. Others, however, have reported

Figure 11-1 An overweight infant who became a lean well-proportioned 12-year-old and a muscular 16-year-old.

Table 11-1 Approximate energy value of common snack foods offered young children

Food	Portion Size	kcal	Food	Portion Size	kcal
Cheese cubes	$\frac{1}{4}$ oz	25	Homogenized milk	3 oz	60
Hard-boiled egg	$\frac{1}{2}$ medium	36	Chocolate milk	3 oz	80
Frankfurter, 5" by $\frac{3}{4}$"	1	133	Cauliflower buds	2 small	2
Pretzel, 3" by $\frac{1}{2}$"	1	20	Green pepper strips	2	2
Potato chips	10	114	Cucumber slices	3 large	2
Popcorn with oil and salt	1 cup	41	Cherry tomato	1	3
Bread stick, $4\frac{1}{2}$"	1	38	Raw turnip slices	2	5
Saltines	1	12	Dill pickle, large	$\frac{1}{3}$	5
Graham cracker	2 squares	55	Apple wedges	$\frac{1}{4}$ medium apple	20
Animal cracker	1	11	Banana	$\frac{1}{2}$ small	40
Brownie, 3" by 1" by $\frac{7}{8}$"	1	97	Orange wedges	$\frac{1}{4}$ medium orange	18
Chocolate cupcake	1	51	Orange juice	3 oz	35
Vanilla wafer	1	18	Grape juice	3 oz	60
Yogurt, plain	$\frac{1}{4}$ cup	40	Lemonade	3 oz	40

From Adams, C.F.: Nutritive value of American foods in common units, Agriculture Handbook No. 456, Washington D.C., 1975, U.S. Department of Agriculture.

that restricted calorie intakes did modify linear growth. Wolff and Lloyd[30] noted children who lost 2% or more of their weight per month grew in length at a less than expected rate. Children who (1) lost less than 2% of their body weight, (2) did not lose, or (3) gained weight grew at a rate faster than expected. Knittle[3] reported that children on a protein-sparing modified fat diet may experience a transient slowed rate of growth but that 6 months after weight reduction height for age is not affected.

The many factors in the etiology of childhood obesity indicate that a multidisciplinary approach may be necessary. The team might consist of a psychologist or behaviorist, a physician, and a dietitian-nutritionist.

CASE STUDY

At the request of her local pediatrician the 2 1/2-year-old daughter of a single parent was seen at the Child Development and Mental Retardation Center at the University of Washington. She needed evaluation and therapy from several professionals. The child was visibly obese. Her weight plotted above the 95th percentile; her length, between the 25th and 50th percentiles; her weight for height, over the 95th percentile.

During the nutrition interview it was reported that she was obviously overfat at 4 months of age. By 14 months of age her mother and grandmother became concerned. When she was 2 years of age, she was often upset because she was "fat." Her mother tried offering her low-calorie foods. She, however, often gorged and sneaked food. The child, according to her diet history, was consuming 1500 to 1700 kcal/day, 75 to 85 kcal/kg, 16 to 18 kcal/cm of height. A diet supplying 850 kcal (9 cal/cm) was prescribed.

The mother and child lived with the mother's male friend and his father. The child was often cared for by her grandmother, and there was no coordination of efforts to control her food or energy intake.

The mother's friend, a rehabilitated drug addict, frequently told the child she was a "fatty" and ugly and then gave her food to keep her quiet. The

Figure 11-2 A previously obese child and her mother exercise as part of a program to control the child's weight.

child's mother did not want to move to her parents' home and doubted that she could "make it" on her own.

In the following 3 months the child lost 2 kg. Her linear growth proceeded in channel. Often when she came to the clinic she was very reluctant to be weighed, stating "I not a fatty; I not ugly." Play therapy for the child and therapy sessions for the mother as well as nutrition counseling were incorporated into the monthly visits.

The child's mother applied for and received a scholarship to a junior college, which carried a monthly stipend, and was able to move to her own apartment and enroll the child in a preschool program that included a variety of daily physical activities. When she had lost 3 kg her weight/height plotted below the 95th percentile, and her suggested energy intake was increased to 10.5 kcal/cm/day (950 to 1000 kcal/day) with a goal of weight maintenance. However, she began to gain weight.

It soon became apparent that each episode of weight gain was associated with psychosocial problems of the mother and that only the continuing counseling and play therapy made implementation of

the plan for maintaining a normal weight possible. Even today, as a school-age child, her diet and weight gains must be carefully monitored. She is, however, no longer classified as obese. Continuing support has been necessary to maintain the gains toward prevention of future obesity.

Parents and their children need continuing support as they implement programs to prevent obesity and face unwitting responses from other members of society. Well-meaning merchants and bankers who provide sweets for children should be encouraged to provide nonfood items as alternatives. Neighbors, relatives, and other children's parents should support weight control programs.

As children grow older, they must learn to exercise willpower in refusing amounts of food that result in a positive energy balance. The children themselves should receive positive reinforcement for control of weight gain. They need continuing support, education, and

Figure 11-3 Weight/height grid of an obese preschooler during and after nutrition counseling and psychosocial intervention.

understanding as they grow older. An 8-year-old boy who has been on a weight control program for 6 years, since obesity was reversed at 27 months of age, expressed the difficulties encountered on such a program. He stated during a recent clinic visit, "It's really hard to control my weight. I'm often hungry. I can't eat as much as the other boys, and my food is different from that of the other children in my class. I don't want to get fat, but I don't like being different." He, however, understands his program and knows he will receive the guidance and support he desires from his family as he assumes control of his own food selection and management of weight control.

FOOD ALLERGIES IN INFANCY AND CHILDHOOD

The most common chronic condition affecting children is allergies. There is no agreement as to the prevalence of food allergies in infants and children. Various investigators have reported incidences that range from 0.3% to 38%, the incidence reported varying with the criteria used for diagnosis and the population studied.[32]

Symptoms of most food allergies appear in the first year of life. However, symptomatic responses to the majority of foods disappear within 9 months.[32] Children whose parents have allergic reactions to food are at a greater risk of having food allergies than are others.

Allergic Responses to Food

Manifestations of allergy result from **antigen antibody** reactions. Any tissue in the body can be the site of an immune reaction, and a single allergen may trigger reactions in several sites in the same individual. Allergic responses to food result in a variety of symptoms that include rhinitis, diarrhea, vomiting, malabsorption, abdominal pain, urticaria, eczema, irritability, and **hyperactivity**. Symptoms are not specific for any food or for allergies alone; they mimic those of other clinical conditions.

Reactions may occur immediately after a food is eaten (usually within 2 hours) or may be delayed, occurring within 4 to 72 hours. Both types of responses may be observed in the same child but to different foods. The type of reaction experienced by different children may vary when the same food is ingested. The immediate reaction is thought to be caused by antigenic properties of intact protein, the delayed reaction by antigenic properties of compounds formed during digestion.

The frequency and severity of symptoms may be influenced by psychological and physiological stress, the quantity of food consumed at one time, and the frequency a food is ingested. Anxiety and worry are known to cause symptoms after ingestion of a food that can be consumed with no problem in the absence of psychological stress. Allergic reactions to nonfood items, such as pollens during hay fever season, may cause allergic symptoms to foods that are normally nonallergenic. Reactions may be cumulative. A food consumed irregularly without any effect may cause symptoms when eaten regularly. Overindulgence in a food that can be consumed in small amounts without problem may cause allergic reactions.

Any food is potentially allergenic. Investigators do not agree on the most important food allergens; however, milk, wheat, eggs, and corn are consistently listed as the most allergenic foods. Other foods to which children are often allergic include chocolate, oranges, soy, legumes, rice, fish, beef, pork, and chicken. Bock found 12% of children from birth to 3 years of age to have allergic reactions to fruit or fruit juice. Oranges, tomatoes, apples, and grapes most frequently caused reactions.[33] Food additives such as flavorings and colors often cause allergic reactions. Diagnosed allergy to one food item often implies allergy to all food in its botanical group. For example, a child allergic to apples is often also allergic to pears.

The allergenicity of food may be reduced by cooking or processing. For example, some individuals allergic to fresh cow's milk tolerate evaporated milk. Others allergic to a raw fruit or vegetable may eat it without reaction when it is cooked.

Diets used in diagnosis

The variability of symptoms makes diagnosis of allergy a challenge for physicians. Skin tests may identify some food allergens but are generally considered unreliable. Diagnoses are made from dietary histories coupled with parents' perception of symptomatic responses to food, food diaries in combination with records of careful observations of symptoms, and elimination and challenge diets.

Detailed dietary histories give the physician indications of the foods and amount commonly consumed. During the interview parents are questioned as to whether they suspect any food of causing symptoms. Parents appear to report immediate reactions well but are often unaware of foods that cause delayed reactions.

Food diaries are often requested. The parents are asked to record every food (including condiments) the child consumes for 1 week and to note every symptom the child manifests each day during that time (see box below). Careful scrutiny of such records gives the physician clues about which foods to suspect.

If dietary histories or diaries indicate specific foods that appear to be allergenic to the child, these foods are restricted from the diet for 1 week or longer. If improvement

Diet/Symptom Diary*

Name _____   Starting Date _____

Day	1	2	3	4	5	6	7
Breakfast Morning snacks Drinks							
Symptoms							
Medicine							
Lunch Afternoon snacks Drinks							
Symptoms							
Medicine							
Dinner Evening snacks Drinks							
Symptoms							
Medicine							

From Bierman, C.W., and Furukawa, C.T.: Pediatr. Rev. 3:213, 1982. Copyright American Academy of Pediatrics, 1982
*List amounts of foods and drinks consumed; symptoms: severity and time; medications dosage and time given.

Table 11-4 Mean and (SD) cholesterol (TC), triglyceride (TG), high (C-HDL) and low (C-LDL) density lipoprotein cholesterol (mg/dl) in 927 fasting school children

Male subjects

Age		White					Black			
	No.	TC	TG	C-HDL	C-LDL	No.	TC	TG	C-HDL	C-LDL
6-7	50	158 (21)	50 (16)	56 (11)	94 (21)	17	158 (31)	49 (15)	60 (15)	93 (26)
8-9	45	158 (20)	57 (25)	56 (10)	92 (18)	18	172 (29)	48 (14)	62 (13)	103 (23)
10-11	60	164 (31)	58 (20)	56 (10)	98 (29)	20	171 (27)	58 (20)	63 (9)	99 (29)
12-13	78	160 (24)	65 (29)	55 (15)	96 (22)	28	167 (38)	59 (21)	55 (13)	102 (39)
14-15	57	155 (29)	69 (29)	48 (10)	96 (27)	23	156 (22)	60 (22)	53 (10)	95 (17)
16-17	68	155 (24)	78 (39)	48 (10)	94 (22)	13	145 (19)	63 (18)	50 (12)	86 (18)
6-11	155	160 (25)	55 (21)	56 (11)	95 (24)	55	167 (29)	52 (17)	62 (12)	98 (26)
12-17	203	157 (25)	70 (33)	51 (12)	96 (23)	64	159 (30)	60 (21)	54 (12)	97 (29)

Female subjects

Age		White					Black			
	No.	TC	TG	C-HDL	C-LDL	No.	TC	TG	C-HDL	C-LDL
6-7	39	161 (16)	71 (35)	49 (9)	101 (19)	16	168 (15)	55 (14)	57 (11)	104 (15)
8-9	40	162 (21)	70 (28)	53 (11)	98 (19)	21	176 (22)	56 (20)	62 (8)	104 (23)
10-11	70	161 (25)	72 (24)	51 (10)	98 (21)	22	160 (22)	69 (36)	53 (10)	99 (20)
12-13	56	161 (25)	73 (24)	52 (10)	98 (20)	32	168 (25)	69 (28)	56 (13)	102 (24)
14-15	56	151 (21)	72 (27)	50 (10)	91 (19)	21	166 (18)	60 (18)	56 (11)	102 (19)
16-17	65	159 (24)	72 (33)	55 (12)	93 (22)	12	152 (24)	62 (19)	54 (10)	89 (30)
6-11	149	161 (22)	71 (28)	51 (10)	99 (20)	59	168 (21)	60 (27)	58 (10)	102 (20)
12-17	177	157 (24)	72 (28)	52 (11)	94 (21)	65	164 (23)	65 (24)	56 (12)	100 (24)

From Morrison, J.A., and others: Pediatrics **62**:990, 1978. Copyright American Academy of Pediatrics, 1978.

Etiological Factors in Atherosclerosis

Cardiovascular disease, considered epidemic in the western world, is responsible for more deaths in the United States than all other causes together. Atherosclerosis is responsible for more than 50% of the deaths resulting from cardiovascular disease.

Atherosclerosis is a major specific type of arteriosclerosis, involving primarily the large elastic and medium-sized arteries. Lipids similar to those circulating in the blood accumulate on the intima of the arteries, to which an accumulation of connective tissue and various blood products are added, and plaques result. Several complications such as hemorrhage, thrombosis, or ulceration can occur in the atherosclerotic lesion and transform plaques into rough, complicated lesions. The plaques narrow the lumen of the arteries and may produce a deficiency of blood flow to some degree. They set the stage for complete occlusion.[82]

Fatty flecks and streaks are present by 3 to 5 months of age in the aortas of all children of all populations. As children age, the number and size of the streaks increase. Studies of animals have suggested that dietary intakes of cholesterol and fatty acids determine whether the fatty deposits are reabsorbed, remain, or develop into atherosclerotic plaques.[83,84]

The average extent of intimal involvement is small in the first 10 years of life. After the first decade the extent of the intimal surface involved by fatty streaks increases rapidly. The lipid in the juvenile fatty streak is predominantly intracellular, and there is minimal connective tissue. Black children have more extensive fatty streaks than do children of other ethnic groups. Females have more extensive streaking than do males. This is true in all populations studied, regardless of the incidence of atherosclerosis. After 25 to 29 years of age, differences appear. Fatty streaks progress through continued lipid accumulation and lead to plaque formation. These fatty streaks contain much of their lipid in the form of extracellular accumulations in areas where intact cells are scanty. An increase in extracellular components of connective tissue also becomes apparent. Fibrous plaques then appear in a significant number of cases.

Autopsies of soldiers who died in the wars in Korea and Vietnam revealed a striking incidence of atherosclerotic plaques in males in their early twenties. Seventy-seven percent of males killed in Korea were found to have evidence of atherosclerosis, ranging from minimal thickening to complete occlusion of one or more of the main artery branches.[85] Autopsies of soldiers killed in Vietnam revealed a lesser but significant incidence of atherosclerosis. Of the casualties autopsied during this war 45% were found to have atherosclerosis, but only 5% had gross evidence of coronary artery involvement.[86]

Autopsy studies of children from the Bogalusa Heart Study found an adverse effect of elevated risk factor levels including serum cholesterol and lipoprotein levels in accelerating the development of fatty streaks and fibrous plaques in adolescence.[87]

Risk Factors Associated with Atherosclerosis

Two hundred and forty six risk factors have been identified for cardiovascular disease. However, the major risk factors include elevated serum levels of low-density lipoprotein cholesterol, cigarette smoking, hypertension, obesity, sedentary life-style, and a family history of heart disease. All risk factors have been found to be independent and continuous variables. There is no arbitrary serum cholesterol level at which the risk of developing cardiovascular heart disease is increased. As the serum cholesterol level is increased, the risk for atherosclerosis increases. Also, the risk of developing atherosclerosis increases as the number of risk factors increases. Two or three risk factors increase the risk for atherosclerosis in an exponential manner. For example, the obese individual with a moderately elevated serum cholesterol level who has hypertension and smokes cigarettes has a higher risk of developing atherosclerosis than the person who has a more elevated serum cholesterol level but is lean, active, and does not smoke.

Elevated serum low-density lipoprotein cholesterol and low serum high-density lipoprotein cholesterol concentrations are clearly risk factors in the etiology of coronary artery disease. Populations that consume diets rich in cholesterol and saturated fats have higher serum cholesterol concentrations and higher incidences of and mortality rates from premature coronary heart disease than populations that consume diets low in cholesterol and saturated fat. The risk of developing premature atherosclerotic heart disease increases in any population group as the serum cholesterol concentration rises.[88] The Framingham study showed that the risk of myocardial infarction for men 30 to 49 years of age increased five times if cholesterol levels were greater than 260 mg/100 ml as compared with less than 220 mg/100 ml.[89]

Effect of dietary intervention

It has been proved that dietary alterations can reduce serum lipids. Reduction in intakes of dietary cholesterol reduces serum lipids from 5% to 8%. Reductions in intakes of saturated fats accompanied by increases in intakes of polyunsaturated fats and reductions in cholesterol can reduce the serum cholesterol by 24%.[90] It has not been possible, however, to establish relationships in individuals between serum cholesterol levels and dietary consumption of fat and cholesterol.

Morrison and others[91] found few significant correlations between dietary lipid and lipoprotein levels in 10-year-old children. However, children in the top quartiles for serum cholesterol ingested more total fat, more saturated fat, and less polyunsaturated fat than those in the lowest quartile. Another study found no significant correlation between serum cholesterol levels and mean daily intakes of total calories, total fat, and sugar.

Anderson, Lifschitz, and Friis-Hansen found serum cholesterol levels during infancy were directly correlated with intakes of saturated fat and inversely related to the ratio of polyunsaturated to saturated fatty acids of the diet. However, they found no relationship between intakes of fat and serum lipid levels in 3- to 4-year-old children.[92]

McGandy and others[95] reduced calories from fat from 39% to 34%, reduced cholesterol consumption from 720 to 380 mg/day, and increased the dietary P/S ratio from 0.2 to 1.2 in children 12 to 18 years of age. Boys whose initial serum cholesterol was 200 mg/100 ml experienced a reduction of 15%. However, those whose initial serum cholesterol was 199 mg/100 ml or less experienced a reduction of only 8.3%.

Recommendations

Many questions remain unanswered. Although there is a proven relationship between serum cholesterol and dietary intakes of fat in populations, no association has been found between dietary habits and serum lipid levels or coronary lesions in individuals within populations. It remains to be proved if reductions in serum lipid concentrations can delay the onset of atherosclerosis. The variability in response of individuals to dietary fat is as yet unexplained, although there is a large body of data that suggests genetic control. There are those who believe that serum lipid disorders originate in childhood and that food habits developed during that time should be patterned to acceptance and selection of diets low in cholesterol and saturated fats and rich in polyunsaturated fats. Others believe that efforts directed toward prevention of atherosclerosis should be focused on the adolescent and young adult. Still others think that dietary intervention should be directed only to susceptible individuals.

There is no difference of opinion that dietary intervention is appropriate for individuals in whom hyperlipoproteinemia has been identified or who have proven coronary artery disease. All agree that obesity and overweight should be discouraged at all ages. The Committee on Nutrition of the American Academy of Pediatrics[93] recommends screening children older than 2 years of age who are at risk because of a family history of hyperlipoproteinemia with at least two serum cholesterol measurements. If high-density lipoprotein cholesterol is not the cause of an elevated serum cholesterol, they recommend that the child be treated with diet or drugs or both. For other children who are not at risk, they recommend a varied diet with selections from each of the major food groups and a moderate decrease in the consumption of saturated fat and cholesterol.

Dietary factors other than fats have been shown to influence cholesterol levels. For example, fiber, especially pectin, has a hypocholesterolemic effect. The source of dietary protein has also been shown to be a factor. It is apparent that until many questions are answered recommendations for modification of dietary intakes of fat and cholesterol should be individualized to the needs of each child and family.

SALT INTAKE

Essential hypertension, another risk factor in cardiovascular heart disease, is also a major health problem affecting 20% of adults over 40 years of age. Epidemiological studies have suggested that as with hyperlipidemia, genetic and environmental factors interact to determine an individual's susceptibility to the disorder. Salt has been implicated as one factor that may cause hypertension.

Success in reducing blood pressure in hypertensive patients with the low-sodium rice diet designed by Kempner caused some researchers to hypothesize that excessive salt intakes could cause hypertension. Dahl[94] became so convinced that salt intakes were important in the development of hypertension that he devoted his life to this research. He studied the effect of salt intakes on thousands of rats, the effect of reduced sodium intake on hypertensive patients, and the relationship of sodium intakes to the incidence of hypertension in populations.

Evidence from Animal Studies

Meneely and others[95] induced hypertension in rats by mixing salt with their food and allowing them to consume as much water and food as they wished. They studied six groups of rats, each of which was fed an increasing amount of salt, and found that as sodium chloride intakes increased, elevations in blood pressures increased. Hypertension developed early in those animals who consumed the highest salt intakes. Although increases in blood pressure of groups of animals were related to the level of salt intakes, individual variations within groups were noted. They later fed diets that included extra amounts of salt to three groups of older animals who had been maintained on the basic food throughout their lives. Elevation in blood pressure did occur, but increases were always less than those of the young animals who ate the same rations.[96]

Dahl and others[97] found that in unselected rats, blood pressure increases in response to high salt intakes ranged from none to gradually increasing blood pressures, including the malignant phase. Some rats died from hypertension within a few months. One fourth of the animals showed no increase in blood pressure. The other animals developed increases in blood pressure that were associated with increasing morbidity and mortality.

In successive generations, rats were inbred and a strain of rats genetically susceptible to salt was developed. It was found that increased salt intakes of these animals during the first 12 to 13 months after weaning produced hypertension that was sustained regardless of later reductions in sodium intakes. Control rats fed low-sodium mixtures developed no hypertension.[98] Dahl, Heine, and Tassinari[99] concluded that salt intakes in infancy and early childhood may be more critical than those in later life to persons genetically determined to be responsive to salt intakes. In 1963 they fed commercially prepared salted infant foods to those rats bred to be genetically sensitive to salt. Five of seven rate developed hypertension, whereas none of the seven control rats who were fed low-sodium diets developed the disorder. At that time they suggested that there may be groups of human infants with similar genetic potentials who are at risk of induced hypertension from salt intakes in early life. They advocated reductions in salt intakes in infancy.

Srinivasan and others[100] found the systolic and diastolic blood pressure levels increased in spider monkeys that were fed salt and salt-sucrose diets as compared with the levels of monkeys fed a control diet. A greater rise was noted in blood pressure of those fed the salt-sucrose diet. They suggested a potentiating effect of sucrose on sodium-induced hypertension.

Studies of Populations

Dahl[94] studied five population groups whose lifetime salt intakes varied from 4 to 26 gm/day and found that as average salt intakes increased the incidence of hypertension increased.

Gleibermann[101] reviewed studies of 27 populations. Sodium intakes had been estimated by urinary excretion of sodium for 24 hours in some and by estimated salt intakes in others. Her statistical analysis of these studies suggested a direct relationship between salt intakes and blood pressure across population lines.

Oliver, Cohen, and Neel[102] found that blood pressure in Yanomamo Indians who add no salt to their diets failed to increase with age but remained low throughout life.

The relationship of salt intakes of individuals to blood pressure has not been established. Data from the HANES I study and from a large population in Connecticut found no relationship between blood pressure and dietary sodium or salt intake.[103,104]

Whitten and Stewart[105] studied two groups of black males, one fed a low level of salt, the other a high level of salt starting at 3 months of age. They found no difference in blood pressure levels of the two groups at 8 months or 8 years of age. Pietinen, Wong, and Altschul[106] found a correlation between sodium excretion and blood pressure of 20- to 40-year-old volunteers who had first-degree relatives who were hypertensive but no correlation between sodium excretion and blood pressure of individuals with no family history of hypertension.

It has been estimated that 18% of the population is hypertensive and that about one third to one half of those individuals are salt sensitive.[107]

Sodium intakes

The sodium intake of infants is relatively low when human milk and commercially prepared infant foods are consumed, relatively high when cow's milk and table foods are eaten. As the transition is made to table foods, salt intakes will reflect family food habits and cultural patterns.

The use of convenience foods and the popularity of fast-food establishments for feeding children past infancy have given the food industry a major role in determining salt intakes of children.[108]

In response to concern about the quantity of salt added to commercially prepared infant foods, in 1971 a subcommittee of the Food Protection Committee of the Food and

Nutrition Board reviewed the studies and recommended that the level of salt added to infant foods be reduced and that the upper limit of salt added to commercially prepared infant foods be 0.25%.[109] However, concern continued until all manufacturers stopped adding salt to commercially prepared infant foods.

Many parents prefer to make their own infant foods from a variety of foods prepared and seasoned for the family. Those who serve the highest sodium intakes to their infants have less education, feed salty snacks, and heavily salt their own food.[110]

Need for sodium

Sodium is an essential nutrient. It functions in the maintenance of water and acid base balance and the regulation of blood volume. It regulates cell membrane and capillary permeability and is a constituent of tissues. It is estimated that total body sodium increases from 240 mEq in the 3.3-kg newborn to 3100 mEq in a 70-kg adult. Requirements are determined by the individual's needs for growth and by losses from the skin and in the urine and stools.[111] Needs for growth are estimated to be 0.5 mEq/kg/day during the first 3 months, 0.2 mEq/kg/day from 3 to 6 months, 0.1 mEq/kg/day from 6 to 12 months, and less than 0.1 mEq/kg/day after the first year. Skin losses depend on the ambient temperature. Stool losses are independent of intake, averaging 5% to 10% in the first year. Because of the variability of losses, Fomon[112] suggests an advisable intake of 8 mEq/day from birth to 4 months of age, 6 mEq/day from 4 to 24 months of age, and 8 mEq/day from 24 to 36 months of age.

Humans adapt to a wide range of sodium intake by varying excretion in relation to intake and nonrenal losses. The Committee on Nutrition of the Academy of Pediatrics[108] has stated that safe limits for normal children appear to be between 8 and 100 mEq/day. They have recommended that moderation be practiced in the trend to decrease sodium intakes of children. Dietary therapy should be individualized for children with identified hypertension and those with family histories of hypertension who may or may not derive benefits from reductions in sodium intakes. It is important to remember that iodized salt is a major source of iodine in the United States. Intakes of children who consume low-sodium diets should be carefully monitored for iodine. A palpable goiter has been noted in two adolescent females whose family had adopted a low-sodium dietary intake because of diagnosed hypertension in the father.

Summary

Obesity, hypertension, and hyperlipoproteinemia increase the risk of cardiovascular disease, as well as other disorders. The multiple etiologies of all three conditions have made it difficult to define the role nutrient intake plays in causing such problems. Dietary intervention is appropriate for children who are overweight or obese or who have diagnosed hyperlipoproteinemia or hypertension.

It has been suggested for the remainder of the population of children that moderation be practiced in the trend to reduce sodium and saturated fat and cholesterol intakes.

Diets of children that must be modified because of food allergies or lactose intolerance should be carefully monitored for the adequacy of nutrient intake. Reducing sucrose intake combined with using noncariogenic foods at snacktime is effective in reducing the incidence of dental caries.

SUGGESTED LEARNING ACTIVITIES

1. Plan a week's menu for a 5-year-old girl who weighs 21 kg and is 109 cm tall. The diet should maintain her weight.
2. Investigate and report on physical activities that are developmentally appropriate to

increase energy expenditure for 2- and 8-year-old girls.

3. Describe how you would counsel the parents of an obese 8-month-old male.

4. Plan a week's menu for a child who is allergic to milk, wheat, eggs, fish, beef, and chocolate. Calculate the energy and nutrients in the menu.

5. Investigate sources in your community of rice flour, potato flour, and other products that can be used in the diet of a child allergic to wheat, rye, and oats.

6. Prepare a class for preschool children on snacks that are noncariogenic.

7. Investigate and report on the races in which one could expect to find a relatively high incidence of postweaning lactose intolerance.

8. Describe children at risk of hyperlipoproteinemia. How would one counsel parents of these children?

9. Investigate the salt content of fast-food menu items.

REFERENCES

Obesity

1. Hammar, S. L., and others: An interdisciplinary study of adolescent obesity, J. Pediatr. 80:373, 1972.
2. Dietz, W. H.: Prevention of childhood obesity. Pediatr. Clin. North Am. 33:823, 1986.
3. Knittle, J. L., and others: Childhood obesity. In Suskin, R. M.: Textbook of pediatric nutrition, New York, 1981, Raven Press.
4. Kalata, G.: Obese children: A growing problem. Science 232:20, 1986.
5. Mullins, A. G.: The prognosis in juvenile obesity, Arch. Dis. Child. 33:307, 1958.
6. Zack, P. M., and others: A longitudinal study of body fatness in childhood and adolescence, J. Pediatr. 95:126, 1979.
7. Lloyd, J. K., Wolff, O. H., and Whelen, W. S.: Childhood obesity, a long-term study of height and weight, Br. Med. J. 2:145, 1961.
8. Forbes, G. B.: Lean body mass and fat in obese children, Pediatrics 34:308, 1964.
9. Angel, J. L.: Constitution in female obesity, Am. J. Phys. Anthropol. 7:433, 1949.
10. Gurney, R.: The hereditary factor in obesity, Arch. Intern. Med. 57:557, 1936.
11. Stunkard, A. J., and others: An adoption study of human obesity, N. Engl. J. Med. 314:193, 1986.
12. Seltzer, C.C., and Mayer, J.: Body build and obesity—who are the obese? J.A.M.A. 189:677, 1964.
13. Berkowitz, R. I. and others: Physical activity and adiposity: A longitudinal study from birth to childhood. J. Pediatr. 106:734, 1985.
14. Dietz, W. H. and Gortmaker, S. L.: Do we fatten our children at the television set? Obesity and television viewing in children and adolescents, Pediatrics 75:807, 1985.
15. Shukla, A., and others: Infantile overnutrition in the first year of life: a field study of Dudley, Worcestershire, Br. Med. J. 4:507, 1972.
16. Sveger, T., and others: Nutrition, overnutrition, and obesity in the first year of life in Malmo, Sweden, Acta Paediatr. Scand. 64:635, 1975.
17. Fisch, R. O., Bilek, M. K., and Ulstrom, R.: Obesity and leanness at birth and their relationship to body habits in later childhood, Pediatrics 56:521, 1975.
18. Yeung, D. L., and others: Infant fatness and feeding practices: a longitudinal assessment, J. Am. Diet. Assoc. 79:531, 1981.
19. Dubois, S., Hill, D. E., and Beaton, G. H.: An examination of factors believed to be associated with infantile obesity, Am. J. Clin. Nutr. 32:1997, 1979.
20. Fomon, S. J., and others: Indices of fatness and serum cholesterol at age eight years in relation to feeding and growth during early infancy. Pediatr. Res. 18:1233, 1984.
21. Shapiro, L. R., and others: Obesity prognosis: A longitudinal study of children from the age of 6 months to 9 years. Am. J. Public Health 74:968, 1984.
22. Committee on Nutrition, American Academy of Pediatrics: Nutritional aspects of obesity in infancy and childhood, Pediatrics 68:880, 1981.
23. Massengale, O. N.: The obese adolescent observations on etiology management prevention, Clin. Pediatr. 4:649, 1965.
24. Hertzler, A. A.: Obesity—impact of the family, J. Am. Diet. Assoc. 79:525, 1981.
25. Bruch, H.: Obesity in childhood. III. Physiologic and psychologic aspects of food intake of obese children, Am. J. Dis. Child. 59:739, 1940.
26. Kahn, E. J.: Obesity in children: identification of a group at risk in a New York ghetto, J. Pediatr. 77:771, 1970.
27. Garn, S. M., Clark, D. C., and Guire, K. E.: Growth, body composition and development of obese and

lean children. In Winick, M., editor: Childhood obesity, New York, 1975, John Wiley & Sons, Inc.

28. Garn, S. M., Hopkins, P. J., and Ryan, A. S.: Differential fatness of low income boys and girls, Am. J. Clin. Nutr. 34:1465, 1981.

29. Griffith, M., and Payne, P. R.: Energy expenditure in small children of obese and nonobese parents, Nature 260:698, 1976.

30. Wolff, O. H., and Lloyd, J. K.: Obesity in childhood, Proc. Nutr. Soc. 32:195, 1973.

31. Pugliese, M. T. and others: Fear of obesity. A cause of short stature and delayed puberty. N. Engl. J. Med. 309:513, 1983.

Food allergies

32. Crawford, L. V., and Herrod, H. G.: Allergy diets for infants and children, Curr. Prob. Pediatr. 11:1, 1981.

33. Bock, S. A.: Prospective appraisal of complaints of adverse reactions to foods during children's first 3 years of life. Pediatrics 75:613, 1987.

34. May, C. D., and Bock, S. A.: A modern clinical approach to food hypersensitivity, Allergy 33:166, 1978.

35. Rowe, A. H., and Rowe, A.: Food allergy, its manifestations and control and the elimination diets: a compendium, Springfield, Ill., 1972, Charles C. Thomas, Publisher

36. Hughes, E. C.: Use of a chemically defined diet in the diagnosis of food sensitivities and the determination of offending foods, Ann. Allergy 40:393, 1978.

Carbohydrate and dental caries

37. Guggenheim, B., and others: The cariogenicity of different dietary carbohydrates tested on rats in relative gnotobiosis with a streptococcus-producing extracellular polysaccharide, Helv. Odontol. Acta 10:101, 1966.

38. Gustafson, B. E., and others: The Vipeholm dental caries study: the effect of different levels of carbohydrate intake on dental caries in 436 individuals observed for five years, Acta Odontol. Scand. 11:232, 1954.

39. Firestone, A. R., Schmid, R., and Mühlemann, H. R.: Effect of the length and number of intervals between meals. Caries Res. 18:128, 1984.

40. Palmer, J. D.: Dietary habits at bedtime in relation to dental caries in children, Br. Dent. J. 130:288, 1971.

41. Tass, E. N.: Is bottle feeding of milk a factor in dental caries? J. Dent. Child. 29:245, 1962.

42. Finn, S. B.: Dental caries in infants, Curr. Dent. Concepts 1:35, 1969.

43. Gardner, D. E., Norwood, J. R., and Eisenson, J. E.: At-will breastfeeding and dental caries, J. Dent. Child. 13:186, 1977.

44. Hankin, J. H., Chung, C. S., and Kau, M. C. W.: Genetic and epidemiologic studies of oral characteristics in Hawaii's schoolchildren: dietary patterns and caries prevalence, J. Dent. Res. 52:1079, 1973.

45. Bagramian, R. A., and Russell, A. L.: Epidemiologic study of dental caries experience and between meal eating patterns, J. Dent. Res. 52:342, 1973.

46. Mirth, D. B., and Bowen, W. H.: Chemotherapy antimicrobials and methods of delivery in microbial aspects of dental caries. In Stiles, H. M., and others, editors: Microbial aspects of dental caries, Washington, D.C., 1976, Information Retrieval.

47. Edgar, W. M., and others: Acid production in plaque after eating snacks: modifying factors in food, J. Am. Dent.Assoc. 90:418, 1975.

48. Clancy, K. L., and others: Snack food intakes of adolescents and caries development, J. Dent. Res. 56:568, 1977.

49. Bowen, W. H., and others: A method to assess cariogenic potential of food stuffs, J. Am. Dent. Assoc. 100:677, 1980.

50. Schachtele, C. F., and Jensen, M. B.: Human plaque pH studies: estimating the cariogenic potential of foods, Cereal Food World 26:14, 1981.

51. Schachtele, C. F.: Changing perspectives on the role of diet in dental caries formation, Nutr. News 42:13, 1982.

Lactose malabsorption and intolerance

52. Simoons, F. J.: The geographic hypothesis and lactose malabsorption, a weighing of the evidence, Dig. Dis. 23:963, 1978.

53. Rosenweig, N. S.: Diet and intestinal enzyme adaptation: implications for gastrointestinal disorders, Am. J. Clin. Nutr. 28:684, 1975.

54. Protein Advisory Council of the United Nations: Low lactase activity and milk intake, N.Y.P.A.G. Bull. 2:2, 1972.

55. Johnson, J. D., Kretchmer, N., and Simons, F. J.: Lactose malabsorption: its biology and history, Adv. Pediatr. 21:197, 1974.

56. Ament, M. E.: Malabsorption syndromes in infancy and childhood, J. Pediatr. 81:685, 867, 1972.

57. Newcomer, A. D., and McGill, D. B.: Lactose tolerance test in adults with normal lactase activity, Gastroenterology 50:340, 1966.

58. Calloway, D. H., Murphy, E. L., and Bauer, D.: Determination of lactose intolerance by breath analysis, Am. J. Dig. Dis. 14:811, 1969.

59. Arvanitakis, C., and others: Lactase deficiency—a comparative study of diagnostic methods, Am. J. Clin. Nutr. 30:1597, 1977.

60. Paige, D. M., and others: Lactose malabsorption in preschool black children, Am. J. Clin. Nutr. 30:1018, 1977.

61. Garza, C., and Scrimshaw, N. S.: Relationship of lactose intolerance to milk intolerance in young children, Am. J. Clin. Nutr. 29:192, 1976.

62. Committee on Nutrition, American Academy of Pediatrics: The practical significance of lactose intolerance in children, Pediatrics 62:240, 1978.

63. Wald, A., and others: Lactase malabsorption in recurrent abdominal pain of childhood, J. Pediatr. 100:65, 1982.

64. Calloway, D. H., and Chenoweth, W. L.: Utilization of nutrients in milk and wheat-based diets by men with adequate and reduced abilities to absorb lactose. I. Energy and nitrogen, Am. J. Clin. Nutr. 26:939, 1973.

65. Bowie, M. D.: Effect of lactose-induced diarrhea on absorption of nitrogen and fat, Arch. Dis. Child. 50:363, 1975.

66. Reddy, V., and Pershad, J.: Lactase deficiency in Indians, Am. J. Clin. Nutr. 25:114, 1972.

67. Stephenson, L. S., and Latham, M. C.: Lactose intolerance and milk consumption: the relationship of tolerance to symptoms, Am. J. Clin. Nutr. 27:296, 1974.

68. Paige, D.M., Bayless, T. M., and Dellinger, W. S.: Relationship of milk consumption to blood glucose rise in lactose intolerant individuals, Am. J. Clin. Nutr. 28:677, 1975.

69. Stephenson, L. S., Latham, M. C., and Jones, D. V.: Milk consumption by black and by white pupils in two primary schools, J. Am. Diet. Assoc. 71:258, 1977.

70. Barillas, C. and Solomons, N. W.: Effective reduction of lactose maldigestion by direct addition of β-galactosidase to milk at mealtime. Pediatrics 79:766, 1987.

Fats

71. Sheikh, M. S. and others: Gastrointestinal absorption of calcium from milk and calcium salts. N. Engl. J. Med. 317:532, 1987.

72. Weidman, K. and others: Diet in the healthy child. Circulation 67:1411, 1983.

73. Wynder, E. L. and others: Summary and recommendations of the conference on blood lipids in children: Optimal levels for early prevention of coronary artery disease. Prev. Med. 12:728, 1983.

74. Consensus Developmental Panel: Lowering blood cholesterol to prevent heart disease. J.A.M.A. 253:2080, 1985.

75. American Academy of Pediatrics, Committee on Nutrition: Prudent life style for children: dietary fat and cholesterol. Pediatrics 78:521, 1986.

76. Harper, A. E.: Dietary goals—a skeptical view. Am. J. Clin. Nutr. 31:310, 1978.

77. Farris, R. P., and others: Influence of milk source on serum lipids and lipoproteins during the first year of life, Am. J. Clin. Nutr. 38:42, 1982.

78. Berenson, G. S., and others: Serum high-density lipoprotein and its relationship to cardiovascular disease risk factor variables in children—the Bogalusa Heart Study, Lipids 14:91, 1979.

79. Morrison, J.A.: Lipids and lipoproteins in 927 school children, ages 6 to 17 years, Pediatrics 62:990, 1978.

80. Berenson, G. S., and others: Dynamic changes of serum lipoproteins in children during adolescence and sexual maturation, Am. J. Epidemiol. 113:157, 1981.

81. Morrison, J. A.: Personal communication.

82. deGroot, I., and others: Lipids in school children, aged 6-17: upper normal limits, Pediatrics 60:437, 1977.

83. Armstrong, M. L., Warner, E.D., and Connor, W. E.: Regression of coronary atheromatosis in rhesus monkeys, Circ. Res. 27:59, 1970.

84. Wissler, R. W., and others: Atherogenesis in the cebus monkey, Arch. Pathol. 74:312, 1962.

85. Enos, W. F., Holmes, R. H., and Beyer, J. C.: Coronary disease among United States soldiers killed in action in Korea, J.A.M.A. 152:1090, 1952.

86. McNamara, J. J., and others: Coronary artery disease in combat casualties in Vietnam, J.A.M.A. 216:1185, 1971.

87. Cresanta, J. L. and others: Prevention of atherosclerosis in childhood. Pediatr. Clin. North Am. 33:835, 1986.

88. Hatch, F. T.: Interactions between nutrition and heredity in coronary heart disease, Am. J. Clin. Nutr. 27:80, 1974.

89. Dawber, T., and others: The epidemiology of coronary heart disease, Proc. Roy. Soc. Med. 55:256, 1962.

90. North, A. F.: Should pediatricians be concerned about children's cholesterol levels? Clin. Pediatr. 14:439, 1975.

91. Morrison, J. A., and others: Parent child association at upper and lower ranges of plasma cholesterol and triglyceride levels, Pediatrics 62:468, 1978.

92. Anderson, G. E., Lifschitz, C., and Friis-Hansen, B. F.: Dietary habits and serum lipid during the first four years of life, Acta Paediatr. Scand. 68:165, 1979.

93. McGandy, R. B.:Adolescence and the onset of atherosclerosis, Bull. N.Y. Acad. Med. 47:590, 1971.

Salt and hypertension

94. Dahl, L. K.: Salt and hypertension, Am. J. Clin. Nutr. 25:231, 1972.
95. Meneely, G. R., and others: Chronic sodium chloride toxicity in the albino rat. II. Occurrence of hypertension and a syndrome of edema and renal failure, J. Exp. Med. 98:71, 1953.
96. Meneely, G. R., and Ball, C. O. T.: Experimental epidemiology of chronic sodium chloride toxicity and the protective effect of potassium chloride, Am. J. Med. 25:713, 1958.
97. Dahl, L. K., and others: Effects of chronic excess salt ingestion: modifications of experimental hypertension in the rat by variations in the diet, Circ. Res. 22:11, 1968.
98. Dahl, L. K.: Effect of chronic excess salt feeding induction of self-sustaining hypertension in rats, J. Exp. Med.114:231, 1961.
99. Dahl, L. K., Heine, M., and Tassinari, L.: High salt content of Western infants' diet: possible relationship to hypertension in the adult, Nature 198:1204, 1963.
100. Srinivasan, S. R., and others: Effects of dietary sodium and sucrose on the induction of hypertension in spider monkeys, Am. J. Clin. Nutr. 33:561, 1980.
101. Gleibermann, L.: Blood pressure and dietary salt in human populations. Ecol. Food Nutr. 2:143, 1973.
102. Oliver, W. J., Cohen, E. L., and Neel, J. V.: Blood pressure, sodium value, and sodium related hormones in the Yanomamo Indians: a "no-salt" culture, Circulation 52:146, 1975.
103. Harlan, W. R. and others: Dietary intake and cardiovascular risk factors. I. Blood pressure correlates: United States 1971-75. Vital and Health Statistics, Series 11, No. 226, DHHS, Pub. No. PHS 83-1676, Public Health Services, Washington, D.C., February 1983, U. S. Government Printing Office.
104. Halden, R. A. and others: Dietary salt intakes and blood pressure, J.A.M.A. 250:365, 1983.
105. Whitten, C. F., and Stewart, R. A.: The effect of dietary sodium in infancy on blood pressure and related factors, Acta Paediatr. Scand. Suppl. 279, 1980.
106. Pietinen, P. I., Wong, O., and Altschul, A. M.: Electrolyte output, blood pressure, and family history of hypertension, Am. J. Clin. Nutr. 32:997, 1979.
107. Select Committee on GRAS Substances. Evaluation of the health aspects of sodium chloride and potassium chloride as food ingredients. SCOGS 12, Bethesda, Maryland. Federation of American Societies for Experimental Biology, Life Science Research Office, 1979.
108. Committee on Nutrition, American Academy of Pediatrics: Sodium intake of infants in the United States, Pediatrics 68:444, 1981.
109. Filer, L. J.: Salt in infant foods, Nutr. Rev. 29:27, 1971.
110. Schaefer, L. J. and Kumanyika: Maternal variables related to potentially high infant-feeding practices. J. Am. Diet. Assoc. 85:433, 1985.
111. Sperotto, G.: Sodium chloride in pediatrics. In Moses, C., editor: Sodium in medicine and health, Baltimore, Md., 1980, Reese Press.
112. Fomon, S. J.: Infant nutrition, Philadelphia, 1974, W. B. Saunders Co.

12

Nourishing the Premature and Low Birth Weight Infant

Mary J. O'Leary

OBJECTIVES

After studying this chapter, the student should:

1. Be aware of the reasons why the premature infant is at greater risk for nutritional problems than the full-term infant.

2. Be aware of the vulnerability of the premature infant to a variety of medical problems that may limit nutrient and energy intake and complicate methods of feeding.

3. Be aware of factors that determine whether the premature infant will receive parenteral or enteral feeds.

4. Recognize that human milk from the infant's mother is an appropriate milk for the low birth weight baby.

5. Know differences between formulas designed for the low birth weight baby and those designed for the full-term infant.

During the past 15 years, there have been many advances in neonatal intensive care. New technologies, better understanding of pathophysiology, and cooperative interactions to regionalize the delivery of perinatal care have all contributed to the increased survival of newborns requiring intensive care. As the prognosis for survival of low birth weight (LBW) neonates improves, attention is being focused on the nutritional support of these infants. Adequacy of postnatal nutrition affects the clinical course of critically ill babies and may influence their long-term developmental outcome. This chapter describes current methods of nutritional support and suggests guidelines for nutritional assessment and manage-

Parts of this chapter are modified from O'Leary, M.J.: Nutritional care of the low birth weight infant. In Krause, M.V., and Mahan, L.K., editors: Food, nutrition, and diet therapy, ed. 7, Philadelphia, 1984, W.B. Saunders Co.

ment of LBW infants who require intensive care.

NUTRITION SERVICES IN NEONATAL CARE

Delivery of Neonatal Care

Practical considerations of limited economic, technical, and human resources prohibit the availability of intensive care facilities in all hospitals. However, so that all infants may be provided equal access to the highest quality care, a regionalized system of perinatal services has evolved over the past 15 years. The regional perinatal network encompasses three levels of neonatal care. The system of classifying nurseries as level I, II, or III, based on the type of care they are capable of providing for newborn infants, has been described in several publications.[1-3]

Level I nurseries provide uncomplicated neonatal care for healthy infants who are products of normal, full-term pregnancies. In addition, level I nursery personnel are trained in early detection of potential complications and use coordinated mechanisms for referral and transport of high-risk infants to level II or level III units. When unexpected problems arise suddenly after birth, care provided in level I nurseries usually consists of stabilization until the infant can be safely transferred.

Level II nurseries also provide a full range of services for normal newborns and expertise in screening and referral of high-risk infants. But these nurseries are also prepared to care for moderately ill neonates or convalescing babies whose immaturity or medical risks preclude discharge.

In contrast, level III nurseries are specifically staffed and equipped to cope with the most serious types of neonatal illnesses and abnormalities. Critically ill infants usually require intensive care and are hospitalized in neonatal intensive care units of level III tertiary care centers. A level III neonatal intensive care unit often assumes a leadership role within its region of influence by setting standards of clinical care, developing educational materials, and providing consultative services to other nurseries. The nutrition specialist on such a unit may, in turn, have a similar opportunity and responsibility to serve as a regional resource for improvement in nutritional care of high-risk newborns.

Role of the Nutritionist

The skills required of the pediatric nutritionist vary according to the clinical status of the newborn infants at each level of neonatal care. The National Research Council Committee on Nutrition of the Mother and Preschool Child has identified specific skills required to provide clinical services at each of the three levels of neonatal care.[4] In general, these skills should enable the nutrition consultant to screen for the various nutrition problems, monitor and assess nutritional progress, and develop and implement management plans.

It is important that nutrition services be coordinated with the physicians, nurses, and pharmacists also involved in the clinical care of these infants. Providing adequate nutrition to intensive care neonates is a challenge that requires the skillful input of several disciplines. Many nutritionists function as members of nutrition support teams that facilitate development of guidelines for safe and effective nutritional management of critically ill neonates.[5]

LBW INFANTS REQUIRING INTENSIVE CARE

Characteristics

The infants cared for in Level III intensive care units typically include those at high medical risk, critically ill babies with serious pediatric or surgical problems, or infants suffering from congenital abnormalities. Many of these infants weigh less than 2500 gm ($5\frac{1}{2}$ pounds) at birth, and are therefore classified as LBW infants. Increasing numbers of infants weighing less than 1500 gm ($3\frac{1}{2}$ pounds) are being admitted to Level III intensive care units. These tiny babies are frequently referred to as very low birth weight (VLBW) infants. The medical status of larger infants may also warrant intensive care. However, the discussion in this chapter will focus on the particular problems and nutritional needs of LBW and VLBW infants who require Level III intensive care (Figure 12-1).

Infants may be LBW because of a shortened period of gestation, which means that they are premature, or because of a retarded rate of growth, which makes them small for gestational age. Whereas the full-term infant is born between 37 and 42 weeks of gestation, a premature infant is born before 37 weeks of gestation. Infants born before 25 weeks of gestation rarely survive. Although the management of VLBW infants who require intensive care has improved dramatically during the past decade, medical science is still unable to meet the metabolic and medical needs of most infants born before the third trimester of pregnancy (earlier than 26 weeks' gestation).

Accurate assessment of gestational age is important in establishing nutritional goals for individual infants and in differentiating the short gestation infant from the small for gestational age infant. This differentiation is determined by the date of the last menstrual period, fetal ultrasound, and clinical assessment. Clinical parameters fall into two broad groups: (1) a series of neurological signs, dependent mainly on postures and tone, and (2) a series of external characteristics that reflect the physical maturity of the infant.[6]

LBW infants may have a variety of clinical problems in the early postnatal period. These problems vary in type and severity depending on such factors as the intrauterine health of the fetus, degree of prematurity, birth-related trauma, and functioning of immature or stressed organ systems. Although a wide range of medical problems may complicate the neonatal

Figure 12-1 Little girl born at 26 weeks' gestation, weighing 650 gm. Her eyes are covered for protection from the photography lights.

course of LBW infants, certain problems occur with such frequency as to be considered typical problems of prematurity. Small, immature infants are at risk for development of the problems listed in Table 12-1. Not all premature infants do, in fact, develop clinical signs of these potential problems. However, medical and nutritional management of high-risk infants must anticipate their occurrence so preventive measures can be taken or effective treatment modalities employed.

Metabolic Reserve

The interruption of the influx of water, energy, and nutrients that occurs at the time of birth presents a greater hazard for the premature infant than for the full-term infant.[7] The premature infant has a smaller metabolic reserve and is physiologically less well prepared to maintain homeostasis. Fat stores are limited because most fetal fat is deposited during the last 6 weeks of gestation. In the premature infant weighing 1000 gm, fat contributes only

Table 12-1 Examples of problems common to premature or LBW infants in the neonatal period

System	Problem
Respiratory	Hyaline membrane disease, also known as respiratory distress syndrome
Cardiovascular	Patent ductus arteriosus
Renal	Fluid and/or electrolyte imbalance
Neurological	Intracranial hemorrhage
Metabolic	Hypoglycemia; hypocalcemia
Gastrointestinal	Hyperbilirubinemia; feeding intolerance; necrotizing enterocolitis
Hematological	Anemia
Immunological	Sepsis; pneumonia; meningitis

1% of total body weight; in contrast, the body of the full-term infant (3500 gm) is about 16% fat.[8] Glycogen reserves are particularly small and are rapidly depleted. Babies who weigh 1000 gm have a glycogen and fat reserve of approximately 110 kcal/kg.[9] With basal metabolic needs of about 50 kcal/kg/day, it is obvious that these babies will rapidly run out of fat and carbohydrate fuel unless adequate nutritional support is established. Depletion time will vary between 2 and 4 days, depending on the volume and concentration of parenteral dextrose that can be tolerated. Obviously, depletion time will be even shorter for premature babies who weigh less than 1000 gm at birth. Energy reserves are depleted most quickly by tiny infants who suffer from intrauterine growth retardation.

It is often difficult, however, to provide adequate nutritional intake during the first several days of life because of immaturity of organ systems and severe medical problems. When adequate dietary intake cannot be achieved and fat and glycogen reserves have been exhausted, the infant will begin to catabolize vital body protein tissue for energy. Heird and others[9] have theoretically estimated the survival time of starved and semistarved infants. Their estimates assume depletion of all glycogen and fat and about one third of body protein tissue at a rate of 50 kcal/kg/day with fluids as intravenous water (no exogenous calories) or 10% dextrose solution. Even at the expense of significant protein tissue catabolism, the projected survival times shown in Table 12-2 are alarmingly short. These numbers are estimates and lack empirical precision, but they do serve to demonstrate the disadvantage of the small infant when faced with inadequate nutritional support.

Premature babies with small metabolic reserves are particularly vulnerable to the hazardous consequences of protein-energy malnutrition. Inadequate intake for even a

Table 12-2 Duration of survival expected in starvation (H_2O only) and semistarvation ($D_{10}W$)

Birth Weight (gm)	Estimated Survival Time (Days)	
	H_2O only	$D_{10}W$
1000	4	11
2000	12	30
3500	32	80

From Heird, W.C., and others: J. Pediatr. 80:351, 1972.

few days may adversely affect their clinical course. For example, immature infants suffering from pulmonary disease may experience weakening of the respiratory muscles, depression of ventilatory drive, and increased difficulty in weaning from mechanical ventilation when protein-energy malnutrition complicates their clinical status.[10] The relationship between protein-energy malnutrition and decreased immune competence is well known and results in increased risk of infection.[11] Cardiac performance of malnourished patients may be depressed, resulting in decreased ability to withstand episodes of stress such as surgery.[12]

Furthermore, malnutrition in critically ill infants may compromise their long-term outcome. Evidence from animal[13] and human[14] studies suggests that protein-energy malnutrition at the critical period of rapid brain growth results in irreversible impairment of brain growth and function. Damage from protein-energy malnutrition includes reduction in the number and size of brain cells. Therefore neonates in general, and LBW infants in particular, are at risk of suffering damaging consequences when protein-energy malnutrition complicates their clinical course.

Need for Fluid, Glucose, and Electrolytes

Because most LBW infants who require intensive care are unable to tolerate enteral feedings in the early neonatal period, intravascular delivery of fluid, glucose, and electrolytes must be established to maintain fluid balance and promote metabolic homeostasis. Immature newborns have an immediate need for fluid to replace ongoing water losses. Since most of these babies are unstable at birth and deprived of oral intake, intravenous (IV) fluid therapy is usually required to prevent dehydration or fluid imbalance. Premature infants become rapidly dependent on an exogenous source of glucose because of limited glycogen stores and decreased capacity for gluconeogenesis. To prevent hypoglycemia and to spare protein tissue, an IV solution containing a measured amount of dextrose is infused as soon as primary postnatal demands for resuscitation and stabilization have been completed. In addition to fluid and glucose administration, most premature newborns require sodium, chloride, and potassium to replace daily losses. In practice, electrolytes are not usually added to the IV solution until the second day of life.

PARENTERAL NUTRITION

Parenteral nutrition is broadly defined as the delivery of nutritive material by some means other than through the intestinal canal. Common usage of the term "parenteral nutrition," however, usually refers to the parenteral delivery of a hyperalimentation solution containing dextrose, amino acids, electrolytes, minerals, vitamins, and trace elements. The osmolarity of this solution increases in proportion to the concentration of dextrose in the infusate and can be markedly hyperosmolar. Infusion of an iso-osmolar lipid emulsion may accompany the delivery of the hyperalimentation solution.

Hyperalimentation fluids can provide all essential nutrients as the sole means of nutritional support. In this case, the term "total parenteral nutrition" is used to signify that no enteral feeds are being given and that all nutritional support occurs by means of a vascular route. In contrast, partial parenteral nutrition refers to the administration of hyperalimentation fluids as a supplement to limited enteral intake. Such a regimen is advantageous for LBW infants who are unable to tolerate full enteral feedings or who are being weaned from total parenteral nutrition to a program of complete enteral nutrition.

Route of Administration

It is possible to provide complete nutritional support to LBW infants by either central or peripheral vascular routes. By placing a catheter in a central blood vessel, it is possible to provide LBW infants with adequate caloric intake to permit positive nitrogen balance and allow normal growth and development.[15,16] Because blood flow through central vessels such as the superior vena cava is very rapid, hyperosmotic hyperalimentation fluids are quickly diluted and inflammation in the wall of the blood vessel is prevented. It is also possible to meet the nutritional needs of some LBW infants by peripheral delivery of parenteral nutrition. When isotonic lipid emulsions are appropriately used, their high caloric density decreases the need for hyperosmotic glucose solutions, such that the osmolarity of the solution entering the peripheral blood vessel is low enough to prevent damage to the vein.

Selecting the peripheral versus the central route of administration involves several considerations that should be individualized according to the unique circumstances of each infant. The principal factors to consider in choosing one technique over another are the caloric needs of the infant[17] and the projected duration of need for parenteral support.[18] Peripheral vein hyperalimentation solutions are usually not as calorically dense as central vein solutions. Peripheral veins are limited to dex-

trose concentrations of less than 10% to 15%, whereas central veins can tolerate concentrations of 20% to 25%. This means that infants who receive central vein nutrition can potentially receive more calories to promote positive nitrogen balance and growth. In the critically ill infant for whom prolonged parenteral therapy is projected and improved physical growth is possible, central vein nutrition is usually the treatment of choice.[18] If minimal stress is present and vessel access is good, the peripheral route of administration is often preferred.[18] This is most desirable for infants who are expected to receive less than 2 to 3 weeks of parenteral nutrition therapy or who receive parenteral nutrition as a temporary supplement to a progressive enteral intake (Figure 12-2).

Consideration of certain practical advantages and potential disadvantages also plays a role in selecting the preferred method of delivery for individual infants. Several of these advantages and disadvantages are listed in Table 12-3. In general, there are more serious technical and infectious complications encountered in central delivery than in peripheral delivery, but both routes have characteristic problems related to the method of administration. Although strict adherence to aseptic technique and to established guidelines for catheter care and maintenance markedly decrease the incidence of these complications, neither method of delivery is benign. Therefore candidates for parenteral nutrition should be carefully selected on the basis of need, and the potential benefits of the nutritional support should be weighed against the risks inherent to the methods of delivery before initiating therapy. The decision to begin parenteral nutrition in infants should occur on an individualized rather than a routine basis.

Indications

The need for parenteral nutrition is clear for those infants who have gastrointestinal problems that preclude or severely limit the use

Figure 12-2 A central venous catheter has been surgically implanted in the superior vena cava. This type of catheter permits delivery of hyperalimentation by a central venous route.

Table 12-3 Advantages and disadvantages of central and peripheral vein parenteral nutrition

	Advantages	Disadvantages
Central	Stable catheter	Infection of blood by means of catheter
	Concentrated dextrose solutions used allowing smaller infusion volume	Venous thrombosis
	Long-term	Hypoglycemia if abruptly discontinued
		Catheter must be surgically placed
		Requires frequent dressing changes
		Catheter dislogment and infusion of fluid into thoracic cavity
Peripheral	Not surgically placed	Catheter unstable; repeated attempts to restart IV may be stressful
	Infection less likely	Depletion of venous access
		Interruption of nutrition when IV out of patient
		Larger volume of infusion

Modified from Dolcourt, J.: Pediatric parenteral nutrition manual, Salt Lake City, Utah, 1983, Primary Children's Medical Center.

of the intestine for nutritional support. Infants with congenital anomalies of the enteric canal are usually unable to receive enteral nutrition until corrective surgical procedures occur. Total parenteral nutrition is indicated for these infants soon after birth and should be continued until recuperation is sufficient to permit oral feedings.[19] The use of total parenteral nutrition in surgical gastrointestinal disorders such as **gastroschisis, omphalocele, tracheoesophageal fistulas, intestinal atresias,** malrotation, and **volvulus** has been shown to greatly decrease the rate of morbidity and mortality in this vulnerable group of babies.[20-22]

Infants with ischemic disease of the intestinal mucosa, such as necrotizing enterocolitis, are also candidates for parenteral nutrition support. If necrotizing enterocolitis results in intestinal resection, total parenteral nutrition meets the infant's nutritional needs until the remaining intestine demonstrates returned function. According to Kerner,[18] a gradual transition from parenteral to enteral feeding can then begin. Partial parenteral nutrition provides supportive therapy while the intestine adapts and gradually compensates for the rapid transit, diminished digestive mass, and inadequate absorptive surface area.[18] Most of these infants are eventually able to tolerate a program of complete enteral nutrition.

Parenteral nutrition may also be indicated for repletion of a malnourished infant.[23] In clinical situations in which prolonged starvation is anticipated, parenteral nutrition may be started prophylactically (e.g., postoperative support).[24] Older infants with intractable diarrhea may be successfully rehabilitated with parenteral feedings as well.[25] In addition, certain situations that do not involve the gastrointestinal tract warrant the use of parenteral nutrition, for example, renal failure, hypermetabolic states, and malignancies.[26]

The need for parenteral nutrition in infants with the aforementioned conditions is clearly indicated. When the technique is applied with proper care, the morbidity and mortality associated with these clinical problems can be significantly reduced. Other clinical situations, however, do not indicate the need for parenteral nutrition support as clearly. Deciding whether or not to give hyperalimentation solutions to a LBW infant for whom feeding is risky rather than prohibitive is a process that is more often ambiguous than clear.

Many VLBW infants demonstrate poor tolerance to enteral feedings in the first few days or even weeks of life. This is related in part to the inadequate mechanical and digestive function of their immature gastrointestinal tract. Mechanical limitations such as poor coordination of intestinal motility and delayed gastric emptying contribute to delayed introduction and slow progression of enteral feeds in VLBW infants.[18] The digestive capacity of the gastrointestinal system is also limited, although it is usually adequate when human milk or specialized formula products are appropriately selected. VLBW infants may also have medical problems that limit their ability to ingest and use enteral nutrients.[18] In general, infants who are medically unstable are often precarious in their tolerance of enteral feeds as well. When LBW infants contract gastrointestinal and other medical problems, some projection of the extent to which these will delay the progression of enteral feeds is important in determining whether parenteral nutrition is appropriate.

Parenteral nutrition in LBW infants is usually indicated when the projected duration of need for parenteral support exceeds the metabolic reserve of the infant. This period varies, as does the metabolic reserve, according to the birth weight and gestational age of the infant, the adequacy of intrauterine growth, and any metabolic stress that is superimposed on basal energy needs. For VLBW infants whose metabolic reserves are severely limited, it is imperative that efforts are made to provide early nutritional support. As shown in Table

12-2, survival time under conditions of starvation and semistarvation diminishes in proportion to decreasing birth weight and gestational age. Because malnutrition complicates the clinical course of these tiny infants and may have irreversible developmental consequences, parenteral nutrition may be indicated for VLBW infants who are unable to tolerate enteral feedings after as little as 2 to 3 days.[27] Even if small amounts of enteral feeds are introduced in the first couple of days of life, immaturity of organ systems and coexisting medical stress often slow oral advancement substantially enough to warrant partial parenteral nutrition as a supplement to enteral feedings until the premature infant can tolerate full enteral volume and calories. When early introduction of any oral feeding is prohibited, the nutritional benefits and potential risks associated with parenteral nutrition should be considered and total parenteral nutrition started if the infant's condition permits catheter placement.

Larger LBW infants with correspondingly larger metabolic reserves may be able to tolerate a slightly longer delay before the need for parenteral nutrition becomes imminent. Still, these infants will begin to catabolize vital body protein tissue and deplete reserves of other essential nutrients within the first week of life if adequate nutritional support is not provided. Assuming somewhat larger stores of fat and glycogen in this population, the key factor in determining whether or not to begin parenteral nutrition is the predicted time lapse before there is adequate enteral intake. For example, a stable infant weighing 2000 gm who is hospitalized to rule out the possibility of **sepsis** (systemic infection) may initially receive IV fluid, glucose, and electrolytes but may not require hyperalimentation fluids if enteral feeds can be initiated within the first 4 to 5 days of life and can then be rapidly advanced. However, another infant of similar size and metabolic reserve who suffers episodes of clinical instability and associated feeding setbacks may benefit from partial parenteral nutrition until enteral feedings are sufficient to maintain homeostasis and promote growth.

Energy Needs

The energy needs of LBW infants who receive parenteral nutrition are usually less than those of infants who are enterally fed because absorptive loss does not occur when nutritional intake bypasses the intestinal tract. Whereas most LBW infants who are enterally fed need approximately 120[28] to 130[7] kcal/kg/day to grow, premature neonates demonstrate adequate growth with parenteral energy intakes of about 70 to 90 kcal/kg/day.[29]

Published studies of LBW infants generally show values for resting caloric expenditure to be about 50 kcal/kg/day, provided that measurements are made under thermoneutral conditions and that the infants are relatively inactive.[30] Provision of 60 kcal/kg/day plus 2 to 2.5 gm protein/kg/day is needed to meet resting metabolic energy needs and to allow nitrogen retention to occur.[31] However, higher energy intakes are required for increased nitrogen retention and growth. When premature infants receive parenteral energy intakes averaging 80 kcal/kg/day compared with 50 kcal/kg/day, greater tissue protein synthesis and weight gain result.[32]

It is often difficult, however, to provide sick LBW infants with adequate energy and other nutrients in the first few days of life. Many of these infants are severely stressed in the early postnatal period and must have fluids restricted to permit normal **diuresis** and to support medical management. These factors can initially limit energy intake to as little as 30 to 40 kcal/kg/day.[33] But as soon as possible, it is important to begin to increase both energy and protein intake so that metabolic homeostasis can be achieved and protein tissue catabolism can be prevented. It is desirable to meet basic nutritional needs for homeostasis before the second week of life. Later, after the infant's medical condition has stabilized, the goal of nutritional management can change from maintenance of homeostasis to the promotion of growth. Guidelines for parenteral energy and protein intake during maintenance and growth phases are shown in Table 12-4.

Hyperalimentation Solutions

Hyperalimentation fluids for parenteral nutrition are complex solutions that must be carefully managed to derive maximal nutritional benefit without exceeding metabolic limitations. These solutions can provide all essential nutrients to promote positive nitrogen balance and growth but must be tailored in their composition to meet the unique needs of each LBW infant. The theoretical and practical considerations involved in the management of hyperalimentation in pediatric patients have been expertly summarized by Kerner[34] and by Lebenthal.[35]

Fluid

Parenteral fluid therapy is required by LBW infants who are unable to tolerate an adequate enteral volume. Infants deprived of a normal oral intake continue to lose basal amounts of fluid that require water replacement.[36] Water requirements are therefore estimated by the sum of the predicted losses. A major route of water loss in LBW infants occurs by evaporation of water through the skin and respiratory tract; this insensible water loss is highest in the smallest and least mature babies.[37] Reasons for the inverse correlation between birth weight and insensible water loss include increased permeability of the skin epidermis to water, larger body surface area relative to body weight, and greater skin blood flow relative to metabolic rate.[38] Water loss through the skin of LBW infants occurs mainly by evaporative heat loss, since sweating is limited in premature infants. Measurements of insensible water loss using direct weighing techniques show that insensible losses vary from about 10 to 60 ml/kg/day, with the higher losses occurring in the smallest babies.[39]

Excretion of urine is another important route of water loss for LBW infants. The range of urine volume that can be excreted is determined by the solute load presented to the kidneys for excretion and by the ability of the kidneys to concentrate the urine.[40] Immature infants are limited in their ability to regulate water balance by means of antidiuretic hormone control and do not achieve maximal concentration or dilution mechanisms until some time after birth.[38] Urine excretion by LBW

Table 12-4   Guidelines for parenteral energy and protein intake during maintenance and growth phases

	Maintenance	Growth
Carbohydrate (dextrose)	60 kcal/kg/day	70-90 kcal/kg/day
Lipid (intravenous fat emulsions)	Begin: 0.5-1 gm/kg/day Increments: 0.25-0.50 gm/kg/day	Maximum 2-3 gm/kg/day
Protein	Begin: 0.5-1 gm/kg/day Increments: 0.5 gm/kg/day Goal: 2-2.5 gm/kg/day	Maximum 2.5-3 gm/kg/day

Modified from O'Leary, M.J.: Parenteral nutrition guidelines for preterm infants, Seattle, 1988, University of Washington Hospital.

babies normally varies between 60 and 125 ml/kg/day, with loss occurring at a rate of about 2 to 5 ml/kg/hour.[41] Fecal water loss on the other hand is small and relatively constant. The stool accounts for only about 10 to 15 ml/kg/day of water lost.[41]

There are two other factors to consider in the estimation of water requirements for LBW infants. First, there is a net loss of fluid when water is retained by tissues during growth. Second, there is a net gain in fluid when water is produced as a by-product of oxidative metabolism. Because the net loss and gain of these fluid components is roughly equal, they do not usually have practical importance in the calculation of actual water requirements for LBW infants.[41]

Several factors can either increase or decrease the fluid requirements of LBW infants by altering fluid losses. For example, radiant warmers[42] and phototherapy lights[43] markedly increase water requirements by increasing insensible fluid losses. On the other hand, heat shields[37] and thermal blankets[44] help to decrease the evaporative water losses of LBW infants. To determine total water requirements, the various environmental and physiological factors that alter fluid losses should be taken into account and the appropriate additions or subtractions should be made according to individual circumstances.

Because of the many variables affecting fluid losses and because of differences among babies depending on birth weight and medical status, it is difficult to establish routine guidelines for fluid management of LBW infants.[36] Many nurseries prefer to determine fluid needs based on individualized criteria. After initial fluid administration of 40 to 80 ml/kg/day, subsequent needs are determined by clinical examination of the patient. Clinical parameters and laboratory data such as urine output and specific gravity, serum electrolyte and blood urea nitrogen, blood pressure, peripheral circulatory status, mucous membrane mois-

ture, and skin turgor aid in individualized fluid management.[41] In addition, serial body weights should be determined on a routine daily basis or more often as clinically indicated. According to the guidelines of Hodson and Truog, total daily fluid administration is generally increased by 10 to 15 ml/kg/day depending on clinical status, laboratory data, and estimates of insensible water loss.[41] Most LBW infants receive 100 to 200 ml of fluid/kg/day by the second week of life, with intakes averaging 120 to 160 ml/kg/day.

The consequences of inadequate fluid intake in LBW infants are serious and include such problems as dehydration, electrolyte imbalances, and hypotension.[45] Fluid excess on the other hand can also be dangerous for the LBW infant. If too much fluid is administered, edema and congestive heart failure with opening of the ductus arteriosus may ensue.[46,47] There are also some indications that intraventricular hemorrhage and **bronchopulmonary dysplasia** are related to excessive fluid administration in the first few days of life.[48,49]

Appropriate fluid intakes in premature infants allow for normal transition of body fluids from fetal to neonatal status. Premature infants have relatively more total body water than do full-term infants, and a greater percentage of this total is extracellular fluid (Table 12-5). A reduction of extracellular water normally occurs in all newborn infants in the first few days of life but appears to be particularly important for LBW infants.[50] This reduction is accompanied by a normal loss of body weight (10% to 15%)[39] and by an improvement in renal function.[51] Failure of changes in fluid dynamics and lack of diuresis in the early neonatal period may complicate the course of respiratory diseases in the LBW infants.[52]

Carbohydrate

Although LBW infants are metabolically dependent on the availability of glucose, there is no absolute parenteral or enteral requirement

Table 12-5 Body water compartments of preterm and full-term infants (expressed as percent of body weight)

	Preterm (%)	Full-term (%)
Total body water	85-90	80
Extracellular fluid	50-55	45

From Hodson, W.A., and Truog, W.E.: Fluid and glucose administration. In Hodson, W.A., and Truog, W.E., editors: Critical care of the newborn, Philadelphia, 1983, W.B. Saunders Co.

for carbohydrate. Glucose can be produced in the body through gluconeogenic pathways or by catabolism of glycogen stores. Enzymes for the endogenous production of glucose are present in LBW infants, but the high incidence of hypoglycemia in these babies when exogenous intake is poor indicates that gluconeogenic mechanisms are immature and that glycogen stores are limited in premature infants.

Dextrose (D-glucose) is the carbohydrate typically chosen for infants receiving parenteral nutrition. Glucose is a good source of energy, providing 3.4 kcal/gm; however, tolerance to glucose infusions is variable in newborns and limited in premature infants. Glucose intolerance characterized by hyperglycemia is common among LBW infants and is most frequently encountered in very immature babies.[53] The reasons for the limited glucose tolerance are still unclear, but possible causes include inadequate insulin production or function and immature hepatic enzyme systems.[54] Hyperglycemia does not occur as often in LBW infants who are receiving an IV infusion of dextrose plus amino acids as it occurs in LBW infants receiving dextrose alone.[55] Amino acids may exert a stimulatory effect on the release of insulin.[54] Hay[56] has summarized several in vitro

studies that support this idea. A recent study in preterm infants showed a higher insulin level in infants receiving amino acid and glucose infusions than in infants receiving only glucose.[57] Other hormonal systems may also play a role in the glucose metabolism of LBW neonates. For example, the higher incidence of hyperglycemia among stressed infants may be associated with the stress-induced release of catecholamines and glucagon.[57]

Hyperglycemia is a hazardous condition for the LBW infant. When serum glucose levels exceed 150 mg/100 ml, glucosuria may follow. Glucosuria causes an osmotic diuresis, which may lead to dehydration, increased serum osmolarity, and potential complications.[58] Administration of glucose is usually monitored by frequent evaluation of serum glucose levels during the initiation of parenteral nutrition and at regular intervals thereafter. Urine may also be checked for glucose. However, urine tests are less reliable than blood tests and should not be relied on to determine therapy.[56]

The first step toward preventing hyperglycemia in LBW infants is to administer an amount of glucose that can be adequately metabolized without exceeding the infant's glucose tolerance. The amount of glucose supplied to the infant is determined not only by the concentration of the solution, but also by the rate at which it is administered. It is important to realize that the glucose load, and not the dextrose concentration alone, determines the amount of glucose that is delivered to an infant. Glucose load may be calculated using the following formula:

$$\text{Glucose load} = \text{mg/kg/minute}$$
$$= \text{mg glucose/ml} \times \text{ml/kg/minute}$$

This formula can be used to adjust fluid volume and dextrose concentration without changing the glucose load.

According to Kerner;[54]

Infants weighing less than 1000 g at birth should initially receive no more than 6 mg glucose/kg/min, and those weighing between 1000 g and 1500 g should not receive more than 8 mg/kg/min. Even with these low glucose loads, hyperglycemia could conceivably occur. After the infant has stabilized and is able to tolerate the initial infusion, the glucose load can be increased slowly with careful monitoring.

This can be accomplished either by advancing the concentration of the dextrose solution or by increasing the fluid volume. Most stable VLBW infants can tolerate daily increments in glucose load of approximately 1.5 to 2 mg/kg/minute, but individual infants demonstrate considerable variation in glucose tolerance. Dextrose infusion in larger LBW and full-term infants can usually be initiated at a rate of 7 to 8 mg/kg/minute and then rapidly increased to 12 to 14 mg/kg/minute without difficulty.[54] Maximum glucose load is determined primarily by the glucose tolerance of the individual infant. High glucose loads with low protein infusions should be avoided because of the risk of fatty infiltration of the liver.[56]

In some preterm infants, particularly those who are extremely immature or very ill, glucose intolerance may persist despite administration of conservative glucose loads. Serious problems can occur as a result of hyperglycemia and inadequate energy intake. Insulin therapy may be indicated if hyperglycemia persists. Continuous insulin infusion has been recommended,[59] but the efficacy is questionable and the actual amount delivered is unknown because of absorption of the insulin to plastic or glass surfaces.[60] In a recent review Pildes[60] recommended subcutaneous administration of insulin in a dose of 0.1 to 0.2 units/kg, given every 6 to 12 hours until glucose levels are stable. One or two doses of insulin are usually sufficient to correct the hyperglycemia. Serum glucose should be measured frequently to prevent hypoglycemia.[60]

Hypoglycemia may occur as a complication of insulin use. Under normal circumstances, it is a concern only when the glucose infusion declines precipitously, which may occur because of complications in delivery such as infiltration at the peripheral intravenous site. Rapid weaning from IV dextrose may also precipitate a hypoglycemic response if adequate energy is not provided by enteral feedings. The dextrose concentration can usually be decreased by 5 gm/100 ml decrements at 12-hour intervals without significant hypoglycemia (e.g., $D_{15}W$ to $D_{10}W$ to D_5W). When a decrease is ordered, serum glucose levels should be checked hourly for at least 3 hours, since rebound hypoglycemia usually occurs within that period.[54]

Dextrose solutions are notoriously hyperosmotic. Because of their high osmolarity, subcutaneous infusions of solutions exceeding 10% to 15% dextrose have a high incidence of skin sloughs. Therefore dextrose used in peripheral vein parenteral nutrition should not exceed this concentration. Although central vein parenteral nutrition concentrations greater than 25% dextrose can be used, concentrations above 25% are usually not necessary. Table 12-6 lists various dextrose concentrations, with their corresponding osmolarities and caloric densities. Since the osmolarity of human blood is approximately 300 mOsm/L, it is apparent that most dextrose solutions are comparatively hyperosmotic.

Protein. The first protein solutions available for IV use were hydrolysates of fibrin and casein. These products successfully supported positive nitrogen balance and growth in infants but were also characterized by certain problems. The protein hydrolysate solutions contained several amino acids as chloride salts. This contributed to the development of hyperchloremic metabolic acidosis in infants receiving parenteral nutrition. Furthermore, the amino acid composition of the protein

Table 12-6　Osmolarity and caloric density of dextrose solutions

Dextrose Solution	Calculated Osmolarity (mOsm/L)	kcal/ml
D_5W*	252	0.17
$D_{7.5}W$	378	0.25
$D_{10}W$	505	0.34
$D_{15}W$	758	0.51
$D_{20}W$	1010	0.68
$D_{25}W$	1263	0.85

*D_5W = 5% dextrose = 5 gm/100ml. Since hydrated dextrose provides 3.4 kcal/gm, 5 gm/100ml × 3.4 kcal/gm = 0.17 kcal/ml.

hydrolysate solutions was inconsistent.[61] During the process of hydrolysis, only about half of the whole proteins were broken down to free amino acids; the remaining nitrogen was present as peptides that were incompletely utilized.[62]

Protein hydrolysates have now largely been replaced by crystalline amino acid solutions. These solutions mimic the amino acid composition of naturally occurring proteins with high biological values, such as casein or egg albumin. Since the amino acid composition of these solutions is known, protein intake is more consistent when free amino acids are infused. Metabolic studies comparing crystalline amino acids and protein hydrolysates show better nitrogen utilization of the amino acid solutions.[63]

Several amino acid solutions are on the market; the products identified in Table 12-7 are among those frequently chosen for use in parenteral nutrition of LBW infants. These solutions were originally designed for use in adults, and although they are acceptable for LBW infants, they are not ideal. These products contain lesser amounts of certain amino acids than are theoretically required and may contain excessive quantities of others. Infusion of mixtures containing high amounts of glycine, for example, may result in plasma glycine levels approximately four times normal postprandial values.[64] Since glycine is a potent **neurotransmitter** inhibitor, hyperglycinemia may have adverse effects on the developing central nervous system. In addition, these products contain little tyrosine and cysteine; these amino acids may be required by premature neonates. In studies in which either cysteine or tyrosine was removed from the diets of premature infants, there was a decreased level of that amino acid in the infant's plasma, as well as impaired nitrogen retention and growth.[65] In the case of cysteine, this may be explained by the low hepatic cystathionase activity of immature infants, such that there is inadequate conversion of methionine to cysteine.[66]

Since taurine is synthesized from cysteine, it too may be required by premature infants. Although the role of taurine has not been fully elucidated, this sulfonic amino acid is involved in a number of physiological functions.[67] For example, taurine is important in neural transmission and in retinal, cardiac, and muscle function in laboratory animals and possibly in humans.[67] It is important to note, however, that although LBW infants may require cysteine, tyrosine, and taurine, many of these infants have received long-term parenteral nutrition with the amino acid preparations listed in Table 12-7 without evidence of nutrient deficiency.

Certain metabolic problems can occur in association with parenteral administration of amino acid solutions. Although preterm infants are at risk for developing metabolic acidosis for a number of reasons, one of these may be the excess quantity of cationic amino acids in most of the currently available amino acid solutions.[68] Metabolism of these positively charged amino acids can lead to production of

Table 12-7   Concentrations of amino acids adjusted to 2% solutions

Amino Acids	Solution (mg/100 ml)			
	Aminosyn	Travasol	Freamine II	Freamine III
Essential				
Leucine	188	124	181	181
Phenylalanine	88	124	113	113
Methionine	80	116	106	106
Lysine	144	116	205	205
Isoleucine	144	96	139	139
Valine	160	92	132	132
Histidine	60	88	56	56
Threonine	104	84	80	80
Tryptophan	32	36	31	31
Nonessential				
*Cysteine	—	—	<5	<5
*Tyrosine	18	8	—	—
*Taurine	—	—	—	—
Alanine	256	414	141	141
Arginine	196	207	73	191
Proline	171	84	224	224
Serine	84	—	118	118
Glycine	256	414	400	280
Glutamate	—	—	—	—

*May be essential for preterm infants.

hydrogen ions in excess of the buffering capacity of small, sick infants. Careful administration of an appropriate amount of protein and frequent monitoring of serum electrolytes and blood pH help to protect against the development of metabolic acidosis. Premature infants receiving crystalline amino acids are also at risk of developing hyperammonemia; this may be related to hepatic immaturity or to hepatic dysfunction that occurs as a result of hepatocellular damage.[69,70] Since the blood ammonia concentration is directly related to the amount of protein infused, protein intake should be reduced when blood ammonia levels are high.[68]

Azotemia, characterized by elevated blood urea nitrogen values, may also occur if the amount of protein delivered to an infant is excessive.

Plasma amino acid patterns reflect the amino acid composition of IV protein solutions.[71] Because the amino acid mixtures shown in Table 12-7 are not ideal, LBW infants receiving these solutions do not have normal plasma amino acid profiles.[72] Abnormal plasma aminograms may be etiologically related to the hepatic dysfunction mentioned earlier. Specific types of abnormal amino acid patterns and their potential consequences have been summarized by Kerner.[72]

Parenteral infusion of amino acid solutions has also been cited as one of the factors related to the development of neonatal cholestasis (prolonged conjugated **hyperbilirubinemia**). Several studies in animals indicate that parenteral infusion of certain amino acids may be related to the development of cholestasis.[73-76] The relationship between cholestasis and the use of total parenteral nutrition in neonates has been recognized since 1971,[77] and has been confirmed by several subsequent reports. The major factors identified with total parenteral nutrition–associated cholestasis are very low birth weight (less than 1500 gm) and the use of total parenteral nutrition for longer than 2 weeks.[78]

Cholestasis can occur, however, in infants who have not received total parenteral nutrition.[79] Studies have shown that factors other than amino acid infusion, duration of total parenteral nutrition, and birth weight are also related to the development of cholestasis. These other factors include the occurrence of severe hyaline membrane disease, hypotension (shock),[78] hypoxemia, prolonged ventilator assistance,[80] intracranial hemorrhage, **patent ductus arteriosus**, sepsis, and gastrointestinal conditions that require surgery.[81] For further information about the causes and consequences of neonatal cholestasis, see the recent reviews by Balistreri[82] and Merritt.[83]

Because there are several potentially serious problems or complications associated with the use of amino acid solutions in LBW infants, efforts are currently being made to develop new solutions. The goal in developing these new products is to design mixtures of amino acids that will more appropriately meet the specific nutrient needs of LBW infants without exceeding the physiologic and metabolic limitations of these immature babies.

Although the ideal reference for the composition of these new amino acid solutions is not yet known, the amino acid profile of human milk[84] and the minimum requirement of amino acids for preterm infants based on oral feeding studies[85,86] have been suggested as guidelines. The new solution has been specifically designed to maintain normal plasma amino acid concentrations in infants and children receiving parenteral nutrition. Normal plasma amino acid patterns were defined as those found in healthy, growing, breast-fed infants. Compared to the amino acid solutions shown in Table 12-7, Trophamine (Kendall McGaw Laboratories) contains more taurine, tyrosine (as N-acetyl-2-tyrosine), histidine, and the dicarboxylic amino acids and less phenylalanine, methionine, and glycine. Cysteine is added separately as cysteine HCl at the time of parenteral use (Table 12-8). In a recent clinical evaluation of LBW infants receiving trophamine, plasma concentrations of all amino acids except phenylalanine were within the 95% confidence limits of the plasma concentrations observed in LBW infants fed sufficient amounts of human milk to result in a rate of weight gain similar to the intrauterine rate.[87] These researchers expressed concern, however, that the LBW infant's ability to use N-acetyl-L-tyrosine and cysteine HCl may be even more limited than that of the full-term infant or older child.[87] Additional clinical evaluations are needed to further support the efficacy of this new amino acid solution for LBW infants. Researchers are expected to continue to test new products, such as Trophamine, and to develop other products that are also designed to meet the unique needs of the LBW infants.

The amount of protein delivered to an infant is determined by the protein load, which is a function of both the concentration of the amino acid solution and the rate at which it is administered. For example, if a 1.5% amino acid solution (e.g., 1.5 gm protein/100 ml) is infused at a rate of 120 mg/kg/day, the infant actually receives 1.8 gm protein/kg/day. Although the initiation and advancement of protein in parenteral nutrition varies with individual circumstances, protein is usually added to the IV solution in the first 2 to 5 days

Table 12-8 Concentrations of amino acids in Trophamine adjusted to a 2% solution

Amino Acid	Concentration in Trophamine Solution (mg/100 ml)
Essential	
Leucine	280
Phenylalanine	97
Methionine	67
Lysine	163
Isoleucine	163
Valine	157
Histidine	97
Threonine	83
Tryptophan	40
Nonessential	
*Cysteine	< 0.7†
*Tyrosine	46 ‡
*Taurine	0.5
Alanine	107
Arginine	243
Proline	137
Serine	77
Glycine	—
Glutamate	100

*May be essential for preterm infants.
†Additional cysteine is added separately as cysteine HCl.
‡Primarily in the form of N-acetyl-L-tyrosine.

of life and is increased every other day or as tolerated. Factors such as glucose tolerance, venous access, and medical condition many influence the decision to start or to advance protein intake. Kerner[72] recommends an initial protein load of 0.5 to 1 gm/kg/day. This may be gradually increased to a maximum of 2 to 2.5 gm/kg/day. Under normal circumstances and with adequate caloric intake, LBW infants achieve positive nitrogen balance at protein levels of 2 to 2.5 gm/kg/day.[88] Provision of protein in excess of actual requirements is discour-

aged, as the additional protein offers no apparent advantage and greatly increases the risk of metabolic complications.[54] Older infants and children may tolerate somewhat higher intakes of protein, but most investigators agree that more than 3 gm/kg/day is not necessary.

Lipid

The first IV fat emulsion (Lipomul) was removed from the market in 1965 because of its association with a "fat-overloading syndrome." There was no IV replacement until 1975 when Intralipid (Kabi-Vitrum Laboratories) was approved for use in the United States. Later, two additional fat emulsions became available for IV use: Liposyn II (Abbott Laboratories) and Travamulsion (Travenol Laboratories). The fat-overloading syndrome has not been associated with any of these newer products.[89]

The composition of these intravenous fat emulsions is shown in Table 12-9. Although Liposyn (Abbott Laboratories) was previously based on safflower oil instead of soybean oil, it was reformulated in 1985 to contain 5% of each of these oils. Concerns about linolenic acid sufficiency[90] and triglyceride clearance[91] using the old Liposyn product should therefore no longer be relevant. All three products now contain adequate amounts of both linoleic and linolenic acid to meet the essential fatty acid needs of LBW infants.

The emulsified fat particles of IV fat emulsions are cleared from the bloodstream in a manner similar to chylomicron metabolism. As summarized by Gryboski and Walker,[26] the enzyme lipoprotein lipase hydrolyzes the IV lipid to free fatty acids. These free fatty acids either circulate, bound to albumin, and are used as an energy source or are reesterified to triglycerides and stored in adipose tissue. If the rate of IV fat administration exceeds the infant's ability to clear the free fatty acids and triglycerides adequately from the bloodstream, hyperlipidemia occurs. Elevated triglyc-

Table 12-9   Ten percent intravenous fat emulsions

	Intralipid	Liposyn II	Travamulsion
Base	Soybean oil	Safflower oil and soybean oil	Soybean oil
Fatty acids			
Linoleic	54%	66%	56%
Oleic	26%	18%	23%
Palmitic	9%	9%	11%
Linolenic	8%	4.2%	6%
Glycerin	2.25%	2.5%	2.25%
Egg phospholipids (emulsifier)	1.2%	1.2%	1.2%
Osmolarity	280 mOsm/L	320 mOsm/L	270 mOsm/L
Caloric value	1.1 cal/ml	1.1 cal/ml	1.1 cal/ml

eride and free fatty acid levels may cause visible lactescence. Although the ability of newborn infants to clear lipid is variable,[92] most infants born at term have clearance rates similar to those of adults.[88] Premature infants, however, often experience impaired lipid tolerance.[89] Infants at particular risk for hyperlipidemia include those who are very premature (less than 32 weeks of gestation), born weighing less than 1500 gm, small for gestational age, septic or acutely ill, or nutritionally depleted.[89] Intravenous fat emulsions can usually be given to these infants by the end of the first week of life, but cautious advancement and careful monitoring are required. The maximum lipid load for infants less than 32 weeks of gestation should not exceed 2 gm/kg/day because of impaired lipid clearance from the circulation and risk of hyperlipidemia.[93]

Since 1980 there has been increasing interest in the use of **heparin** to improve the lipid clearance of LBW infants receiving intravenous fat emulsions. Heparin stimulates the release of the enzymes lipoprotein lipase and hepatic lipase into the circulation and therefore stimulates intravascular lipolysis of fat. Studies have shown that intravenously infused lipids are cleared from the circulation more efficiently when heparin is used.[93-96] Continuous infusions of low heparin doses are preferred over bolus doses of larger amounts of heparin.[96] Although studies have demonstrated an increase in serum-free fatty acid concentrations in response to heparin administration,[94-97] other studies did not report adverse effects on bilirubin binding to albumin.[96] More studies are needed to determine the clinical risks and benefits of heparin use in LBW infants before routine recommendations can be made.

The impaired lipid tolerance characteristic of many LBW infants may be related in part to a lack of exogenous carnitine. Carnitine facilitates the mechanism by which fatty acids are converted to acyl-carnitine derivatives to permit transport across the mitochondrial membrane. Once inside the mitochondria, β-oxidation of the fatty acids can occur. There is no carnitine in any of the solutions currently used in total parenteral nutrition regimens. Plasma levels and urinary excretion of carnitine rapidly decrease in premature newborns if exogenous carnitine is not given[98,99] (e.g., no human milk or cow's milk-base formula). Results of studies of newborn[100,101] and preterm[102] infants receiving short-term total parenteral nutrition with carnitine supplementation show an increase in fatty acid oxidation and ketogenesis. The effect of carnitine supplementation in preterm infants receiving long-term total parenteral nutrition is not yet known. However, one recent study did show enhanced lipid utilization in preterm infants receiving oral L-carnitine during long-term parenteral nutrition.[103] Further studies are needed before a specific need for exogenous carnitine in preterm infants receiving total parenteral nutrition can be established.

One important reason for administering IV fat emulsions to LBW infants is to provide energy in a concentrated form. The caloric density (1.1 kcal/ml) of the 10% emulsions allows a substantial number of calories to be delivered with only a moderate increase in fluid volume. Intralipid and Liposyn II are also available as 20% solutions (2 kcal/ml), but use of these concentrated products should be limited to infants who are severely fluid restricted.[84] The low osmolarities of these preparations (shown in Table 12-9) make it possible, in some cases, to deliver sufficient calories for growth by a peripheral route rather than obligating a central mode of delivery.

Another significant reason for IV fat administration is to prevent essential fatty acid deficiency. The essential fatty acid needs of humans are usually expressed as the requirement for linoleic acid. Daily requirements are estimated to be 1% to 2% of total calories.[104] For example infants receiving Intralipid, which contains 54% linoleic acid, require about 2% to 4% of total calories as Intralipid. Premature infants who do not receive exogenous fat can quickly develop essential fatty acid deficiency. Biochemical evidence of essential fatty acid deficiency has been noted in neonates as early as 2 days after initiation of fat-free total parenteral nutrition;[105] clinical signs of the deficiency do not appear until somewhat later. Risk of essential fatty acid deficiency is higher in more immature infants, and the degree of essential fatty acid deficiency increases with

the duration of fat-free parenteral nutrition.[106] Under normal circumstances, LBW infants should receive 0.5 to 1 gm/kg/day of an IV fat emulsion as early as possible, at least by the end of their first week of life, to avoid essential fatty acid deficiency.[104]

Attempts to meet essential fatty acid needs by infusion of plasma[105] or by cutaneous application of oils rich in polyunsaturated fatty acids[108] are probably not effective.

Intravenous fat emulsions can be administered separately by peripheral vein, or they can be infused along side the hyperalimentation solution through a Y or a T connector placed close to the peripheral or central vein infusion site.[109] Under no circumstances should other solutions or medications be mixed with the IV fat, since this results in instability of the fat droplets. Generally, these products should be infused over 24 hours,[110] and the rate of infusion should not exceed 0.15[111] to 0.25[110] gm/kg/hour.

Some nurseries recommend that a dose of IV fat be given to check for allergic reactions, fever, and the like.[89] However, **hypersensitivity** reactions are rare in pediatric patients, and this testing is usually unnecessary.[109] In general, 0.5 to 1 gm/kg/day may be used as an initial load for LBW infants and may be increased as tolerated by 0.25 to 0.5 mg/kg/day to a maximum of 2 to 3 gm/kg/day.[110] The lipid load should not exceed 40% to 50% of the total calories. Rate of advancement and maximal total dose are determined by the infant's ability to metabolize the IV lipid preparation. Tolerance should be monitored by periodic measurements of serum triglyceride and free fatty acid levels.[112] If these levels are elevated, the IV fat load should be adjusted accordingly. In particular, serum triglyceride levels should be kept below 150 mg/100 ml.[110]

It is important that hyperlipidemia be prevented or rapidly ameliorated in LBW infants receiving IV fat emulsions. If allowed to persist, the elevated blood lipids may provoke complications: displacement of albumin-bound bilirubin by plasma free fatty acids, and alteration of pulmonary function.[113] Recent studies indicate that macrophage, leukocyte, and macrocyte function are not impaired by use of an appropriate amount of IV fat in LBW infants.[114-116]

Free fatty acids released during the hydrolysis of IV fat emulsions can compete with bilirubin for albumin binding sites. If bilirubin is displaced, the increase in free or unbound bilirubin can potentiate the risk of kernicterus. In practice, this is an uncommon problem if IV fat administration is started during the second week of life (when the bilirubin level is less than half the potential exchange level for the individual infant) and if the lipid is infused slowly over 24 hours. In a study at Stanford University where these conditions were applied to 29 premature infants, the fatty acid/serum albumin molar ratio was well below 6.0,[118] which is considered to be the safe limit for LBW neonates.[119]

Hyperlipidemia resulting from the infusion of IV fat emulsions has been reported to affect pulmonary function. There have been several reports of fat accumulation in the pulmonary microcirculation of infants who receive IV fat emulsions.[120-122] The significance of these accumulations has been questioned because pulmonary fat deposition can also occur in infants who receive no IV fat and because no adverse clinical effects have been reported. Intravenous fat infusion has also been associated with hypoxemia in infants; decreased arterial oxygen tension (PaO_2) occurs in preterm infants and seems to be related to increased serum triglyceride concentrations.[123] However, a recent study reported no detrimental effects on oxygenation in preterm infants with severe respiratory distress syndrome provided the IV fat load did not exceed 0.5 to 1 gm/kg/day (the dosage needed to prevent essential fatty acid deficiency).[124] Increased pulmonary vascular resistance has also been reported in LBW infants receiving IV fat, but the clinical significance of this is not yet clear.[125]

Although the association between lipid infusion and pulmonary changes is important to consider, it should not prohibit the use of IV fat emulsions in LBW infants with respiratory disease. Cautious use of IV fats in amounts needed to meet essential fatty acid requirements are usually appropriate. Prevention of essential fatty acid deficiency may be particularly important for infants with respiratory disease. An association between essential fatty acid deficiency and altered fatty acid composition of pulmonary surfactant phospholipids has been reported, suggesting that this alteration may diminish lung function and contribute to the pathophysiology of respiratory distress syndrome.[126]

There is also some indication that IV fat, in addition to dextrose solutions, may benefit the infant with respiratory disease. Parenteral nutrition regimens that include half the nonprotein calories as fat have lower carbon dioxide production and minute ventilation compared with regimens in which dextrose alone is the nonprotein calorie source.[127] High glucose loads may aggravate ventilator weaning or precipitate pulmonary failure.[128]

Carbohydrate loads that are proportionately high compared with poor intakes of fat and protein are also associated with fatty infiltration of the liver.[89] This kwashiorkor-like picture improves when fat is included in the diet. In a study of total parenteral nutrition in protein-depleted rats, fatty infiltration of the liver was avoided when a regimen of 75% carbohydrate and 25% fat was used.[129]

Electrolytes. Sodium, potassium, and chloride are supplied by total parenteral nutrition solutions; the usual requirements for these elements are listed in Table 12-10. Actual requirements, however, are variable depending on such factors as clinical status, renal function, state of hydration, and the use of diuretics.[130] Very immature infants may be limited in their ability to conserve sodium and may require up to 9 mEq/kg/day to maintain a nor-

Table 12-10 Recommended daily intakes of electrolytes for parenteral nutrition solutions

Element	Daily Amount
Sodium	2-4 mEq/kg
Potassium	2-3 mEq/kg
Chloride	2-3 mEq/kg

From Poole, R.L.: Electrolyte and mineral requirements. In Kerner, J.A., Jr., editor: Manual of pediatric parenteral nutrition. Copyright © 1983, John Wiley & Sons, Inc., New York.

mal serum sodium concentration (135 to 140 mEq/L).[131] Although 2 to 3 mEq/kg/day is the usual amount of potassium needed to maintain a normal serum level (3.5 to 5 mEq/L),[130] occasionally VLBW infants require as much as 8 to 10 mEq/kg/day of potassium.[132] Excess chloride intake is more common than inadequate intake; hyperchloremia in infants is manifested as metabolic acidosis. The incidence of this acidosis can be decreased by altering the amounts of chloride salts in parenteral nutrition solutions; for example, sodium and potassium can be supplied as acetate or phosphate salts, rather than exclusively as chloride salts.[130] Serum electrolyte levels should be routinely monitored; they are checked initially on a daily basis and later two or three times per week. Urine sodium and specific gravity may be helpful tests if there is a serum abnormality.[41]

Minerals. The recommended magnesium intake for an LBW infant on a parenteral nutrition regimen is 0.25 to 0.5 mEq/kg/day at some centers,[130] and 0.5 to 1 mEq/kg/day at others. Although most infants are able to maintain homeostasis at this level of intake, some infants who have problems such as impaired renal function, inflammatory bowel disease, or losses related to diuretic use may have increased magnesium needs.[130]

Calcium and phosphorus are important components of pediatric parenteral nutrition regimens. Low intake of calcium and phosphorus by LBW infants receiving total parenteral nutrition can result in poor bone mineralization.[135] Several cases of rickets have been reported in premature infants receiving total parenteral nutrition.[134-135] Rickets is most likely to occur in infants who are born very prematurely and receive total parenteral nutrition for extended periods. Immature infants who receive only about 2 mEq of calcium/kg/day for 2 weeks or more should be regarded as at risk for **osteopenia** of prematurity and should be monitored accordingly. The concentrations of calcium and phosphorus in the parenteral infusate may need to be cautiously increased to maintain mineral homeostasis.

Calcium and phosphorus should be added to the parenteral nutrition solutions of LBW infants on an ongoing basis; they should not be discontinued simply because serum calcium levels are normal. Serum calcium levels can be maintained in a normal range at the expense of bone demineralization. Also, these levels can be normal or even high when hypophosphatemia is present. It is generally recommended that premature infants receiving total parenteral nutrition be followed for the development of osteopenia or rickets by monitoring serum calcium, phosphorus, and alkaline phosphatase levels, as well as by radiographical bone studies.

Although recommendations for parenteral calcium and phosphorus for full-term infants vary from 0.5 to 1.5 mEq of calcium/kg/day, and 0.5 to 2 mmol of phosphorus/kg/day,[130] most preterm infants have higher calcium and phosphorus needs. During the final weeks of gestation, the fetus normally receives 120 to 160 mg/kg/day of elemental calcium by means of active transport mechanisms across the placenta.[111] Phosphorus is delivered in the fetus in approximately a 2:1 ratio of calcium to phosphorus. Since 1 mEq of calcium is equivalent to about 20 mg of elemental calcium, it is apparent that premature infants on typical parenteral nutrition regimens containing about 2 mEq of calcium/kg/day receive less than one third of the amount of calcium that would have been received in utero.

Hypercalciuria is a common occurrence in preterm infants receiving typical parenteral nutrition regimens.[137] Increased IV phosphorus intake has been shown to decrease this calciuria in preterm infants on total parenteral nutrition.[138] In addition, by correcting the hypophosphatemia in these infants, the renal filtration load could have decreased with the improved incorporation of calcium in bone.[138]

In the past, it was difficult to add enough IV calcium and phosphorus to the parenteral solution to approach intrauterine accretion rates without precipitation of the minerals.[133] However, studies have now shown that the concentrations of calcium and phosphorus can be increased without precipitation by favorably altering certain properties of the hyperalimentation solution (i.e., pH, temperature, amino acid product and concentration, type of calcium salt, dextrose concentration, and the order in which calcium and phosphate are added to the solution).[139-142] Although alternating 12-hour infusions of high-calcium and high-phosphorus solutions has been suggested as a means of administering increased minerals without coprecipitation,[143] recent studies have shown that this practice is inappropriate.[138,144-145]

One study has shown that up to 120 mg of calcium/kg/day and 55 mg of phosphate/kg/day can be successfully delivered by selected parenteral nutrition solutions.[139] Although this may be possible for some premature infants, the concentrations of calcium and phosphorus needed to achieve such intakes by VLBW infants who are fluid restricted may exceed the limit of solubility for these minerals.[140] In a more recent study in which infants received 60 mg of calcium/100 ml and 46.5 mg of phosphorus/100 ml in parenteral nutrition solutions,

minimal stress to calcium and phosphorus homeostatic mechanisms was reported without increasing urinary calcium excretion.[145]

Vitamins. Multivitamin preparations for IV administration are essential for use in total parenteral nutrition therapy.[146] They are required for the prevention of vitamin deficiency states, for maintenance of good nutritional status, and in some cases, for rehabilitation of patients with vitamin depletion. Although IV vitamin administration is clearly necessary, the specific requirements for vitamins in total parenteral nutrition are not well known. Because precise data describing IV vitamin needs of preterm infants are not yet available, the Recommended Dietary Allowances (which provide reference ranges for vitamin intake for healthy, full-term infants who are enterally fed) are currently used as general guidelines. It is likely, however, that premature infants have higher needs for some vitamins because they have smaller body stores, greater losses, and higher intrinsic needs than full-term infants. Furthermore, the parenteral vitamin needs of LBW infants are probably different from their enteral requirements.

Kerner[147] has summarized several reasons why parenteral vitamin requirements might differ from oral recommendations. First, there are potential interactions between vitamins in multivitamin preparations or between vitamins and the amino acid or dextrose components of hyperalimentation solutions that may alter the effectiveness of specific vitamins.[142,147] Second, parenteral nutrients are generally infused from plastic or glass containers containing room air; thus vitamins may adhere to tubing and containers or may be subject to oxidative destruction.[122,147-149] Other factors that might affect parenteral vitamin requirements include degradation of vitamins secondary to phototherapy or sunlight exposure,[150] increased urinary excretion,[151] underlying disease states,[147] and impaired synthesis, activation, or storage of vitamins related to bypassing the enteric canal.[147]

At present the multivitamin preparation approved for IV use in infants and children in the United States is MVI-Pediatric (Armour Pharmaceutical Company). Table 12-11 shows the vitamin content of MVI-Pediatric compared to the recommendations of the Nutrition Advisory Group of the American Medical Association[152] for children under 11 years of age. According to the current MVI-Pediatric package insert, the daily dose for infants weighing less than 1 kg should not exceed 30% of the contents of one vial. The recommended daily dose for infants weighing 1.0 to 3.0 kg is 65% of the contents of one vial. Infants and children weighing 3 kg or more and up to 11 years of age can usually receive the full contents of one vial unless clinical or laboratory studies indicates the need for increasing or decreasing the dosage. Several recent studies have evaluated the use of MVI-

Pediatric in preterm infants receiving parenteral nutrition.[153-155] The importance of limiting the percentage of the vial given to LBW infants has been well documented.[153-156]

Additional research is needed to clarify the specific vitamin requirements of LBW infants receiving parenteral nutrition and to continue to improve our ability to meet those requirements. Low blood levels of retinol have recently been reported in VLBW infants receiving parenteral nutrition.[157] This may be related to losses resulting from light exposure or adherence to plastic infusion sets.[157] Controversy currently exists regarding the appropriate means of meeting the vitamin E requirements of LBW infants without causing either decreased or elevated levels of vitamin E in serum.[156-158] Johnson and co-workers[159] have recommended that serum levels of vitamin E in VLBW infants be kept between 1 to 3 mg/100 ml to prevent clinical consequences of prolonged serum elevations of vitamin E. Consequences of prolonged vita-

Table 12-11   Vitamin content of MVI-Pediatric* compared with the AMA/NAG Recommendations for children under 11 years of age

Vitamin	AMA/NAG Recommendations[152]	MVI-Pediatric (per 5 ml)
A (IU)	2,300.0	2,300.0
D (IU)	400.0	400.0
E (IU)	7.0	7.0
K (μg)	200.0	0.2
C (μmg)	80.0	80.0
Thiamine (mg)	1.2	1.2
Riboflavin (mg)	1.4	1.4
Pyridoxine (mg)	1.0	1.0
Niacin (mg)	17.0	17.0
Pantothenic acid (mg)	5.0	5.0
Folic acid (μg)	140.0	140.0
B_{12} (μg)	1.0	1.0
Biotin (μg)	20.0	20.0

*Product Information, Armour Pharmaceutical Company, Kankakee, Ill., 1985.

min E deficiency have also been reported. Several recent studies have documented a relationship between vitamin E deficiency and neurologic abnormalities in infants and children with chronic cholestasis.[160,161]

Trace elements. LBW infants receiving total parenteral nutrition require the addition of trace elements to their hyperalimentation solutions. The small quantities of trace elements that are present as contaminants in hyperalimentation solutions or as normal components of blood products (which infants may receive as a result of the need for transfusions) cannot be depended on to meet trace element needs. Premature infants are at particular risk for development of trace element deficiency states because of low body stores, increased losses, and increased requirements for growth.[162]

Although further research is needed to establish precise requirements of all trace elements in total parenteral nutrition, the recommendations of an expert panel of the American Medical Association[163] are used as guidelines (Table 12-12). Larger quantities of certain trace elements may be required in some cases. For example, one study showed that preterm infants receiving parenteral nutrition needed intakes of 438 μg zinc/kg/day and 63 μg of copper/kg/day to achieve intrauterine accumulation rates.[164] These dosages are significantly higher than the AMA recommendations shown in Table 12-12. Furthermore, the main route for zinc loss in infants fed intravenously is via the kidneys.[164] The extent of these losses appears to depend largely on the particular amino acid solution used in the parenteral infusate.[165]

In contrast to zinc, loss of copper by parenterally fed infants is relatively low.[164] Concern exists about the potential hepatotoxicity of copper when administered intravenously.[165] Infants in whom liver function or bile excretion is compromised (e.g., those with cholestasis) should receive reduced or intermittent copper supplementation.[165]

Very little data currently exist regarding the parenteral requirements of the preterm infant for chromium and manganese. A recent review by Casey and Hambidge supported the IV guidelines shown in Table 12-12.[165] There is increasing evidence that selenium should also be added to hyperalimentation fluids. Selenium concentrations in blood fall rapidly when infants receive total parenteral nutrition without added selenium.[166] For this reason, and because preterm infants are particularly vulnerable to oxidative stressors, it has been recommended that selenium be supplied intravenously to the preterm infant at a rate of 1 to 2 μg/kg/day from the initiation of total parenteral nutrition. Although infants receiving parenteral nutrition originally for short periods of time may not require additional iodine, infants receiving long-term total parenteral nutrition may need supplemental iodine. Thyroid func-

Table 12-12 Suggested daily intake of essential trace elements

Trace Element	Daily Amount* (μg/kg)
Zinc	300†
	100‡
Copper	20
Chromium	0.14-0.2
Manganese	2-10

From Nutrition Advisory Group of the American Medical Association, Department of foods and Nutrition: JAMA 241:2051, 1979. Copyright 1979, American Medical Association.
*Limited data are avaiable for infants weighing less than 1500 gm. Their requirements may be higher because of low body stores and increased requirements for growth.
†Premature infants up to 3000 gm body weight. Thereafter, the recommendations for full-term infants apply.
‡Full-term infants and children up to 5 years old.

tion should be monitored and, if necessary, 1 μg/kg/day can be added to the hyperalimentation fluids.[165]

The iron requirements of preterm and full-term infants are discussed on pp. 45–46. It is not common to add iron to total parenteral nutrition solutions because allergic reactions may occur and because of reports of incompatibility between iron-dextran preparations and hyperalimentation solutions.[162] However, recent reports have shown that iron can be both safely and effectively added to hyperalimentation solutions.[167] Although effective, this practice should be limited to situations in which IV iron is clearly needed. Intravenous administration of iron may be indicated for LBW infants who have inadequate muscle mass for intramuscular injection and who require 2 or more months of total parenteral nutrition.

CASE 1

A 26-week-gestation infant weighing 750 gm at birth was admitted to a neonatal intensive care unit shortly after birth. The baby developed severe hyaline membrane disease and required assisted ventilation with oxygen needs of 85% to 90%. An umbilical arterial catheter was placed to aid in ventilatory management; fluid, glucose, and electrolytes were also infused through this line. The initial solution contained 10% dextrose; this was started at a range of 70 ml/kg/day and was increased to 12.5% dextrose at a rate of 110 ml/kg/day by day 3 of life. Dextrostix measurements simultaneously increased from 60 to 80 mg/100 ml to 180 to 240 mg/100 ml; serum glucose measurements confirmed hyperglycemia. The dextrose infusion was subsequently reduced to 9% dextrose at a rate of 100 ml/kg/day. Blood sugar levels normalized, and the glucose load was then gradually increased without further difficulty. Because the serious nature of the infant's medical condition prohibited the introduction of enteral feedings in the first week of life and because metabolic reserves were presumed to be meager, parenteral nutrition was started on day 3 of life. At this time, the infant had lost 60 gm and

weighed 9% less than birth weight. The initial hyperalimentation order included (1) rate: IV + hyperalimentation = 4.2 ml/hour (IV at keep-open rate of 1.5 ml/hour and hyperalimentation at rate of 2.7 ml/hour), (2) 8% dextrose, and (3) amino acid: 0.5 gm/kg/day. All electrolytes, minerals, and trace elements were added to the 250 ml bottle in quantities that provided appropriate amounts to be delivered in 96 ml/kg/day of hyperalimentation solution. Intralipid was ordered on day 7 of life at an initial load of 0.5 gm/kg/day. Tolerance to all components of the hyperalimentation solution was routinely monitored as intake was advanced.

TRANSITION FROM PARENTERAL TO ENTERAL NUTRITION

The transition from total parenteral to enteral nutrition should occur slowly. Infants who receive total parenteral nutrition have a relatively low digestive mass and delayed gastrointestinal growth compared with infants who receive enteral stimuli.[168] These effects are more pronounced in infants who receive total parenteral nutrition for prolonged periods of time. Studies in animals and humans have documented pancreatic hyposecretion, intestinal mucosal atrophy, and decreased parietal cell mass during total parenteral nutrition.[169,170] These effects are reversible on resumption of enteral feedings. Advancement of enteral feedings should, however, be gradual to allow time for adaptive increases in enzymes involved in digestion and metabolism and for establishment of mechanisms necessary for absorption of nutrients.[171,172]

It is desirable to initiate enteral feedings in LBW infants as early as possible. Even in small amounts, these feedings act to stimulate gastrointestinal enzymatic development and activity, promote bile flow, and increase small intestinal villous growth.[173] Infants who are not ready for advancement of enteral feeding but could tolerate a very small, constant amount of an appropriate type of milk benefit from this gastrointestinal stimulation. Later transition from parenteral to enteral nutrition may also be easier for these infants.

Preterm infants have poor gastrointestinal motility as a result of motor immaturity of the gastrointestinal tract. For this reason, most preterm infants are more likely to tolerate initial enteral feedings when small volumes are given. Specific guidelines for initiation and advancement of enteral feedings are given on pp. 336–339.

When making the transition from parenteral to enteral nutrition, it is important to adjust both sources of nutrition so the infant's net intake of fluid and specific nutrients remains appropriate. In general, this is accomplished by slowly increasing the volume of the enteral feeding as tolerated while decreasing the volume of the parenteral infusate. Most clinically stable, growing preterm infants benefit from maintaining a total fluid intake of about 150 to 160 ml/kg/day, a total energy intake of about 120 to 130 kcal/kg/day, and a total IV plus oral protein intake of about 3 gm/kg/day.[107] It is usually appropriate to decrease or to discontinue administration of IV fat emulsions when approximately half of the infant's total intake is derived from an appropriate milk source. At this point the amount of fat contained in that volume of milk is sufficient to meet the infant's requirements for essential fatty acids. Continuing to give 2 to 3 gm IV fat/kg/day in addition to milk that contains about 50% of its total calories from fat may cause the infant's net fat intake to exceed 60% of total calories. Once the infant is tolerating more than 75% of total feedings from an enteral source, it is usually appropriate to discontinue the parenteral infusate and substitute IV dextrose until complete volume and nutrient needs can be provided by the enteral route.

CASE 2

An infant born at 28 weeks of gestation developed necrotizing enterocolitis during his fourth week of life. The necrotic damage to the small intestine necessitated surgical removal of 30 cm of bowel, encompassing the distal ileum and the ileocecal valve. After 8 days of total parenteral nutrition, it was decided that enteral feedings could be introduced and cautiously advanced. An elemental formula (e.g., Pregestimil) was chosen to facilitate digestion and absorption of nutrients. The initial volume was 1 ml/hour fed by oral gastric gavage on a continuous drip schedule; this provided 25 ml/kg/day, given a body weight of 960 gm. The composition and infusion rate of the parenteral nutrients remained unchanged until day 3 of enteral feedings when the oral volume was increased to 2 ml/hour. At this point, the volume of the parenteral infusate was decreased to provide a total daily volume of 150 to 160 ml/kg/day. The concentrations of parenteral nutrients were adjusted to meet the goals of the nutritional therapy (e.g., to provide 2.5 to 3 gm protein/kg/day and at least 90 kcal/kg/day). Enteral volume was slowly increased in small amounts to allow time for morphological and functional adaptation of the remaining small bowel and to guard against the volume-induced dumping syndrome. Full enteral volume was not achieved until 28 days after the reintroduction of enteral feeds; at this time the infant weighed 1150 gm and was able to tolerate a continuous orogastric infusion of 8 ml/hour.

ENTERAL NUTRITION

Nutrient Requirements

Essential nutrients should be supplied to LBW infants in quantities sufficient to maintain homeostasis without unnecessary weight loss or tissue catabolism and yet not excessively to avoid potential toxicity and superfluous fat deposition. The exact quantities of nutrients required to meet these goals are still being defined. In general, the nutrient requirements of premature infants are higher than those of full-term babies because of low nutrient stores as a result of shortened gestation, decreased retention and utilization of nutrients related to physiological and metabolic limitations, and increased needs associated with stress, illness, and use of certain medications. In addition, a greater portion of the total nutrient intake of preterm infants is needed for synthesis of new tissue and for more rapid growth.[174] The most recent statement of the American Academy of Pediatrics, Committee on Nutrition,[175] provides an excellent summary of the enteral nutrient requirements of LBW infants.

Energy. Sinclair and others[28] have estimated that 75 kcal/kg/day are required to meet maintenance energy needs, compared with 120 kcal/kg/day to provide adequate energy for growth as shown in Table 12-13. However, energy needs may be increased by stress and rapid growth or decreased in a neutral thermal environment and when absorptive loss is eliminated with parenteral nutrition. To estimate the energy needs of individual infants, it is important to consider the dynamic biological and environmental factors that alter their needs (Table 12-14). To evaluate the accuracy of the

Table 12-13   Energy requirements of low birth weight infants

	kcal/kg/day
Basal metabolic rate	50
Activity	15
Cold stress	10
TOTAL MAINTENANCE	75
Specific dynamic action	8
Fecal loss	12
Growth	25
TOTAL ADDITIONAL REQUIREMENTS	45
TOTAL ENERGY NEEDS FOR GROWTH	120

From Sinclair, J., and others: Pediatr. Clin. North Am. 17:863, 1970.

Table 12-14   Factors to consider in estimating the energy requirements of LBW infants

Factor	Comment
Weight	Small babies may have: High absorptive losses High heat losses caused by a lack of subcutaneous fat insulation and a large body surface area
Classification	Small for gestational age infants often have: High basal metabolic rate Rapid growth rate
Postnatal age	Energy requirements may diminish with increasing postnatal age.
Physiological stress	Infants who experience: Hypermetabolic states (e.g. fever) Malabsorptive problems (e.g., short bowel syndrome) Labored breathing (e.g., chronic lung disease) will have increased energy needs.
Environmental stress	Circumstances that increase: Fluid losses (e.g., radiant warmers) Energy expenditure (temperature instability) will also increase energy needs.
Type of feeding	Enterally fed babies require more calories for growth than parenterally fed infants Inappropriate selection of a formula can increase absorptive loss.
Method of feeding	Some LBW infants expend more energy while learning to nipple feed.
Growth	Energy intake must be increased to support rapid catch-up growth and new tissue synthesis.

estimate, it is important to consider the infants' growth progress in relation to their average energy intakes. Some premature infants may require at least 130 to 150 kcal/kg/day to sustain an appropriate rate of growth, especially during their catch-up growth phase (p. 25). To achieve these caloric intakes in babies with limited capacities to tolerate large fluid volumes, it may be necessary to concentrate the feedings to provide more than 20 kcal/oz.

Protein. Gastric, pancreatic, and intestinal enzymes responsible for protein hydrolysis are present in neonates, including premature babies.[176] Active transport of amino acids in the small intestine of the infant is not well understood, but because there is active transport in fetal life, such mechanisms are presumed to be well developed.[176] Feeding studies corroborate the biochemical finding that neonates can digest and absorb an adequate quantity of dietary protein.[177]

Although much attention has been directed toward determining the protein requirement of LBW infants, this is still a controversial subject. At the core of the controversy are basic questions concerning optimal postnatal growth and tissue composition changes of premature babies. Answers to these questions and data from direct clinical investigations are needed to establish precise protein requirements.

One approach to estimating the protein needs of preterm infants considers the goal to be the intrauterine rate of protein accumulation.[7] A reference fetus model is used to determine the amount of protein that would need to be ingested to match the quantity of protein that is deposited into newly formed fetal tissue.[136,178] To achieve these fetal accretion rates, additional protein must be supplied to compensate for intestinal losses and obligatory losses in urine and skin. Table 12-15 shows the advisable intakes for protein using this factorial method. Obviously, the advisable protein intake for enterally fed infants (3.5 to 4 gm/kg/day) exceeds the recommendation for parenterally fed babies (2 to 2.5 gm/kg/day).

Although 3.5 to 4 gm/kg/day of protein is apparently well tolerated by stable infants who are growing rapidly, there are no clinical data to prove that this much protein is needed. In fact, this quantity may exceed the metabolic capacity of very immature babies or may stress the sick infant.

Another approach to estimating the protein needs of preterm infants considers the effect that the quality or type of protein fed may have on the quantitative requirement. Whey-predominant proteins of high biological value for the preterm infant (e.g., human milk protein) support sustained growth in quantities less than advisable intake estimates.[179] LBW infants who ingest adequate calories and whey-predominant protein at 2.25 gm/kg/day show steady gains in weight and length,[180] although their rate of growth may be slow compared with intrauterine growth curves.[181] It can be argued that a slower rate of growth is normal for many preterm infants living in an extrauterine environment.

Several studies have shown that premature infants tolerate whey better than casein. Premature babies fed whey-predominant proteins experience less metabolic acidosis and have more normal plasma amino acid patterns than those fed casein-predominant proteins.[180,182–184] Whey protein is also more soluble in gastric acid secretions and may be more easily digested by the premature infant. Avoiding gastric curd formation probably averts the potential for lactobezoar development.[185] Furthermore, the amino acid composition of whey protein differs from that of casein and may be more appropriate for the premature infant. The premature infant has a limited ability to convert methionine to cystine as a result of little or no activity of the enzyme cystathionase. Whey protein contains more cystine and less methionine than does casein and may be more suitable for the immature baby during the first weeks of life. Because of the preference by preterm infants for whey protein, more whey (in the form of β-lactaglobulin) has

Table 12-15 Estimated requirements and advisable intakes for protein (grams) as derived by the factorial method

Body Weight of Infant	Tissue Increment Per Day	Dermal Loss Per Day	Urine Loss Per Day	Intestinal Absorption (% Intake)	Estimated Requirement Per Day (gm)	Advisable Intake		
						Per Day (gm)	Per kg* (gm)	Per 100 kcal†(gm)
800-1200 gm	2.32	0.17	0.68	87†	3.64	4.0	4.0	3.1
1200-1800 gm	3.01	0.25	0.90	87	4.78	5.2	3.5	2.7

From Ziegler, E.E., Biga, R.L., and Fomon, S.J.: Nutritional requirements of the premature infant. In Suskind, R.M., editor: Textbook of pediatric nutrition. New York, Copyright 1981, Raven Press.
*Assuming body weight of 1000 and 1500 gm, respectively, for the 800-1200 and 1200-1800 gm infants.
†Assuming energy intake of 130 kcal/kg/day.

329

been added to the premature formulas to simulate the amount present in human milk, resulting in a 60:40 whey/casein ratio.

In addition to the amount and type of protein, the distribution of protein calories (relative to carbohydrate and fat) affects the protein requirement. It is desirable that protein comprise 7% to 16% of total calories.[186] Feedings with less than 7% may limit growth; those with more than 16% may cause azotemia and acidosis.

Lipid. LBW infants need an adequate amount of dietary fat to help meet their high energy needs for growth, to provide essential fatty acids, and to assist in absorption of other important nutrients such as the fat-soluble vitamins and calcium. However, neonates in general and premature and small-for-gestational age infants in particular are relatively inefficient in digestion and absorption of lipid.

Fat digestion is compromised by low levels of lipase, the pancreatic enzyme responsible for the hydrolysis of dietary fats.[187] In addition, LBW infants, especially those who are very premature, have a relatively low concentration and an altered composition of bile salts. Their bile acid pool falls below the critical micellar concentration and is therefore insufficient to solubilize most long-chain lipids for absorption.[188] Because medium-chain triglycerides require few or no bile salts for absorption, these fats have been added to the new premature formulas in varying quantities. When medium-chain triglycerides are added to vegetable oils, there is improved fat absorption in LBW infants, resulting in alleviation of steatorrhea, increased weight gain, enhanced calcium absorption, and improved nitrogen retention.[189]

The composition of dietary fat also plays a role in the digestion and absorption of lipid. Full-term and preterm infants show better digestion and absorption of fats from human milk than from cow's milk or standard infant formulas, in part because of the presence of two human milk lipases and in part because

of the unique fatty acid composition of human milk fat.[175,190] Furthermore, vegetable oils are absorbed more efficiently by LBW infants than saturated animal fats.[191]

Vegetable oils containing polyunsaturated fatty acids contain linoleic acid; medium-chain triglyceride oil does not. Adequate intake of this essential fatty acid is important; at least 3% of the total enteral calories is required.[192] However, an excessively high intake of polyunsaturated fatty acids may have adverse effects. Because the fatty acid composition of the red blood cell membrane is primarily determined by the fatty acid composition of the diet, infants fed large amounts of polyunsaturated fatty acids have increased erythrocyte susceptibility to oxidative destruction. It is recommended that commercial formulas fed to LBW infants not contain more than about 12% linoleic acid to prevent hemolytic anemia.

The percentage of total calories as fat relative to carbohydrate and protein is another important consideration. It is desirable that fat comprise 30% to 55% of total calories[186]; fat intake greater than 60% of calories may lead to ketosis. Furthermore, a diet high in fat and low in protein may yield more fat deposition than is desirable for the growing LBW infant.

Carbohydrate. Lactose is the predominant carbohydrate in almost all mammalian milks. There is physiological concern that the premature infant's ability to digest lactose may be marginal; intestinal lactase activity develops during the third trimester of gestation but does not achieve maximal activity until term.[193] Premature infants fed high-lactose formulas or human milk might be expected to experience fermentative diarrhea secondary to incomplete lactose digestion and absorption; however, this is not a common problem beyond the first few days of life.[194]

Sucrose is another disaccharide commonly found in commercial infant formula products. Because sucrase activity is present at 70% of newborn levels early in the third trimester,[193] sucrose is well tolerated by most premature infants. Both sucrase and lactase are sensitive to changes in the intestinal milieu, however, and babies afflicted by diarrhea, receiving antibiotic therapy, or suffering from undernutrition may develop a temporary intolerance to lactose and sucrose.

Glucose polymers are an increasingly common carbohydrate in the diets of LBW infants. The polymers, composed mainly of chains of 5 to 9 glucose units linked together, are used to achieve the iso-osmolality of certain specialized formulas. Glucosidase enzymes for digestion of glucose polymers are active in small preterm infants.[195]

Human milk and standard infant formulas contain approximately 40% of the total calories as carbohydrate. An appropriate intake of carbohydrate is desirable; 35% to 65% of total calories as carbohydrate is the recommended range.[186] Too little carbohydrate may lead to hypoglycemia, while too much carbohydrate may provoke an osmotic diuresis or loose stools.

Vitamins and minerals. Premature infants require all of the vitamins and minerals that are essential for full-term infants; however, LBW babies have increased requirements for several of these as a result of poor body stores and physiological immaturity. The most recent statement of the Committee on Nutrition of the American Academy of Pediatrics summarizes the current recommendations regarding vitamin and mineral needs of LBW infants.[110] (Requirements for certain of these vitamins and minerals and recommendations for their supplementation are discussed in the following section.)

Premature infants who are growing rapidly require increased intakes of *calcium, phosphorus,* and *vitamin D* for optional bone mineralization. As discussed on p. 41, the fetus accumulates 120 to 150 mg calcium/kg/day and about 75 mg phosphorus/kg/day during the final weeks of gestation; the premature infant is deprived of this important intrauterine mineral deposition. Inadequate dietary intakes can result in osteopenia of prematurity.[196] This disease is characterized by demineralization of growing bones and is documented by radiological evidence of "washed-out" bones in preterm infants. Very immature babies are particularly susceptible to osteopenia and may develop bone fractures or florid rickets[197] if dietary deficiency is prolonged.

The pathophysiology of osteopenia of prematurity is not completely understood. However, there is increasing evidence that a deficiency of calcium and phosphorus is the primary cause of the disease, regardless of the intake of vitamin D. This subject has been recently reviewed by Greer and Tsang.[198]

Osteopenia of prematurity is most likely to occur in preterm infants who have bronchopulmonary dysplasia (a chronic lung disease), are fed human milk that is not supplemented with calcium and phosphorus, or are fed standard infant formulas. First, preterm infants with bronchopulmonary dysplasia are often at risk for osteopenia because of low dietary intake and high urinary losses. These infants often have a history of total parenteral nutrition for more than 2 to 3 weeks. As discussed on p. 321, standard hyperalimentation solutions usually contain inadequate amounts of calcium and phosphorus to meet the high needs of preterm infants. In addition, infants with bronchopulmonary dysplasia are often fluid restricted and therefore may receive limited amounts of calcium and phosphorus-containing enteral feedings. Increased urinary losses of calcium and phosphorus also occur secondary to furosemide diuretic therapy.

Second, although human milk contains fully adequate amounts of calcium and phosphorus for healthy full-term infants, it does not contain sufficient quantities of these minerals to meet the greater needs of preterm infants. The smallest and most immature infants have the highest risk of developing osteopenia of prematurity when fed unsupplemented human milk. These infants develop a relative hypercalciuria, apparently because of inadequate phosphorus intake for bone utilization of calcium.[199]

The third problem occurs when small preterm infants are fed standard infant formulas designed for full-term infants, instead of the premature infant formula products that are specifically designed to meet the particular nutrient needs of preterm infants. Table 12-16 compares the advisable intakes for calcium and phosphorus (based on intrauterine accretion rates) with the amounts contained in preterm and mature human milk, standard infant formulas, and premature infant formula products. It is apparent that human milk and standard infant formulas do not provide enough calcium and phosphorus to match advisable intake recommendations. Since intestinal absorption of calcium from standard formulas can be as low as 40% to 60% of intake levels in LBW infants, the amount of calcium retained by the premature infant may only be one fourth to one fifth of the amount that would have been received in utero. Calcium and phosphorus supplements should be given to preterm infants who are fed either standard infant formulas or human milk. Preterm infants who receive supplements have greater retention of calcium and phosphorus and improved bone mineralization.[200,201] Recommendations for supplementation of human milk are discussed on p. 342.

As shown in Table 12-16, the three premature infant formula products available in the United States contain more calcium and phosphorus than the three standard infant formula products. Several studies have reported the results of feeding premature infant products to VLBW infants (most weighing 1200 to 1600 gm).[202-205] Additional research is needed to determine ideal calcium and phosphorus concentrations and relative ratio in these products. At present, additional calcium and phosphorus supplements are not usually given to preterm infants who receive the majority of their milk feedings from premature infant formula products. The appropriate use of premature infant formulas is discussed in more detail on page 343.

It has been suggested that LBW infants have immature vitamin D hydroxylation pathways and that this may contribute to the development of osteopenia of prematurity. However, in a study of preterm infants of 32 to 37 weeks of gestation, the administration of oral vitamin D_3 increased serum 1,25-dihydroxyvitamin D concentrations at 5 days of age[206]; this finding indicates that vitamin D is well absorbed and metabolized in preterm infants. Furthermore, serum 1,25-dihydroxyvitamin D levels were found to be elevated in LBW infants with rickets.[207] After feeding a standard infant formula supplemented with calcium and phosphorus, there was resolution of the rickets and serum 1,25-dihydroxyvitamin D concentrations fell to normal levels.[207] These findings appear to show that rickets of prematurity is caused by calcium and phosphorus deficiency, rather than by a deficiency in vitamin D metabolism, and that the elevation of 1,25-dihydroxyvitamin D reflects a compensatory mechanism to achieve maximal calcium and phosphorus absorption.[133] In contrast, there has been one report of rickets in preterm infants in whom 1,25-dihydroxyvitamin D levels were low despite adequate intakes of vitamin D_3.[208] Since resolution of the rickets was achieved with 1,25-dihydroxyvitamin D supplementation, it is possible that a relative unresponsiveness of the intestine to the action of vitamin D may be an additional factor contributing to rickets of prematurity.[208]

Available data are not yet sufficient to establish a precise requirement for vitamin D. Ziegler, Biga, and Fomon[7] have suggested an advisable intake of 600 IU of vitamin D per day. Greer and Tsang[198] have suggested that 400 IU of vitamin D per day is adequate for most preterm infants. According to the Ameri-

Table 12-16 Advisable intakes for calcium, phosphorus, protein, sodium, and vitamin D compared with selected feedings

	Advisable Intake		Human Milk		Standard	Premature		
	1 kg Body Wt.	1.5 kg Body Wt.	Preterm	Mature	Enfamil Similac SMA	Enfamil Premature	Premie SMA	Similac Special Care
Calcium (mg/100 kcal)	160	140	40	43	66-75	117	94	180
Phosphorus (mg/100 kcal)	108	95	18	20	47-58	59	50	90
Protein (gm/100 kcal)	3.1	2.7	2.3 (range 1.9-2.8)	1.5	2.2	3.0	2.5	2.7
Sodium (mEq/100 kcal)	2.7	2.3	1.5 (range 0.9-2.3)	0.8	1-1.4	1.7	1.7	2.2
Caloric density (kcal/100 ml)			73	67	81	81	81	81
Vitamin D (IU/day)*	600	600	?	4†	70-75	396	76	180

Data from Brady, M. S., and others: Formulas and human milk for premature infants, J. Am. Diet. Assoc. 81:547, 1982; and Lemons, J. A., and others: Pediatr. Res. 16:113, 1982. Data updated (1988) to show current concentrations of nutrients in formula products.

*At 120 kcal/kg/day for an infant weighing 1 kg.

†Refer to page 50 for discussion of vitamin D needs of full-term infants with adequate exposure to sunlight.

can Academy of Pediatrics,[110] there is no evidence that administration of the active vitamin D metabolites (25-hydroxy and 1,25-dihydroxy-vitamin D) to LBW infants is necessary or advisable.

Preterm infants are particularly susceptible to *iron* deficiency because they have reduced iron stores associated with premature birth. Although iron stores are sufficient to permit expansion of the blood volume to nearly twice its initial size (i.e., until birth weight has doubled), they drop rapidly after about 2 months of age as active erythropoiesis resumes. Iron deficiency anemia may develop by 3 months postnatal age if iron supplementation is not provided. In contrast, full-term infants do not usually deplete their proportionately larger iron stores until after 4 to 6 months of age.

The iron intake currently recommended for premature infants is 2 mg/kg/day; this is twice the amount recommended for full-term infants. It is possible that VLBW infants, especially those weighing less than 1000 gm, may require somewhat more iron. The iron needs of these infants have been reviewed by Oski.[210] Most premature infant formulas contain low levels of iron (less than 0.5 mg/kg/day when providing 120 kcal/kg/day). LBW infants fed these products need iron supplements by about the time they are 2 months of age. Similarly, the iron content of human milk does not meet the requirements of the premature infant, despite the enhanced absorption of iron from human milk. For infants receiving human milk or premature infant formula without added iron, oral ferrous sulfate drops are an effective supplement. Larger premature infants (weighing 2 kg or more) who are fed standard formula fortified with iron receive 1.8 to 2 mg elemental iron/120 kcal and do not require additional supplementation.

Most authorities agree that iron supplementation in LBW infants should be initiated at least by the time birthweight has doubled (which usually occurs by 2 months of age).

However, whether or not to introduce iron supplements at an earlier time has been a controversial issue. The controversy has focused on two principal concerns: hemolytic anemia and decreased host resistance to infection. Hemolytic anemia rarely occurs if an appropriate amount of iron is ingested by an infant whose vitamin E intake is adequate and whose polyunsaturated fatty acid intake is controlled. In vitro studies indicate that exogenous iron may decrease host resistance to infection through saturation and inactivation of certain antibacterial, iron-binding proteins in serum and human milk.[211] However, in vivo studies do not support in vitro findings that ordinary iron supplementation predisposes infants to infection.[212]

Lundstrom, Siimes, and Dallman[213] suggest that iron supplements of 2 mg/kg/day, started at 2 weeks of age, are both safe and effective for LBW infants. Therefore current recommendations for iron supplementation in LBW infants permit iron as early as 2 weeks of age, but not later than about 2 months of age.

LBW infants may require more *vitamin E* than full-term infants, probably a result of poor vitamin E absorption and low body stores. Impaired absorption of vitamin E by premature infants was described in the early 1970s[209]; however, fat blends in current premature infant formulas are markedly improved, resulting in better absorption of both fat and vitamin E. Still, the premature infant is born with poor vitamin E stores relative to the full-term baby. When supplemented with 30 IU vitamin E per day, most premature infants show plasma tocopherol levels within the desired range.[7] By comparison, nonsupplemented infants are more likely to demonstrate biochemical signs of vitamin E deficiency (e.g., lower hemoglobin concentrations, higher reticulocyte counts, and more fragile red cells in weak solutions of hydrogen peroxide). The advisable intake of vitamin E in LBW infants is 30 IU day.[7]

An important function of vitamin E is its protection of biological membranes against oxidative breakdown of lipids. Requirements for vitamin E increase when the level of polyunsaturated fatty acids in the diet is high. The polyunsaturated fatty acids gradually produce a change in the composition of the fatty acids in cellular and intracellular membranes. The membranes then become more susceptible to oxidative damage, which increases the requirement for the antioxidant effect of vitamin E. Because iron is a biological oxidant, a diet high in either iron or polyunsaturated fatty acids increases the risk of vitamin E deficiency. A premature infant suffering from vitamin E deficiency may experience oxidative destruction of red blood cells or hemolytic anemia.

Several studies in the early 1970s indicated that premature infants were at high risk for hemolytic anemia.[209] However, the formula products used in these studies were high in polyunsaturated fatty acids and iron and contained fat blends that resulted in poor absorption of vitamin E. The combination of high polyunsaturated fatty acid content and high levels of the oxidant iron in the face of vitamin E deficiency resulted in red blood cell hemolysis by membrane destruction. Since that time, the composition of premature infant formulas has been favorably changed to correct these problems. Therefore hemolytic anemia associated with vitamin E deficiency is rarely a problem today when careful attention is paid to the composition of the diet.

Since the dietary requirement for vitamin E depends on the polyunsaturated fatty acid content of the diet, the recommended intake of vitamin E is commonly expressed as a ratio of vitamin E to polyunsaturated fatty acids. The Committee on Nutrition of the American Academy of Pediatrics recommends that milk fed to premature infants provide at least 0.6 mg D-α-tocopherol per gram of polyunsaturated fatty acid (or 1 IU vitamin E per gram of polyunsaturated fatty acid).[192] Both human milk and the new premature infant formulas have vitamin E/polyunsaturated fatty acid ratios well above this recommendation.

Premature infants may have higher *folic* acid needs than full-term infants. Although serum folate levels are high at birth, they decrease dramatically soon thereafter.[214] This may reflect the high utilization of folic acid by the premature infant for DNA and tissue synthesis. Because the preterm baby grows more rapidly than the full-term infant, he or she may have a higher intrinsic need for folic acid.

A mild form of folic acid deficiency manifested by low serum folate concentrations and hypersegmentation of **neutrophils** is not unusual in premature infants. Megaloblastic anemia is much less commonly observed. A daily supplement of 50 to 70 μg is effective in preventing neutrophil hypersegmentation and low serum folate concentrations.[214] Ziegler, Biga, and Fomon[7] recommended an advisable intake of 60 μg/day.

The minimum daily *sodium* requirement for LBW infants has been estimated to be approximately 1.6 mEq/kg/day.[215] However, actual sodium requirements may be much higher for LBW infants who experience excessive sodium losses. LBW infants, especially those born at less than 33 weeks of gestation, have immature renal systems and are consequently limited in their ability to conserve sodium. Below this gestational age the glomerular filtration rate exceeds the limited tubular sodium resorption capacity, and excess sodium is lost.[216] Actual sodium needs of immature infants may be as high as 5 mEq/kg/day during the first 2 weeks of life for infants of less than 30 weeks of gestation and 4 mEq/kg/day for those born between 30 and 35 weeks of gestation.[216] Infants who suffer additional sodium losses through the gastrointestinal tract (e.g., diarrhea or malabsorption related to extreme immaturity)[217] or as a result of diuretic therapy may have sodium needs as high as 8 to 9 mEq/kg/day.[131]

High renal and gastrointestinal losses of sodium contribute to the susceptibility of LBW infants to **hyponatremia** in the neonatal period. Up to 30% of infants weighing less than 1300 gm at birth may be hyponatremic during the first weeks of life.[218] Other factors that contribute to the development of hyponatremia include increased sodium needs related to rapid rates of growth and poor dietary intake resulting from consumption of small volumes of milk.

Although LBW infants are clearly vulnerable to hyponatremia, routine sodium supplementation of enterally fed infants is not recommended.[192] Individual infants vary in their ability to conserve sodium, and it is difficult to predict whether babies will become hyponatremic or maintain normal serum sodium levels. However, it is important to monitor the sodium status of all LBW infants by frequent assessment of serum and urinary sodium concentrations. Milk can be supplemented with sodium if repletion becomes necessary.

When to Begin Enteral Feedings

The decision to begin enteral feeding in LBW infants is often difficult and involves consideration of the degree of prematurity, history of perinatal insults, current medical condition, functioning of the gastrointestinal tract, and several other individualized concerns. Because of the complexity of these factors, the choice of optimal timing of feeding must be personalized for each LBW infant and altered according to the variable course of each baby. Consideration of the factors listed in Table 12-17 may facilitate the decision to start or to delay enteral feedings.

Methods of Feeding

Once it has been decided that enteral feedings will be initiated, the optimal enteral feeding technique must be selected. LBW infants can be fed either by gastric gavage (Figure 12-3) or by bottle nipple (Figure 12-4). These methods of feeding LBW infants have been reviewed by Benda.[219] Mothers who choose to breast-feed their premature infants should begin as soon as the infants are ready to begin nippling.[220,221] Although a discussion of how to nurse a preterm infant is beyond the scope of this chapter, excellent information is available in articles by Meier and Pugh,[220] Meier and Anderson,[221] and Neifert and Seacat.[222]

Techniques. Oral gastric gavage feeding is often chosen for infants unable to suck because of immaturity or insults to their central nervous system. Infants less than 32 to 34 weeks of gestational age, regardless of birth weight, may be expected to have poorly coordinated sucking and swallowing activity related to their developmental immaturity and consequently have difficulty with nipple feeding.[219] The major risks of the oral gastric gavage technique include aspiration and gastric distention. Because of weak or absent cough reflexes and poorly developed respiratory muscles, the tiny baby may not be able to dislodge milk from the upper airway, causing reflex bradycardia or airway obstruction. However, with electronic monitoring of vital functions and proper positioning in the infant during feeding, the danger of aspiration from regurgitation of stomach contents is minimized. Gastric distention and vagal nerve stimulation with resultant bradycardia are potential problems when oral gastric feedings are delivered on an intermittent bolus schedule.[219] Elimination of the distention and vagal bradycardia may occasionally require the use of an indwelling tube for continuous gastric gavage feedings, instead of the usual intermittent technique. Continuous drip feedings may benefit the tiny, immature infant whose small gastric capacity and slow intestinal motility sometimes impede the tolerance of larger-volume bolus feeds. Nasogastric tubes are more stable in their replacement than oral gastric tubes and are preferred for babies on continuous drip feeding with tube changes every 8

Table 12-17 Factors to consider before feeding by an enteral route

Factors to Consider	Comments
Perinatal	
Perinatal asphyxia	If the condition is severe, enteral feedings should be withheld during the first 48 hours of life and possibly longer, depending on respiratory status.
Apgar scores	Wait 24 to 48 hours before feeding if Apgar scores are less than about 3. Consider clinical condition of the infant and neurological status in determining when to feed.
Respiratory status	

Ventilated baby with RDS	Consider feedings when
	    Ventilatory settings are consistent and show improvement.
	    Blood gases are adequate.
	    Episodes of apnea and bradycardia are mild and relatively infrequent.
	    Low risk for pneumothorax.
	Note that infants with tachypnea (rapid respiratory rate) and retractions are vulnerable to aspiration of milk.

Medical status	
Vital signs	Heart rate, respiratory rate, temperature, blood pressure, color, and tone should be adequate for each infant.
Acute illness (such as sepsis)	Acutely ill babies are medically unstable and less likely to tolerate enteral feedings. Once the acute phase has passed and the infant is responding to treatment, enteral feedings should be reconsidered.
Gastrointestinal tract	
Anomalies	Certain anomalies prohibit the use of enteral feedings (e.g., gastroschisis, omphalocele) until surgically repaired.
Patency	The inability to pass a feeding tube or the occurrence of vomiting or distention in response to enteral feedings may indicate inadequate patency of the gastrointestinal tract. Intestinal obstructions (e.g., atresia, stenosis, volvulus) may prohibit enteral feedings before surgical relief.
Functioning	Signs that indicate a functioning gastrointestinal tract should be present (e.g., normal bowel sounds, ability to pass stools).

Risk of necrotizing enterocolitis	Factors that may increase the risk for necrotizing enterocolitis include
	    Immaturity (<32 weeks' gestation)
	    VLBW (<1500 gm)
	    Episodes of hypoxia (asphyxia, respiratory disease)
	    Inadequate perfusion of the gastrointestinal tract
	    Patent ductus arteriosus
	    Possibly the presence of an umbilical arterial catheter (UAC-line)

Equipment/procedures	Intubation, extubation, etc., may be temporary barriers to enteral feedings. Any procedure that is stressful to the infant may warrant *temporary* withholding of enteral feedings.

Figure 12-3 Growing premature infant is being fed by oral gastric gavage.

hours. But because newborns are obligate nose breathers, more frequent replacement of nasogastric tubes may compromise the nasal airway in LBW infants and cause a deterioration in respiratory function.

In the past, transpyloric gavage feeding was occasionally used for LBW infants. The goal of this method was to circumvent the often slow gastropyloric motility of the immature infant by passing the feeding tube through the stomach and pylorus and locating its tip within the duodenum or jejunum. Advantages of transpyloric feeding included the elimination of the pylorus as a barrier for adequate propulsion of milk and a reduced chance of aspiration. But there were several disadvantages as well. Transpyloric feedings were associated with decreased fat absorption, diarrhea, dumping syndrome, alteration of the intestinal microflora, contamination of the feeding system, intestinal perforation, and bilious fluid in the stomach.[223] Transpyloric tubes also required considerable expertise in their placement and x-ray films to determine the location of the catheter tip. Because of the problems inherent in using this technique, transpyloric feeding is now rarely used to feed LBW infants.

Nipple feeding may be attempted in infants whose gestational age is greater than 32 to 34 weeks.[219] The ability to nipple feed is usually indicated by evidence of an established sucking reflex and sucking motion. Because sucking requires considerable effort by the infant, any stress from other causes will diminish sucking ability.[219] Nipple feeding therefore should be offered only when the infant is minimally stressed and has sufficient maturity and strength for a sustained sucking effort.

Volume and schedule. The appropriate amount of milk to be fed to LBW infants depends, in part, on their estimated stomach capacity. The undistended stomach volume varies with the size of the infant and may be as small as 2 to 3 ml in the 800 gm newborn or about 40 ml in the 4000 gm newborn. The gastric capacity of neonates increases with postnatal age; therefore this is a practical concern during the early period of introduction

Figure 12-4   A mother feeds her premature infant using a small, soft "premie" nipple.

to enteral feeds. Another important consideration in determining enteral volume is the gastrointestinal motility of LBW infants. Preterm
infants have poor gastrointestinal motility as a
result of motor immaturity of their gastrointestinal tract. This is the most limiting factor
in advancing enteral volume and may be a persistent problem for some premature infants.
Because individual babies vary in their ability to move food through the gastrointestinal
canal, all premature infants receiving enteral
feeds must be monitored by regular measurements of feeding tolerance.

A suggested feeding schedule is shown in
Table 12-18. These recommendations should
be tailored to meet the fluid needs and feeding
tolerances of individual infants. Some VLBW
infants may not tolerate increases in volume as
large or as often as described in Table 12-18.
Infants weighing less than 1000 gm may not
tolerate an increase in total volume of more
than 20 ml/kg every other day. Such infants
would therefore require 2 or more weeks to
work up to full enteral feeds. Infants weighing

between 1000 and 1500 gm may be able to tolerate daily volume increments of 20 ml/kg/day.
The feeding volume and schedule must be individualized.

Although neonatal intensive care nurseries
vary in their approach to initiating enteral feedings, most nurseries introduce small enteral volumes and increase volume cautiously. There
is no documented advantage to feeding formula that is diluted to one-fourth or one-half
strength.

TOLERANCE OF FEEDINGS

LBW infants are susceptible to feeding
intolerance. Their esophageal motility is poor,
and their gastroesophageal sphincter is relatively incompetent, resulting in frequent regurgitation of food into the esophagus. Small gastric capacity, delayed gastric emptying time,
and poorly coordinated intestinal motility may
be additional problems. The overall result of
this mechanical immaturity is a tendency, most
apparent in the smallest infants, toward frequent abdominal distention, gastric residu-

Table 12-18   Enteral feeding schedule for low birth weight infants

	First Feeding	Subsequent Feedings (12-72 hr)	Final Feeding Schedule	Total Volume (ml/kg/day)
Fluid	Sterile water	Human milk or formula	Human milk or formula	
Weight				
Up to 1000 gm				
Amount	1 ml	Gradually increase by 0.5-1 ml to maximum 3-5 ml	6-12 ml	120-150
Frequency	1 hr	2 hr	2 hr	
1001-1500 gm				
Amount	2-3 ml	Gradually increase by 1 ml to maximum 7-10 ml	18-28 ml	150
Frequency	2 hr	2 hr	3 hr	
1501-2000 gm				
Amount	4-5 ml	Gradually increase by 2 ml to maximum 12-15 ml	28-37 ml	150
Frequency	2 hr	2-3 hr	3 hr	
2000-2500 gm				
Amount	10 ml	Gradually increase by 5 ml to maximum 20 ml	37-50 ml	150
Frequency	3 hr	3 hr	3-4 hr	

Modified from Avery, G.B., and Fletcher, A.B.: Nutrition. In Avery, G.B., editor: Neonatology: pathophysiology and management of the newborn, Philadelphia, 1981, J.B. Lippincott Co.

als, and regurgitation, even in the absence of any recognized food intolerances or systemic illness.[219]

All LBW babies receiving enteral nutrition should be consistently monitored for signs of feeding intolerance; these indicators of feeding intolerance have been reviewed by Benda.[219] Vomiting of feedings usually signals that the infant is unable to retain that amount of milk. When not associated with other signs of a systemic illness or obstruction, vomiting may indicate a too rapid increase in feeding volumes or excessive volume for the infant's size and maturity.[219] It is possible that simply reducing the volume will eliminate the vomiting. However, if vomiting persists despite a reduction of intake, or if it is apparent that the infant is ill, it may be advisable to interrupt the feedings until the infant's condition has stabilized.

Abdominal distention may be caused by feeding excessive volumes, bowel obstruction, excessive swallowing of air, mask ventilation, paralytic ileus, or sepsis. Clinical examination, as well as intermittent measurement of abdominal circumference, will aid in the early detection of distention. A distended abdomen often indicates the need for interruption of feeding until the cause of the distention is determined and the abdomen is once more soft and nondistended.

Gastric residuals are measured by aspiration of the stomach contents and should be routinely checked before each bolus gavage feeding and intermittently in all continuous drip feedings.[224] Whether a residual is significant depends in part on its volume in relation to the total volume of the feeding; a residual whose volume is more than about 20% of the total feeding might be a sign of feeding intolerance. When interpreting the significance of a gastric residual, however, it is important to consider that residual in light of other concurrent signs of feeding intolerance and the pattern of residuals established for that infant. Gastric residuals that are bloody or bilious are more alarming than those that appear to be undigested milk.

The frequency and consistency of bowel movements require constant attention when feeding LBW infants. Furthermore, routine testing of stools for reducing substances is a useful procedure that promptly detects incomplete absorption of sugars by the intestine. Although the presence of gross blood can be detected by simple inspection, occult blood is not always visible and should be investigated by a specific assay to detect small amounts of blood in the stool.

Necrotizing enterocolitis. Several authors have suggested that aggressive enteral feedings in the early days of life may be a cause of necrotizing enterocolotis. Necrotizing enterocolotis is a disease of complex multifactorial pathogenesis related to gut hypoperfusion, ischemia, and mucosal damage. Early enteral feedings in susceptible infants, especially when volumes are rapidly increased and hypertonic formulas are fed, may predispose to necrotizing enterocolitis by contributing to mucosal damage.[225] When bacteria invade the damaged mucosa of the infant's intestine, bowel necrosis may result.

Feedings may also provide substrate for intestinal bacterial growth.

Although enteral feedings may play a part in the pathogenesis of necrotizing enterocolitis, evidence concerning the role of feeding is primarily circumstantial, particularly as the disease has been reported in a number of infants before enteral feeding was begun.[226] Other factors associated with the development of necrotizing enterocolitis include birth asphyxia, arterial hypoxemia from respiratory disease, gut ischemia secondary to a patient ductus arteriosus, or aortic catheters. Enteral feeding is not singularly responsible for the pathogenesis of necrotizing enterocolotis; however, a conservative approach to enteral feeding may be warranted in LBW infants, particularly when other risk factors for the development of the disease are present.

Composition of Feedings

Human milk. Although human milk is considered the ideal food for healthy, full-term infants,[227] there has been controversy over the optimal milk for premature neonates.[228] Some studies have demonstrated that LBW infants fed banked human milk do not grow as rapidly as LBW infants fed infant formulas.[229,230] However, banked human milk, collected during the mature stage of lactation from mothers who have delivered full-term infants, does not provide enough protein and minerals to support intrauterine rates of growth in preterm infants.[231]

More recent studies show that premature infants fed their own mothers' milk grow more rapidly than infants fed banked milk. When adequate volumes of milk from mothers who deliver early are fed to their healthy LBW infants, these babies are able to attain intrauterine rates of weight gain.[232,233] Furthermore, nutritional status as measured by plasma total protein and albumin concentrations is better in LBW infants fed their own mothers milk than in those fed banked breast-milk.[234] This is accomplished without indications of stress to the developing metabolic or excretory systems. Whether resumption of the intrauterine rate of weight gain is appropriate is a separate issue; the fact remains that milk from mothers who deliver early can support rates of growth similar to those achieved by infant formulas.[231]

The different rates of growth in premature infants fed preterm versus mature human milk can be attributed to the unique nutrient composition of preterm human milk. During the first month of lactation, the milk from mothers who deliver prematurely appears to contain more energy and higher concentrations of protein and certain minerals than milk from a more mature stage of lactation.[235-238] It has been suggested that preterm milk more closely approximates the nutritional needs of LBW infants than does other breast-milk.[239]

In addition to nutrient concentration, several other factors contribute to the widely held opinion that preterm mother's milk for her own infant is the feeding choice for the LBW baby. Human milk contains certain growth factors that apparently play an important role in the proliferation and differentiation of cells in body tissues of infants. For example, epidermal growth factor in human milk is known to exert a trophic effect on the developing intestinal epithelium of premature infants.[240,241] Other factors in human milk that have been shown to insulate cellular growth in infants include nerve growth factor, certain enzymes, and interferons.[242] The physiological role of other factors present in human milk, such as prostaglandins and certain hormones, is not yet clear.[243]

Human milk protein is whey predominant, with an amino acid composition that favors the LBW infant. The presence of lipase and amylase[244] in human milk contributes to the premature infant's ability to digest fat and carbohydrate and to derive the maximum caloric benefit of the feeding. The renal solute load of human milk is appropriately low (90 mOsm/L)

and does not interfere with water balance in the LBW infant.

Two anti-infective factors in human milk favor its choice for immature babies: (1) maternal immune factors, notably secretory IgA, lysozyme, and leucocytes,[245-247] and (2) antibacterial factors that cause acidification of the infant's gut and promote the establishment of a vigorous lactobacillus flora.[248] These agents may provide protection from infection for the developing gut mucosa.[249]

There is, however, one well-documented problem associated with feeding human milk to LBW infants. First, human milk, whether preterm, term, or mature, does not meet the calcium and phosphorus needs for normal bone mineralization in infants born prematurely.[250] Despite increased calcium absorption found in preterm infants receiving human milk, the total calcium content of the milk is deficient for the growing preterm infant and may lead to a decrease in bone mineralization.[251,252] Preterm infants who receive their own mothers' milk can develop hypophosphatemia and hypercalciuria (although serum calcium values are usually normal), presumably as a result of low dietary phosphorus intake. For these reasons calcium and phosphorus supplements are recommended for rapidly growing LBW infants predominantly fed human milk (p. 321).

Currently two products are available that contain calcium and phosphorus (among other nutrients); these products are called human milk fortifiers and are designed to be added to expressed breast-milk fed to premature and LBW infants. Similac Natural Care (Ross Laboratories) is available in liquid form, whereas Enfamilk Human Milk Fortifier (Mead Johnson Nutritional Division) is available in powdered form. Both products contain protein, carbohydrate, fat, vitamins, and minerals in addition to calcium and phosphorus. Although the importance of supplementing expressed breast milk with calcium and phosphorus has been well established, the specific needs for supplementation of preterm infants with additional

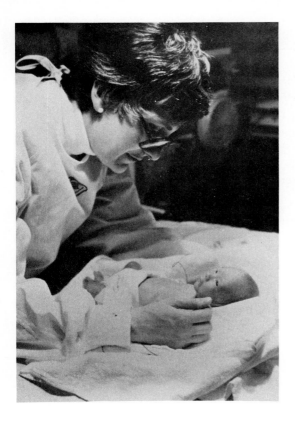

Figure 12-5 A mother interacts with her premature infant who is now 10 weeks old.

nutrients are not yet clear. Recent studies have looked at growth, nutrient balance, and metabolism in small preterm infants fed fortified human milk.[253-256] Additional studies are needed before specific recommendations can be made regarding the need for routine supplementation of human milk with these other nutrients. However, preterm infants who are fed a small total daily volume of human milk usually do receive a multivitamin supplement (guidelines on p. 348). Since vitamins are contained in the human milk fortifier products, infants who receive breast-milk plus a fortifier usually do not need additional vitamin supplementation.

Providing breast-milk for a premature infant can be a positive experience for a mother, who is otherwise confronted by the many stresses associated with separation from her baby in intensive care. Since many preterm infants are neither strong enough nor mature enough to nurse at their mothers' breasts in the early neonatal period, mothers usually express their milk for several days and sometimes several weeks before nursing can be established. Several factors related to the technique of expression, storage, and transport of milk must be considered to ensure that the breast milk provided is appropriate for feeding.

Formulas. New formula preparations have been developed to meet the unique nutrient and physiological needs of growing LBW infants. The quantity and quality of nutrients contained in these products promote growth at intrauterine rates. When fed to stable premature infants who are growing rapidly, these specialized formulas are usually tolerated without metabolic consequences. Studies of stable babies weighing 1200 gm or more indicate that these formulas are safe and promote weight gain, fat absorption, nitrogen retention, and bone mineralization.[200] When fed to VLBW babies who are stressed and have not yet sustained a steady weight gain, premature formulas should be used cautiously.

Generally, formulas are introduced in very small amounts. Gradual increases in volume are made over several days according to the feeding tolerance of the individual infant (p. 339). There is no proven advantage to feeding formula that has been diluted with water.[257] If dilute formula feedings (one-fourth or one-half strength) are used, they should not be fed for prolonged periods of time because of the risks of undernutrition.

The specialized new premature infant formulas differ in many aspects from standard cow's milk–base formulas. Table 12-19 summarizes these differences and identifies some of the advantages of feeding premature infant formulas to LBW infants. Refer to Table 12-20 for

Table 12-19 Comparison of premature versus standard formulas for feeding LBW infants

Element	Premature Formulas*	Standard Formulas†
	Designed, tested in premature infants	Designed, tested in full-term infants
Energy	24 kcal/oz	20 kcal/oz
Protein	Whey casein; 60:40	Whey/casein; 60:40‡
Fat	Part medium-chain triglycerides; part long-chain fats	100% long-chain fats
Carbohydrate	Part glucose polymers; part lactose	100% lactose
Calcium and phosphorus	Fortified to meet needs of premature	*Not* fortified to meet needs of premature
Iron	Not fortified§	Available with or without added iron
Osmolality	Iso-osmolar (300 mOsm/kg H_2O)	Iso-osmolar

From O'Leary, M.J.: Nutritional care of the low birth weight infant. In Krause, M.V., and Mahan, L.K., editors: Food, nutrition, and diet therapy, ed. 7, Philadelphia, 1984, W.B. Saunders, Co.
* Enfamil Premature (Mead Johnson), Premie SMA (Wyeth Laboratories), and Similac Special Care (Ross Laboratories).
† Enfamil (Mead Johnson), and SMA (Wyeth Laboratories).
‡ Similac (Ross Laboratories) contains whey/casein; 18:82. Although the other standard formulas contain whey/casein; 60:40, they are not designed to meet the other unique nutrient and physiological needs of LBW infants.
§ Similac Special Care (Ross Laboratories) has recently been made available with or without iron fortification.

a summary of the composition of human milk and that of premature and standard infant formulas.

Selection of Feedings

Choice of an optimal feeding for an LBW infant is complicated by the fact that no ideal feeding exists. The extrauterine environment represents an abrupt change for the preterm infant, and most of these babies require a period of adjustment before tolerance to any enteral feeding can be established.

There may be some advantage in feeding sterile water as the first feeding after birth, since animal evidence indicates that pulmonary damage from aspiration of water is less than that of either 5% glucose in water or milk.[258] Following the first feeding, human milk or formula may be introduced in slowly increasing amounts.

During the initial period of feeding, premature infants are often still adjusting to enteral nutrition and may be experiencing concurrent stress, weight loss, and diuresis. The primary goal of enteral feeding during this initial period is to facilitate tolerance to the milk provided. Aggressive nutritional support from the onset of enteral feeding often meets with failure, since babies appear unable to assimilate a large volume of nutrients until adjustment has been established. Supplementation of enteral feedings with parenteral fluids is often required until adequate oral volume is tolerated.

Selection of a milk with the characteristics listed on p. 345 may facilitate tolerance to enteral feedings during this period of adjustment. Human milk and premature infant formulas are the most commonly used feedings that meet these criteria. After the initial period of adjustment, the goal of enteral feeding changes to provide complete nutrition to promote growth and rapid organ development. All essential nutrients should be provided in quantities that support sustained growth in all parameters.

In general, infants weighing less than about 2 kg require special attention with respect to their nutritional needs. Whenever mother's milk is available, it is preferred feeding. When breast-milk is not available, premature infant formulas are the usual choice for infants weighing less than 2 kg; standard formulas are usually the more appropriate choice for larger preterm babies. The decision to change from premature to standard formula will vary in timing depending on such factors as the infant's growth history, energy requirements, volume limitations, and discharge plans. Preterm infants with certain medical problems such as chronic lung disease and short bowel syndrome may require specialized formulas for a longer period of time. Criteria that promote tolerance to enteral feeding are shown in the box below.

Dietary Manipulations

It is occasionally desirable to increase the energy content of the formulas fed to small infants. This may be appropriate when the infant is not growing at a desirable rate and is already ingesting a maximum volume of fluid.

**Criteria that Promote Tolerance
to Initial Enteral Feedings**

1. Nutrient composition that is readily digestible and absorbable
2. Whey/casein 60:40
3. Low renal solute load
4. Iso-osmolality (300 mOsm/kg water)

From O'Leary, M.J.: Nutritional care of the low birth weight infant. In Krause, M.V., and Mahan, L.K., editors: Food, nutrition, and diet therapy, ed. 7, Philadelphia, 1984, W.B. Saunders Co.

Concentration of formulas. One approach to providing hypercaloric formulas is to subtract water, thereby concentrating all nutrients, including energy. Concentrated infant formulas (24 kcal/oz or more) are available to hospitals as ready-to-feed nursettes. When using such concentrated formulas, however, it is important to consider the infant's fluid intake and fluid losses in relation to the renal solute load of the concentrated feeding to ensure that positive water balance is maintained.[259]

Caloric supplements. Another approach to increasing the energy content of formulas fed to preterm infants is the use of caloric supplements such as medium-chain triglyceride oil (Mead Johnson) and glucose polymers such as Polycose (Ross Laboratories). These supplements increase the caloric density without marked alterations in solute load or osmolality; however, they do alter the relative distribution of total calories from protein, carbohydrate, and fat. Because adding even small amounts of medium-chain triglyceride oil or Polycose adversely dilutes the percentage of protein calories while altering the percentage of calories from fat and carbohydrate, adding these supplements to human milk or standard 20 kcal/oz formula is not advised.

When a high-energy formula is needed first add appropriate amounts of medium-chain triglyceride oil to a 24 kcal/oz base (either full-strength premature infant formula or a concentrated standard formula), to a maximum of 60% of total calories as fat and a minimum of 7% of total calories as protein. If more energy is needed for sustained growth, glucose polymers may then be added. When preterm infants who weigh more than 2 kg are given fat and carbohydrate supplements, these are usually given in the form of common vegetable oil and table sugar. Unless these infants have a particular problem with fat absorption or osmotic load, more specialized caloric supplements are usually unnecessary.

Table 12-20   Composition of human milk, premature infant formulas, and standard formulas

		Protein		Carbohydrate	
	Caloric density	Whey/ Casein	Total Calories (%)	Type	Total Calories (%)
Human milk					
Mature	20 kcal/oz (0.67 kcal/ml)	60:40	7	Lactose	38
Premature	22 kcal/oz (0.73 kcal/ml)	60:40		Lactose	
Premature infant formulas					
Similac Special Care	24 kcal/oz (0.81 kcal/ml)	60:40	11	Lactose/ glucose polymers 50:50	42
Premature Enfamil	24 kcal/oz	60:40	12	40:60	42
Premie SMA	24 kcal/oz	60:40	10	50:50	42
Standard formula					
Similac	20 kcal/oz	18:82	9	Lactose	43
SMA	20 kcal/oz	60:40	9	Lactose	41-43
Enfamil	20 kcal/oz	60:40	9	Lactose	41

Table 12-20,   *cont'd.*

	Type	Fat Total Calories (%)	Calcium (mg/L)	Phosphorus (mg/L)	Renal (mOsm/L)	Gastrointestinal (mOsm/kg H$_2$O)
Human milk						
Mature	Human milk fat	55	340	169	75	300
Premature	Human milk fat		293	134		300
Premature infant formulas						
Similac Special Care	MCT/soy/ coconut 50:30:20	47	1462	731	162	300
Premature Enfamil	40:40:20	44	950	470	220	300
Premie SMA	Coconut/ safflower/ oleo/soy/ MCT 27:25: 20:18:10	48	750	400	175	300
Standard formula						
Similac	Coconut and soy oils	48	510 520	390 438	110-120	285
SMA	Corn coconut, and/or soy, oleo safflower oils	48-51	420	310	105	250
Enfamil	Coconut and soy oils		460	345	97	285

From O'Leary, M.J.: Nutritional care of the low birth weight infant. In Krause, M.V., and Mahan, L.K., editors: Food, nutrition, and diet therapy, ed. 7, Philadelphia, 1984, W.B. Saunders Co. Data updated: 1988.

Vitamin and Mineral Supplementation

The vitamin and mineral requirements of preterm infants are not precisely known. Estimates (called advisable intakes) take into account intrauterine accretion rates, full-term infants' needs, and the unique physiological demands of LBW infants. Although these advisable intakes lack precision, they do serve as guidelines until more precise empirical data are available. Ziegler, Biga, and Fomon[7] have reported advisable intakes for vitamins and minerals by premature infants. Table 12-21 compares the vitamin recommendations for preterm versus full-term babies.

Multivitamin supplementation for preterm infants is sometimes recommended. The type, quantity, and frequency of supplementation vary with individual body weight and predominant feeding (Table 12-22). Preterm infants who weigh less than 2000 gm and are fed Similac Special Care (Ross Laboratories) or Enfamil Premature (Mead Johnson) formulas do not need an additional multivitamin supplement because the concentrations of vitamins in these formulas are already sufficient to meet preterm needs.

Oral vitamin and mineral supplementation should be delayed until the infant has tolerated full-strength formula or breast-milk for at least 48 hours at a volume sufficient to provide calories for both maintenance and growth. Because common liquid vitamin preparations have very high osmolarities, it is suggested that the supplements be administered in divided doses and mixed with the iso-osmolar milk before feeding. This minimizes the possible adverse effects of vitamin supplementation, such as increased gastric residuals and regurgitation.

Table 12-21 Advisable intakes of vitamins for preterm and full-term infants

Vitamin	Preterm	Full-Term (Up to 12 Months)
Vitamin A (IU)	500	500
Vitamin D (IU)	600	400
Vitamin E (IU)	30	4
Vitamin K (μg)	15	15
Vitamin C (mg)	60	20
Thiamine (mg)	0.2	0.2
Riboflavin (mg)	0.4	0.4
Niacin (mg)	5	5
B$_6$ (mg)	0.4	1.5
B$_{12}$ (μg)	1.5	—
Folic acid (μg)	60	50
Pantothenic acid (mg)	2	—
Biotin (μg)	12	—

From Ziegler, E.E., Biga, R.L., and Fomon, S.J.: Nutritional requirements of the premature infant. In Suskind, R.M., editors: Textbook of pediatric nutrition. New York, Copyright, 1981, Raven Press.

CASE 3

Infant John was a 30-week-gestation baby who weighed 1080 gm at birth. He was admitted to the neonatal intensive care unit with severe respiratory disease; although he was weaned from the ventilator by 4 weeks of age, he developed chronic lung disease and continued to require oxygen by hood. After $2\frac{1}{2}$ weeks of total parenteral nutrition through an umbilical arterial catheter, John's respiratory status was stable enough to permit the introduction of enteral feeds. Premature formula feedings were initiated at full strength, but in small amounts, and John was gradually weaned from the hyperalimentation solution to a regimen of complete enteral nutrition by 36 weeks of gestational age (still 4 weeks before due date). At that time he weighed 1360 gm and received 17 ml of 24 kcal/oz premature infant formula every 2 hours. This provided a total enteral volume of 150 ml/kg/day and a total caloric intake of 120 kcal/kg/day. Vitamin supplements in addition to the particular premature formula product were not needed; however, iron supplementation was started after John was tolerating full enteral volume and had reached 37 weeks of gestational age. Daily measurements of body weight and weekly measure-

Table 12-22 Suggested schedule for vitamin-mineral supplementation based on body weight and predominant feeding

| Type of Supplement | Human Milk | Premature Formulas | | | Standard Formulas |
		Similac Special Care (Ross)	Enfamil Premature (Mead Johnson)	Premie SMA (Wyeth)	Similac, Enfamil, SMA
Less than 1.8 to 2 gm infant					
Premature vitamin compound*		←——— No ———→		Yes	Usually not fed to infants less than 1.8-2 kg
Human milk fortifier	Yes				
Iron ‡	← Prematures: yes, when (1) body weight has doubled,————————→ and/or (2) infant is 2 weeks to 2 months of age				
More than 1.8 to 2 gm infant					
Standard multivitamin compound†		← Usually not fed to infants more than → 1.8 to 2 kg			Yes†
Human milk fortifier	No				
Iron	← Prematures: yes, when (1) body weight has doubled,→ and/or (2) infant is 2 weeks to 2 months of age				No, if receiving formula with iron.

* In-house preparation based on Ziegler's advisable intakes for prematures. (0.6 cc t.i.d)
† 1 ml per day for infants who ingest less than 0.5 ml per day of standard formula; 0.5 ml per day for infants who ingest more than 0.5 L but less than 1 L per day. Infants who consume about 1 L of standard formula per day do not need additional vitamin supplementation.
‡ If Similac Special Care with Iron (Ross Laboratories) is fed, then additional iron supplementation is unnecessary.

ments of occipital frontal circumference and length were plotted on a growth grid on an age-corrected basis. During the next 2 weeks, bolus feedings were increased as the infant grew to maintain a total enteral volume of 150 ml/kg/day and a caloric intake of 120 kcal/kg/day. However, John failed to grow at an adequate rate, and his growth curves were slow as compared with the reference curves on the growth grid. John was a fussy baby with chronic lung dis-

ease, and he obviously expended considerable energy in his labored effort to breathe. Furthermore, John received theophylline (a medication that increases basal metabolic rate). Because of John's high energy expenditure and his extra energy needs for catch-up growth, it was decided to increase his total caloric intake. Volume was limited to 150 ml/kg/day; thus it was decided to add medium-chain triglyceride oil and glucose polymers to the formula to achieve a total caloric intake of 140 kcal/kg/day. John tolerated this modification of the formula and his rate of growth increased. By 16 weeks of age, John's age-corrected growth curves were approaching the 50th percentile of the reference curves and the rate of gain was beginning to taper off. The caloric density of his formula was gradually decreased to 24 kcal/oz. John continued to be followed by regular anthropometric measurements to ensure that his energy and nutrient intake adequately met his needs for normal growth and development.

NUTRITIONAL ASSESSMENT

Growth

All neonates typically lose some weight after birth. This is particularly true for LBW infants who are born with more extracellular water than full-term infants and who may benefit from some degree of fluid loss. However, postnatal weight loss should not be excessive. LBW infants who lose more than about 15% to 20% of their birth weight can be expected to suffer from dehydration as a result of inadequate fluid intake or tissue wasting as a result of poor energy intake. During the first month after birth, the growth grid of Dancis, O'Connell, and Holt[260] is commonly used to assess weight progress. This grid has the advantages of depicting daily weight changes and actual growth curves; disadvantages include a small sample size to generate growth data that are now about 40 years old. The curves should not, therefore, be interpreted to represent optimal growth, particularly for VLBW infants in modern neonatal intensive care units. Although very sick infants who weigh less than 1000 grams may have growth curves similar to those reported by Dancis[260] for that weight group, larger infants who are clinically stable and who are predominantly fed by mouth are able to achieve rates of weight gain more rapidly than of those reported 40 years ago.[262]

Intrauterine growth curves have also been developed using birth weight data of infants born at successive weeks of gestation.[261] These curves do not depict the initial period of postnatal weight loss and are probably unrealistic goals for VLBW infants in the early neonatal period. Once the infant's condition stabilizes and full nutrient intake is possible, many infants are able to grow at a rate that parallels these curves (i.e., gain of 20 to 30 gm/day).

As soon as preterm infants have regained their birth weight and are starting to grow, it is very important to begin weekly measurement of body length and head circumference. Length measurements should be made by two trained persons using an appropriate lengthboard in order to achieve measurements that are both accurate and precise. Reliable growth data must be available in order to make appropriate judgements regarding the adequacy of an infant's growth progress.

Two growth grids are available that depict growth in weight, length, and head circumference for infants between 28 weeks gestational age and 1 to 2 years corrected age.[263,264] These grids were both published in the early 1970s and are based on data collected before or during the 1960s. Neither of these grids should be regarded as a growth standard, since the data source is about 30 years old and the curves are drawn from cross-sectional birth weight data (less than 40 weeks of gestation),[263,264] and from data of studies on full-term infants.[264] However, since reference growth curves for preterm infants based on a large sample of longitudinal data are not yet available, these two grids are still useful. The grids for full-term infants from birth to 3 years of age from the National Center for Health Statistics (refer to pp. 18–20 in Chapter 1) can also be used for preterm infants after 40 weeks gestation, as long as age is corrected (or adjusted) for prematurity. For example, at 3 months postnatal age, the growth parameters of a premature infant born at 32 weeks of gestation can be compared with those of a 1-month baby born at term. When using growth grids, age should be adjusted for prematurity until at least 1 to 2 years corrected age.

Laboratory Indices

Several laboratory measurements have been used as indicators of nutritional status in children and adults. However, these measurements are difficult to interpret in premature infants. Reference ranges for most laboratory parameters based on data from studies on healthy, enterally fed preterm infants are not yet available. At present, laboratory indices are primarily used to evaluate the nutritional status of preterm infants who receive parenteral nutrition.

NEURODEVELOPMENTAL OUTCOME

From the preceding discussion it is apparent that we are now able to meet the metabolic and nutritional needs of premature and LBW infants in a manner sufficient to sustain life and to promote growth and development. With adequate nutritional support and recent advances in neonatal intensive care technology, more tiny, immature infants are surviving than ever before. Survival for infants of 1001 to 1500 gm birth weight improved significantly during the 1970s.[265] During this same period, survival rates nearly doubled for extremely small babies of 501 to 1000 gm birth weight.[265] Since the mid 1970s, there has been a dramatic and continuing reduction in neonatal mortality, particularly for VLBW infants. More infants born very early in gestation are surviving to be discharged home than was the case even in the early 1980s.[266]

With increased survival of VLBW infants, there is increased concern for the short- and long-term neurodevelopmental outcome for these babies. Many questions are asked about the quality of life awaiting infants who received neonatal intensive care.

Surviving LBW infants, particularly those with birth weights less than 800 gm, have an increased risk of developing central nervous system handicapping conditions of varying severity and functional impairment.[263] The neurodevelopmental outcome of LBW infants has been recently summarized by Bennett.[266] But in spite of this risk, the majority of these premature babies reach school age without evidence of any disability (Figure 12-6). It is not always apparent which infants will be undamaged and which will suffer major or minor handicapping conditions. The sometimes poor correlation, in an individual case, between neonatal course and developmental outcome makes neonatal survival decisions extremely difficult. All premature and LBW infants merit

Figure 12-6 Same child as in Figure 12-5. Here she is a healthy $2\frac{1}{2}$-year-old.

personalized and sensitive screening and assessment, with intervention strategies employed as appropriate.

Summary

Both parenteral and enteral nutrition can be effective in nourishing premature and LBW infants. The selection of one technique over another and the choice of specific nutritional goals should follow general guidelines such as those suggested in this chapter. However, these guidelines must be flexible to accommodate the range of individual variation. Clinical judgment of the unique needs of a particular infant may warrant a more tailored approach.

SUGGESTED LEARNING ACTIVITIES

1. Review the chart of an infant in a neonatal intensive care unit who is receiving total parenteral nutrition. Describe the conditions that made total parenteral nutrition the appropriate method of feeding. Calculate the energy and nutrient intake for the past 24 hours.
2. Describe how the transition is made from total parenteral nutrition to enteral feeding in a premature infant.
3. Discuss the advantages and potential problems of human milk as the sole feeding for a premature infant.
4. Describe differences in commercially prepared formulas for full-term infants and those for premature infants.
5. Describe appropriate vitamin supplementation for the premature infant on enteral feedings.
6. Investigate the long-term prognosis for growth and development of premature and low birth weight babies.

REFERENCES

1. Committee on Perinatal Health: Toward improving the outcome of pregnancy, New York, 1976, The National Foundation–March of Dimes.
2. Committee on Fetus and Newborn: Guidelines for perinatal care, Evanston, Ill., 1983, American Academy of Pediatrics; and Washington, D.C., 1983, American College of Obstetricians and Gynecologists.
3. Committee on Fetus and Newborn, American Academy of Pediatrics: Level II neonatal units, Pediatrics 66:810, 1980.
4. Committee on Nutrition of the Mother and Preschool child, Food and Nutrition Board: Nutrition services in perinatal care, Washington, D.C., 1981, Assembly of Life Sciences, National Research Council.
5. Poole, R. L., and Kerner, J. A., Jr.: Establishing a nutrition support team for an intensive care nursery, Nutr. Support Serv. 3:35, 1983.
6. Dubowitz, L. M. S., and others: Clinical assessment of gestational age in the newborn infant, J. Pediatr. 77:1, 1970.
7. Ziegler, E. E., Biga, R. L., and Fomon, S. J.: Nutritional requirements of the premature infant. In Suskind, R. M., editor: Textbook of pediatric nutrition, New York, 1981, Raven Press.
8. Widdowson, E. M.: Growth and composition of the fetus and newborn. In Assali, N. S., editor: Biology of gestation, vol. II, New York, 1968, Academic Press, Inc.
9. Heird, W. C., and others: Intravenous alimentation in pediatric patients, J. Pediatr. 80:351, 1972.
10. Doelkel, R. D., and others: Clinical semistarvation: depression of hypoxic ventilatory response, N. Engl. J. Med. 295:358, 1976.
11. Chandra, R. K.: Immunodeficiency in undernutrition and overnutrition, Nutr. Rev. 39:225, 1981.
12. Abel, R. M., and others: Malnutrition in cardiac surgery patients, Arch. Surg. 111:45, 1976.
13. Dobbing, J.: The later growth of the brain and its vulnerability, Pediatrics 53:2, 1974.
14. Rosso, P., Hormazabal, J., and Winick, M.: Changes in brain weight, cholesterol, phospholipid, and DNA content in marasmic children, Am. J. Clin. Nutr. 23:1275, 1970.
15. Dudrick, S. J., Wilmore, D. W., and Vars, H. M.: Long-term total parenteral nutrition with growth in puppies and positive nitrogen balance in patients, Surg. Forum, 18:356, 1967.
16. Dudrick, S. J., and others: Long-term total parenteral nutrition with growth, development, and positive nitrogen balance, Surgery 64:134, 1968.
17. Ziegler, M., and others: Route of pediatric parenteral nutrition: proposed criteria revision, J. Pediatr. Surg. 15:472, 1980.
18. Kerner, J. A., Jr.: Indications for parenteral nutrition in pediatrics. In Kerner, J. A., Jr., editor: Manual of pediatric parenteral nutrition, New York, 1983, John Wiley & Sons, Inc.

19. Jewett, T. C., Jr., and Lebenthal, E.: Recent advances in gastrointestinal tract surgery in children. In Gluck, L., editor: Current problems in pediatrics, vol. 9, Chicago, 1978, Year Book Medical Publishers, Inc.

20. Dudrick, S. J., Copeland, E. M., III, and MacFadyen, B. V., Jr.: Long-term parenteral nutrition: its current status, Hosp. Pract. 10:47, 1975.

21. Firor, H. V.: Technical improvements in the management of omphalocele and gastroschisis, Surg. Clin. North Am. 55:129, 1975.

22. Stohert, J. C., Jr., and others: Esophageal atresia and tracheosophageal fistula: preoperative assessment and reduced mortality, Ann. Thorac. Surg. 28:54, 1979.

23. Heird, W. C., and Winters, R. W.: Parenteral nutrition in pediatrics. In Schneider, H. A., Anderson, C. E., and Cowisin, D. B., editors: Nutritional support of medical practice, New York, 1977, Harper & Row, Publishers, Inc.

24. Filler, R. M.: Parenteral support of the surgically ill child. In Suskind, R. M., editor: Textbook of pediatric nutrition, New York, 1981, Raven Press.

25. Sunshine, P., Sinatra, F. R., and Mitchell, C. H.: Intractable diarrhea of infancy, Clin. Gastroenterol. 6:445, 1977.

26. Gryboski, J., and Walker, W. A.: Parenteral nutrition. In Gryboski, J., and Walker, W. A., editors: Gastrointestinal problems in the infant, Philadelphia, 1983, W. B. Saunders Co.

27. Ziegler, E. E.: Nutritional management of the premature infant, Perinatology-Neonatology, p. 11, July/Aug., 1985.

28. Sinclair, J., and others: Supportive management of the sick neonate: parenteral calories, water and electrolytes, Pediatr. Clin. North Am. 17:863, 1970.

29. Cashore, W. J., Sedaghatian, J. R., and Usher, R. H.: Nutritional supplements with intravenously administered lipid, protein hydrolyzate, and glucose in small premature infants, Pediatrics 56:88, 1975.

30. Mestyan, J., Jarai, I., and Fekete, M.: The total energy expenditure and its components in premature infants maintained under different nursing and environmental conditions, Pediatr. Res. 2:161, 1968.

31. Anderson, T.L., and others: A controlled trial of glucose versus glucose and amino acids in premature infants, J. Pediatr. 94:115, 1981.

32. Zlotkin, S. H., Bryan, M. H., and Anderson, G. H.: Intravenous nitrogen and energy intakes required to duplicate in utero nitrogen accretion in prematurely born human infants, J. Pediatr. 99:115, 1981.

33. Kerner, J. A., Jr.: Caloric requirements. In Kerner, J. A., Jr., editor: Manual of pediatric parenteral nutrition, New York, 1983, John Wiley & Sons, Inc.

34. Kerner, J. A., Jr., editor: Manual of pediatric parenteral nutrition, New York, 1983, John Wiley & Sons, Inc.

35. Lebenthal, E., editor: Total Parenteral Nutrition, New York, 1986, Raven Press.

36. Kerner, J. A., Jr.: Fluid requirements. In Kerner J. A., Jr., editor: Manual of pediatric parenteral nutrition, New York, 1983, John Wiley & Sons, Inc.

37. Fanaroff, M., and others: Insensible water loss in low-birth-weight infants, Pediatrics 50:236, 1972.

38. Oh, W.: Fluid and electrolyte management. In Avery, G. B., editor: Neonatology, pathophysiology, and management of the newborn, Philadelphia, 1981, J. B. Lippincott Co.

39. Friis-Hansen, B.: Changes in body water compartments during growth, Acta Paediatr. Scand. (suppl. 110) 46:1, 1957.

40. Bell, E. F., and Oh, W.: Water requirement of premature newborn infants, Acta Paediatr. Scand. Suppl. 305:21, 1983.

41. Hodson, W. A., and Truog, W. E.: Parenteral nutrition. In Hodson, W. A., and Truog, W. A., editors: Critical care of the newborn, Philadelphia, 1983, W. B. Saunders Co.

42. Wu, P. Y. K., and Hodgman, J. E.: Insensible water loss in premature infants, Pediatrics 54:704, 1974.

43. Oh, W., and Karechi, H.: Phototherapy and insensible water loss in the newborn infant, Ann. J. Dis. Child. 124:230, 1972.

44. Marks, K. A., Friedman, Z., and Maisels, M. J.: A simple device for reducing insensible water loss in LBW infants, Pediatrics 60:223, 1977.

45. Harkavey, K. L.: Water and electrolyte requirements of the very-low-birth-weight infant, Perinatal Press 6:47, 1982.

46. Bell, E. F., and others: Effect of fluid administration on the development of symptomatic patent ductus arteriosus and congestive heart failure in premature infants, N. Engl. J. Med. 302:598, 1980.

47. Stevenson, J. G.: Fluid administration in the association of patent ductus arteriosus complicating distress syndrome, J. Pediatr. 90:257, 1977.

48. Goldberg, R. N., and others: The association of rapid volume expansion and intraventricular hemorrhage in the preterm infant, J. Pediatr. 96:1060, 1980.

49. Brown, E. R., and others: Bronchopulmonary dysplasia: possible relationship to pulmonary edema, J. Pediatr. 92:982, 1978.

50. Friis-Hansen, B.: Water distribution in the fetus and newborn infant, Acta Paediatr. Scand. Suppl. 305:7, 1983.

51. Oh, W., Oh, M. A., and Lind, J.: Renal function and blood volume in newborn infants related to placental transfusion, Acta Paediatr. Scand. 56:197, 1966.

52. Spitzer, A. R., Fox, W. W., and Delivoria-Papadopoulos, M.: Maximum diuresis—a factor in predicting recovery from respiratory distress syndrome and the development of bronchopulmonary dysplasia, J. Pediatr. 98:476, 1981.

53. Miranda, L. E. V., and Dweck, H. S.: Perinatal glucose homeostasis: the unique character of hyperglycemia and hypoglycemia in infants of very-low-birth-weight, Clin. Perinatol. 4:351, 1977.

54. Kerner, J. A., Jr.: Carbohydrate requirements. In Kerner, J. A., Jr., editor: Manual of pediatric parenteral nutrition, New York, 1983, John Wiley & Sons, Inc.

55. Chance, G. W.: Results in very-low-birth-weight infants (<1300 gm birth weight). In Winters, R. W., and Hasselmeyer, E. G., editors: Intravenous nutrition in the high risk infant, New York, 1975, John Wiley & Sons, Inc.

56. Hay, W. W.: Justification for total parenteral nutrition in the premature and compromised newborn. In Lebenthal, E., editor: Total parenteral nutrition, New York, 1986, Raven Press.

57. Hanning, I., and Andronikou, S.: Parenteral nutrition effect on serum insulin in the preterm infant, Pediatrics 80:693, 1987.

58. Jacobs, W. C., Lazzara, A., and Martin, D. J.: Parenteral nutrition in the neonate, Chicago, 1980, Abbott Laboratories, Hospital Products Division.

59. Vaucher, Y. E., Walson, P. D., and Morrow, G., Ill: Continuous insulin infusion in hyperglycemic, very-low-birth-weight infants, J. Pediatr. Gastroenterol Nutr. 1:211, 1982.

60. Pildes, R. S.: Neonatal hyperglycemia, J. Pediatr. 109:905, 1986.

61. Heird, W. C.: Total parenteral nutrition. In Lebenthal, E., editor: Textbook of gastroenterology and nutrition in infancy, New York, 1981, Raven Press.

62. Fischer, J. E.: Parenteral and enteral nutrition, Disease-a-Month 24:23, 1981.

63. Hooley, R. A.: Parenteral nutrition—general concepts. Part II. Nutr. Support Serv. 1:41, 1981.

64. Heird, W. C.: Panel report on nutritional support of pediatric patients, Am. J. Clin. Nutr. 34:1223, 1981.

65. Snyderman, S. E.: The protein and amino acid requirements of the premature infant. In Jonxis, J. H. P., Visser, H. K. A., and Troelstra, J. A., editors: Metabolic process in the fetus and newborn infant, Baltimore, 1971, Williams & Wilkins.

66. Gaull, G. E., and others: Milk protein quantity and quality in low-birth-weight infants. III. Effects on sulfur amino acids in plasma and urine, J. Pediatr. 90:356, 1977.

67. Rassin, D. K., Raiha, N. C. R., and Gaull, G. E.: Protein and taurine nutrition in infants. In Lebenthal,

E., editor: Textbook of gastroenterology and nutrition in infancy, vol. 1, New York, 1981, Raven Press.

68. Seashore, J. H.: Metabolic complications of parenteral nutrition in infants and children, Surg. Clin. North Am. 60:1239, 1980.

69. Heird, W. C., and others: Hyperammonemia resulting from intravenous alimentation using a mixture of synthetic L-amino acids: a preliminary report, J. Pediatr. 81:162, 1972.

70. Poley, J. R.: Liver and nutrition: hepatic complications of total parenteral nutrition. In Lebenthal, E., editor: Textbook of gastroenterology and nutrition in infancy, New York, 1981, Raven Press.

71. Abitbol, C. L., and others: Plasma amino acid patterns during supplemental intravenous nutrition of low-birth-weight infants, J. Pediatr. 86:766, 1975.

72. Kerner, J. A., Jr.: Protein requirements. In Kerner, J. A., Jr., editor: Manual of pediatric parenteral nutrition, New York, 1983, John Wiley & Sons, Inc.

73. Zahavi, I., Shaffer, E. A., and Gall, D. G.: Total parenteral nutrition-associated cholestasis: Acute studies in infant and adult rabbits, J. Pediatr. Gastroenterol. and Nutr. 4:622, 1985.

74. Bucuralas, J. C., and others: Amino acids are potent inhibitors of bile acid uptake by liver plasma membrane vesicles isolated from suckling rats, Pediatr. Res. 19:1298, 1985.

75. Merritt, R. J., and others: Cholestatic effect of intraperitoneal administration of tryptophan to suckling rat pups, Pediatr. Res. 18:904, 1984.

76. Graham, M. F., and others: Inhibition of bile flow in the isolated perfused rat liver by a synthetic parenteral amino acid mixture: Associated net amino acid fluxes, Hepatology 4:69, 1984.

77. Peden, V. H., Witzleben, C. L., and Skelton, M. A.: Total parenteral nutrition: Letter to the Editor, J. Pediatr. 78:180, 1971.

78. Dosi, P. C., and others: Perinatal factors underlying neonatal cholestasis, J. Pediatr. 106:471, 1985.

79. Rager, R., and Finegold, M. J.: Cholestasis in immature newborn infants: is parenteral nutrition responsible? J. Pediatr. 86:264, 1975.

80. Usmani, S. S., and others: Conjugated hyperbilirubinemia (CH): A predictor of perinatal mortality and poor neurological outcome, Pediatr. Res. 18:353 A, 1984.

81. Bell, R. L., and others: Total parenteral nutrition-related cholestasis in infants, J. Parenter. and Enteral Nutr. 10:356, 1986.

82. Balistreri, W. F.: Neonatal cholestasis, J. Pediatr. 106:171, 1985.

83. Merritt, R. J.: Cholestasis associated with total parenteral nutrition, J. Pediatr. Gastroenterol. Nutr. 5:9, 1986.

84. Hornchen, H., and Neubrand, W.: Amino acids for parenteral nutrition in premature and newborn infants, use of mother's milk–adapted solution, J. Parenter. Ent. Nutr. 4:294, 1980.

85. Holt, L. E., Jr., and Snyderman, S. E.: The amino acid requirements of children. In Nyham, W. L., editor: Amino acid metabolism and genetic variation, New York, 1967, McGraw-Hill Book Co.

86. Fomon, S. J., and Filer, L. J., Jr.: Amino acid requirements for normal growth. In Nyham, W. L., editor: Amino acid metabolism and genetic variation, New York, 1967, McGraw-Hill Book Co.

87. Heird, W. C., and others: Pediatric parenteral amino acid mixture in low-birth-weight infants, Pediatr. 81:41, 1988.

88. Anderson, T. L., and others: A controlled trial of glucose versus glucose and amino acids in premature infants, J. Pediatr. 94:947, 1979.

89. Kerner, J. A., Jr.: Fat requirements. In Kerner, J. A., Jr., editor: Manual of pediatric parenteral nutrition, New York, 1983, John Wiley & Sons, Inc.

90. Byrne, W. J.: Intralipid® or Liposyn® — comparable products? J. Pediatr. Gastroenterol. Nutr. 1(1):7, 1982.

91. Cooke, R. J., and Burckhart, G. J.: Hypertriglyceridemia during the intravenous infusion of a safflower oil–based fat emulsion, J. Pediatr. 103:959, 1983.

92. Griffin, E. A., Bryan, M. H., and Angel, A.: Variations in Intralipid tolerance in newborn infants, Pediatr. Res. 17:478, 1983.

93. Berkow, S. E., and others: TPN with Intralipid in premature infants receiving TPN with Heparin. J. Pediatr. Gastroenterol. Nutr. 6:581, 1987.

94. Zaidan, H., and others: Effect of continuous heparin administration on Intralipid clearing in very-low-birth-weight infants, J. Pediatr. 101:599, 1982.

95. Zaidan, H., and others: Lipid clearing in premature infants during continuous heparin infusion: Role of circulating lipases, Pediatr. Res. 19:23, 1985.

96. Spear, M. L., and others: Effect of heparin dose and infusion rate on lipid clearance and bilirubin binding in premature infants receiving IV fat emulsions, J. Pediatr. 112:94, 1988.

97. Spear, M. L., and others: The effect of fifteen hour fat infusions of varying dosage on bilirubin binding to albumin, J. Parenter. Ent. Nutr. 9:144, 1985.

98. Penn, D., and others: Effect of nutrition on tissue carnitine concentrations in infants of different gestational ages, Biol. Neonate 47:130, 1985.

99. Yu-Yan Yeh, Cooke, R. J., and Zee, P.: Impairment of lipid emulsion metabolism associated with carnitine insufficiency in premature infants, J. Pediatr. Gastroenterol. Nutr. 4:495, 1985.

100. Orzali, A., and others: Effect of carnitine on lipid metabolism in the newborn, Biol. Neonate 43:146, 1983.

101. Orzali, A., and others: Effect of carnitine on lipid metabolism in the neonate. II. Carnitine addition to lipid infusion during prolonged total parenteral nutrition, J. Pediatr. 104:436, 1984.

102. Schmidt-Sommerfeld, E., Penn, D., and Wolf, H.: Carnitine deficiency in premature infants receiving total parenteral nutrition: effect of L-carnitine supplementation, J. Pediatr. 102:931, 1983.

103. Helms, R. A., and others: Enhanced lipid utilization in infants receiving oral L-carnitine during long-term parenteral nutrition, J. Pediatr. 109:984, 1986.

104. Holman, R. T.: Essential fatty acid deficiency. In Holman, R. T., editor: Progress in the chemistry of fats and other lipids, vol. 9, Elmsford, New York, 1968, Pergamon Press, Inc.

105. Friedman, Z., and others: Rapid onset of essential fatty acid deficiency in the newborn, Pediatrics 58:640, 1976.

106. Cooke, R. J., Zee, P., and Yeh, Y-Y.: Essential fatty acid status of the premature infant during short-term fat-free parenteral nutrition, J. Pediatr. Gastroenterol. Nutr. 3:446, 1984.

107. Levy, J. S., Winters, R. W., and Heird, W. C.: Total parenteral nutrition in pediatric patients, Pediatr. Rev. 2:99, 1980.

108. Hunt, C. E., and others: Essential fatty acid deficiency in neonates: inability to reverse deficiency by topical application of EFA rich oil, J. Pediatr. 92:603, 1978.

109. Dolcourt, J.: Pediatric parenteral nutrition manual, Salt Lake City, 1983, Primary Children's Medical Center.

110. American Academy of Pediatrics, Committee on Nutrition: Nutritional needs of low-birth-weight infants, Pediatr. 75:976, 1985.

111. Gustafson, A., and others: Nutrition in low-birth-weight infants. II. Repeated intravenous injections of fat emulsion, Acta Paediatr. Scand. 63:177, 1974.

112. Schreiner, R. L., and others: An evaluation of methods to monitor infants receiving intravenous lipids, J. Pediatr. 94:197, 1979.

113. American Academy of Pediatrics, Committee on Nutrition: Use of intravenous fat emulsions in pediatric patients, Pediatr. 68:738, 1981.

114. Stunk, R. C., and others: Normal macrophage function in infants receiving Intralipid by low-dose intermittent administration, J. Pediatr. 106:640, 1985.

115. Usmani, S. S., and others: In vitro effect of Intralipid on polymorphonuclear leucocyte function in the neonate, J. Pediatr. 109:710, 1986.

116. Padel, S., Shor, R., and Passwell, J. H.: Effect of Intralipid on the phagocytic and microbicidal capacity of human monocytes in culture, J. Pediatr. Gastroenterol. Nutr. 6:575, 1987.

117. Starinsky, R., and Shafir, E.: Displacement of albumin-bound bilirubin by free fatty acids: implications for neonatal hyperbilirubinemia, Clin. Chim. Acta 29:311, 1970.

118. Kerner, J. A., Jr., and others: Monitoring intravenous fat emulsions in neonates with fatty acid/serum albumin molar ratio, J. Parenter. Ent. Nutr. 5:517, 1981.

119. Andrew, G., Chan, G., and Schiff, D.: Lipid metabolism in the neonate. II. The effect of Intralipid on bilirubin binding in vitro and in vivo, J. Pediatr. 88:279, 1976.

120. Hertel, J., Tygstrup, I., and Anderson, G. E.: Intravascular fat accumulation after Intralipid infusion in the very low-birth-weight infant, J. Pediatr. 100:975, 1982.

121. Dahms, B., and Halpin, T. C.: Pulmonary arterial lipid deposit in newborn infants receiving intravenous lipid infusion, J. Pediatr. 97:800, 1980.

122. Schulman, R. J., Langston, C., and Schanler, R. J.: Pulmonary vascular lipid deposition after administration of intravenous fat to infants, Pediatr. 79:99, 1987.

123. Pereira, G. R., and others: Decreased oxygenation and hyperlipemia during intravenous fat infusions in premature infants, Pediatrics 66:26, 1980.

124. Adamkin, D. H., Gelke, K. N., and Wilkerson, S. A.: Influence of IV fat therapy on tracheal effluent phospholipids and oxygenation in severe respiratory distress syndrome, J. Pediatr. 106:122, 1985.

125. Lloyd, T. R., and Boucek, M. M.: Effect of Intralipid on the neonatal pulmonary bed: An echographic study, J. Pediatr. 108:130, 1986.

126. Friedman, Z., and Rosenberg, A.: Abnormal lung surfactant related to essential fatty acid deficiency in a neonate, Pediatr. 69:855, 1979.

127. Askanazi, J., and others: Nutrition for the patient with respiratory failure: glucose vs. fat, Anesthesiology 54:373, 1981.

128. Askanazi, J., and others: Effect of total parenteral nutrition on gas exchange and breathing patterns, Crit. Care Med. 7:125, 1979.

129. Buzby, G. P., and others: Manipulation of TPN caloric substrate and fatty infiltration of the liver, J. Surg. Res. 31:46, 1981.

130. Poole, R.L.: Electrolyte and mineral requirements. In Kerner, J. A., Jr., editor: Manual of pediatric parenteral nutrition, New York, 1983, John Wiley & Sons, Inc.

131. Committee on Nutrition, American Academy of Pediatrics: Sodium intake of infants in the United States, Pediatrics 68:444, 1981.

132. Kerner, J. A., Jr., and Sunshine, P.: Parenteral alimentation, Semin. Perinatol. 3:417, 1979.

133. Kerner, J. A., Jr.: Metabolic complications. In Kerner, J. A., Jr., editor: Manual of pediatric parenteral nutrition, New York, 1983, John Wiley & Sons, Inc.

134. Leape, L. L., and Valaes, T.: Rickets in low-birth-weight infants receiving total parenteral nutrition, J. Pediatr. Surg. 11:665, 1976.

135. Winslow, C., and others: Rickets in very-low-birth-weight infants: growth exceeding mineral intake, Clin. Res. 28:897A, 1980.

136. Ziegler, E. E., and others: Body composition of the reference fetus. Growth 40:329, 1976.

137. Atkinson, S. A.: Calcium and phosphorus requirements of low birth weight infants: a nutritional and endocrinological perspective, Nutr. Rev. 41:69, 1983.

138. Chersex, P., and others: Calciuria in parenterally fed preterm infants: role of phosphorus intake, J. Pediatr. 107:794, 1985.

139. Eggert, L. D., and others: Calcium and phosphorus compatibility in parenteral nutrition solutions for neonates, Am. J. Hosp. Pharm. 39:49, 1982.

140. Poole, R., Ryp, C., and Kerner, J. A., Jr.: Calcium and phosphorus in neonatal TPN solutions, J. Parenter. Ent. Nutr. 5:580, 1981.

141. Venkataraman, P. S., Brissie, E. O., and Tsang, R. C.: Stability of calcium and phosphorus in neonatal parenteral nutrition solutions, J. Pediatr. Gastroenterol. Nutr. 2:640, 1983.

142. Poole, R. S.: Problems with preparation of parenteral nutrition solutions. In Kerner, J. A., Jr.: Manual of pediatric parenteral nutrition, New York, 1983, John Wiley & Sons, Inc.

143. Knight, P. J., Buchanan, S., and Clatworthy, W.: Calcium and phosphate requirements of preterm infants who require hyperalimentation. J. A. M. A. 243:1244, 1980.

144. Hoehn, G. J., and others: Alternate day infusions of calcium and phosphate in very low birth weight infants: wasting of the infused mineral. J. Pediatr. Gastroenterol. Nutr. 6:752, 1987.

145. Koo, W. W. K., and others: Parenteral nutrition for infants: effect of high versus low calcium and phosphorus content, J. Pediatr. Gastroenterol. Nutr. 6:96, 1987.

146. American Medical Association, Department of Foods and Nutrition: Multivitamin preparations for parenteral use; a statement by the Nutrition Advisory Group, J. Parent. Ent. Nutr. 3:258, 1979.

147. Kerner, J. A., Jr.: Vitamin requirements. In Kerner, J. A., Jr., editor: Manual of pediatric parenteral nutrition, New York, 1983, John Wiley & Sons, Inc.

148. Moorhatch, P., and Chiou, W. L.: Interaction between drugs and plastic intravenous fluid bags, Am. J. Hosp. Pharm. 31:149, 1974.

149. Howard, L., and others: Vitamin A deficiency from long-term parenteral nutrition, Ann. Int. Med. 93:576, 1980.

150. Bhaka, J., Mims, L. C., and Roesel, R. A.: The effect of phototherapy on amino acid solutions containing multivitamins, J. Pediatr. 96:284, 1980.

151. Greene, H. L.: Vitamins in total parenteral nutrition, Drug Intell. Clin. Pharm. 6:355, 1972.

152. Nutrition Advisory Group: Guidelines for multivitamin preparation for parenteral use. Chicago, 1975, American Medical Association. Reprinted in J. Parenter. Ent. Nutr. 3:260, 1979.

153. Moore, M. C., and others: Evaluation of a pediatric multiple vitamin preparation for total parenteral nutrition in infants and children. I. Blood levels of water soluble vitamins, Pediatr. 77:530, 1986.

154. Greene, H. L., and others: Evaluation of a pediatric multiple vitamin preparation for total parenteral nutrition. II. Blood levels of vitamins A, D, and E, Pediatr. 77:539, 1986.

155. MacDonald, M. G., and others: The potential toxicity to neonates of multivitamin preparations used in parenteral nutrition. J. Parenter. Ent. Nutr. 11:169, 1987.

156. Green, H. L., and Phillips, B. L.: Vitamin dosages for premature infants: reply to letter to editor, Pediatr. 81:173, 1988.

157. Kerner, J. A., and others: High serum vitamin E levels in premature infants receiving MVI-pediatric. J. Pediatr. Perinatol. Nutr. 1:75, 1987.

158. Phillips, B., Franck, L. S., and Greene, H. L.: Vitamin E levels in premature infants during and after intravenous multivitamin supplementation, Pediatr. 80:680, 1987.

159. Johnson, L., and others: Relationship of prolonged pharmacologic levels of vitamin E to incidence of sepsis and necrotizing enterocolitis in infants with birth weight 1,500 gm or less, Pediatr. 75:619, 1985.

160. Sokol, R. J., and others: Frequency and clinical progression of the vitamin E deficiency neurologic disorder in children with prolonged neonatal cholestasis, Am. J. Dis. Ch. 139:1211, 1985.

161. Alvarez, F., and others: Vitamin E deficiency is responsible for neurologic abnormalities in cholestatic children, J. Pediatr. 107:422, 1985.

162. Kerner, J. A., Jr.: Trace element requirements. In Kerner, J. A., Jr., editor: Manual of pediatric parenteral nutrition, New York, 1983, John Wiley & Sons, Inc.

163. Nutrition Advisory Group, American Medical Association, Department of Foods and Nutrition: Guidelines for essential trace element preparations for parenteral use, J. A. M. A. 241:2051, 1979.

164. Zlotkin, S. H., and Buchanan, B. E.: Meeting zinc and copper intake requirements in the parenterally fed preterm and full-term infant, J. Pediatr. 103:441, 1983.

165. Casey, C. E., and Hambidge, K. M.: Trace minerals. In Tsang, R. C., editor: Vitamin and mineral requirements in preterm infants. New York, 1985, Marcel Dekker, Inc.

166. Amin, S., and others: Selenium in premature infants, Nutr. Metab. 24:331, 1980.

167. Wan, K. K., and Tsallas, G.: Dilute iron dextran formulation for addition to parenteral nutrition solutions, Am. J. Hosp. Pharm. 37:106, 1980.

168. Kerner, J. A., Jr.: The transition from parenteral to enteral feedings. In Kerner, J. A., Jr., editor: Manual of pediatric parenteral nutrition, New York, 1983, John Wiley & Sons, Inc.

169. Feldman, E. J., and others: Effects of oral and venous nutrition on intestinal adaptation after small bowel resection in the dog, Gastroenterology 70:712, 1976.

170. Kotler, D. P., and Levine, G. M.: Reversible gastric and pancreatic hyposecretion after long-term total parenteral nutrition, N. Engl. J. Med. 300:241, 1979.

171. Greene, H.L., and others: Comparison of the adaptive changes in disaccharidase, glycolytic enzyme and fructose diphosphatase activities after intravenous and oral glucose in normal men, Am. J. Clin. Nutr. 28:1122, 1975.

172. Alpers, D. H.: Protein synthesis in intestinal mucosa: the effect of route of administration of precursor amino acids, J. Clin. Invest. 51:167, 1972.

173. Heird, W. C.: Nutritional support of the pediatric patient. In Winters, R. W., and Greene, H. L., editors: Nutritional support of the seriously ill patient, New York, 1983, Academic Press.

174. Brady, M. S., Gresham, E. L., and Rickard, K.: Nutritional care of the low-birth-weight infant requiring intensive care, Perinatal Press 2:125, 1978.

175. American Academy of Pediatrics, Committee on Nutrition: Nutritional needs of low-birth-weight infants, Pediatr. 75:976, 1985.

176. Lebenthal, E., Lee, P. C., and Heitlinger, L. A.: Impact of development of the gastrointestinal tract on infant feedings, J. Pediatr. 102:1, 1983.

177. Feinstein, M. S., and Smith, C. A.: Digestion of protein by premature infants, Pediatrics 7:19, 1951.

178. Ziegler, E. E., and others: Body composition of the reference fetus, Growth 40:329, 1976.
179. Gross, S. J., and others: Growth and biochemical response of premature infants fed human milk or modified infant formula, N. Engl. J. Med. 308:237, 1983.
180. Raiha, N. C. R., and others: Milk protein quantity and quality in low-birth-weight infants. I. Metabolic responses and effects on growth, Pediatrics 57:659, 1976.
181. Fomon, S. J., and Ziegler, E. E.: Protein intake of premature infants: interpretation of data, J. Pediatr. 90:504, 1977.
182. Rassin, D. K., and others: Milk protein quantity and quality in low-birth-weight infants. II. Effects of selected alphatic amino acids in plasma and urine. Pediatrics 59:407, 1977.
183. Gaull, G. E., and others: Milk protein quantity and quality in low-birth-weight infants: III. Effects on sulfur amino acids in plasma and urine, J. Pediatr. 90:348, 1977.
184. Rassin, D. K., and others: Milk protein quantity and quality in low-birth-weight infants. IV. Effects on tyrosine and phenylalanine in plasma and urine, J. Pediatr. 90:357, 1977.
185. Schriener, R. L., and others: Lack of occurrence of lactobezoars with predominantly whey protein formulas, Am. J. Dis. Child. 136:437, 1982.
186. Avery, G. B., and Fletcher, A. B.: Nutrition. In Avery, G. B., editor: Neonatology, Philadelphia, 1981, J. B. Lippincott Co.
187. Lebenthal, E., and Lee, P. C.: Development of functional response in the human exocrine pancreas, Pediatrics 66:556, 1980.
188. Katz, L., and Hamilton, J. R.: Fat absorption in infants of birth weight less than 1300 grams, J. Pediatr. 85:608, 1974.
189. Tantibhedhyangkul, P., and Hashim, S. A.: Medium chain triglyceride feeding in premature infants: effects on fat and nitrogen absorption, Pediatrics 55:359, 1975.
190. Hernell, O., Blackberg, L., and Olivecrona, T.: Human milk lipases. In Lebenthal, E., editor: Gastroenterology and nutrition in infancy, New York, 1981, Raven Press.
191. Hanna, F. M., Navarette, D. H., and Hsu, F. A.: calcium–fatty acid absorption in infants fed human milk and prepared formula simulating human milk, Pediatrics 45:216, 1970.
192. Committee on Nutrition, American Academy of Pediatrics: Nutritional needs of low-birth-weight infants, Pediatrics 60:519, 1977.
193. Antonowicz, I., and Lebenthal, E.: Developmental pattern of small intestinal enterokinase and disaccharidase activities in the human fetus, Gastroenterology 72:1299, 1977.
194. MacLean, W. C., and Fink, B. B.: Lactose malabsorption by premature infants: magnitude and clinical significance, J. Pediatr. 97:383, 1980.
195. Cicco, R., and others: Glucose polymers tolerance in premature infants, Pediatrics 67:498, 1981.
196. Steichen, J. J., Gratton, T. L., and Tsang, R. C.: Osteopenia of prematurity: the cause and possible treatment, J. Pediatr. 96:528, 1980.
197. Tsang, R. C.: The quandary of vitamin D in the newborn infant, Lancet 18:1372, 1983.
198. Greer, F. R., and Tsang, R. C.: Calcium, phosphorus, magnesium and vitamin D requirements for the preterm infant. In Tsang, R. C., editor: Vitamin and Mineral Requirements in Preterm Infants. New York, 1985, Marcel Dekker, Inc.
199. Rowe, J., and others: Hypophosphetemia and hypercalciuria in small premature infants fed human milk: Evidence for inadequate dietary phosphorus, J. Pediatr. 104:112, 1984.
200. Day, G. M., and others: Growth and mineral metabolism in very-low-birth-weight infants. II. Effects of calcium supplementation on growth and divalent cations, Pediatr. Res. 9:568, 1975.
201. Greer, F. R., Steichen, J. J., and Tsang, R. C.: Calcium and phosphate supplements in breast milk–related rickets, Am. J. Dis. Child. 136:581, 1982.
202. Shenai, J.P., Reynolds, J. W., and Babson, S. G.: Nutritional balance studies in very-low-birth-weight infants: enhanced nutrient retention rates by an experimental formula, Pediatrics 66:233, 1980.
203. Curran, J. S., and others: Results of feeding a special formula to very-low-birth-weight infants. J. Pediatr. Gastroenterol. Nutr. 1:327, 1982.
204. Chan, G. M., Mileur, L., and Hansen, J-W.: Effects of increased calcium and phosphorus formulas and human milk on bone mineralization in preterm infants, J. Pediatr. Gastroenterol. Nutr. 5:444, 1986.
205. Rowe, J. C., and others: Achievement of in utero retention of calcium and phosphorus accompanied by high calcium excretion in very-low-birth-weight infants fed a fortified formula, J. Pediatr. 110:581, 1987.
206. Glorieux, F. J., and others: Vitamin D metabolism in preterm infants: serum calcitriol values during the first five days of life, J. Pediatr. 99:640, 1981.
207. Steichen, J. J., and others: Elevated serum 1,25-dihydroxyvitamin D concentrations in rickets of very-low-birth-weight infants, J. Pediatr. 99:293, 1981.
208. Seino, Y., and others: Plasma active vitamin D concentration in low-birth-weight infants with rickets

and its response to vitamin D treatment, Arch. Dis. Child. 56:629, 1981.

209. Melhorn, D. K., and Gross, S.: Vitamin E-dependent anemia in the premature infant. I. Effects of large doses of medicinal iron, J. Pediatr. 79:569, 1971.

210. Oski, F. A.: Iron requirements of the premature infant. In Tsang, R. C., editor: Vitamin and Mineral Requirements in Preterm Infants. New York, 1985, Marcel Dekker, Inc.

211. Committee on Nutrition, American Academy of Pediatrics: Relationship between iron status and incidence of infection in infancy, Pediatrics 62:246, 1978.

212. Baltimore, R. S., Shedd, D. G., and Pearson, H. A.: Effect of iron saturation on the bacteriostasis of human serum: in vivo does not correlate with in vitro saturation, J. Pediatr. 101:519, 1982.

213. Lundstrom, U., Siimes, M. A., and Dallman, P. R.: At what age does iron supplementation become necessary in low-birth-weight infants? J. Pediatr. 91:878, 1977.

214. Shojania, A. M., and Gross, S.: Folic acid deficiency and prematurity, J. Pediatr. 64:323, 1964.

215. Heird, W. C., and Anderson, T. L.: Nutritional requirements and methods of feeding low-birth-weight infants. In Gluck, L., editor: Current problems in pediatrics, Chicago, 1977, Year Book Medical Publishers, Inc.

216. Al-Dahlan, J., and others: Sodium homeostasis in term and preterm infants. I. Renal aspects, Arch. Dis. Child. 58:335, 1983.

217. Al-Dahlan, J., and others: Sodium homeostasis in term and preterm neonates, Arch. Dis. Child. 58:343, 1983.

218. Roy, R. N., and others: Late hyponatremia in very-low-birth-weight infants (1.3 kg), Pediatr. Res. 10:526, 1976.

219. Benda, G. I.: Modes of feeding low-birth-weight infants, Semin. Perinatol. 3:407, 1979.

220. Meier, P., and Pugh, E. J.: Breastfeeding behavior of small preterm infants. Matern. Child Nurs. p. 396, Nov-Dec 1985.

221. Meier, P., and Anderson, G. C.: Responses of small preterm infants to bottle- and breastfeeding, Matern. Child Nurs. p. 97, Mar-Apr 1987.

222. Neifert, M., and Seacat, J.: Practical aspects of breastfeeding the premature infant. Perinatol.-Neonatol. p. 24, Jan-Feb 1988.

223. Schriener, R. L.: Continuous and bolus feeding techniques in the low-birth-weight infant: benefits and complications. In Report of 79th Ross Conference on Pediatric Research: Feeding the neonate weighing less than 1500 grams—nutrition and beyond, Columbus, Ohio, 1979, The Conference.

224. Murphy, M.: Guidelines for nasogastric residuals, Neonatal Network, April:35, 1983.

225. Egan, E. A.: Neonatal necrotizing enterocolitis. In Lebenthal, E., editor: Textbook of gastroenterology and nutrition in infancy, New York, 1981, Raven Press.

226. Krouskop, R. W., Brown, E. G., and Sweet, A. Y.: The relationship of feeding to necrotizing enterocolitis, Pediatr. Res. 8:109, 1974.

227. Committee on Nutrition, American Academy of Pediatrics: Breastfeeding, Pediatrics 62:591, 1978.

228. Fomon, S. J., Ziegler, E. E., and Vasquez, H. D.: Human milk and the small premature infant, Am. J. Dis. Child. 131:463, 1977.

229. Davies, D. P.: Adequacy of expressed breast milk for early growth of preterm infants, Arch. Dis. Child. 52:296, 1977.

230. Tyson, J. E., and others: Growth, metabolic response, and development in very-low-birth-weight infants fed banked human milk or enriched formula. I. Neonatal findings, J. Pediatr. 103:95, 1983.

231. Gross, S.J.: Growth and biochemical response of preterm infants fed human milk or modified infant formula, N. Eng. J. Med. 308:237, 1983.

232. Jarvenpaa, A. L., and others: Preterm infants fed human milk attain intrauterine weight gain, Acta Paediatr. Scand. 72:239, 1983.

233. Chessex, P., and others: Quality of growth in premature infants fed their own mothers' milk, J. Pediatr. 102:107, 1983.

234. Atkinson, S. A., Bryan, M. H., and Anderson, G. H.: Human milk feeding in premature infants: protein, fat, and carbohydrate balances in the first two weeks of life, J. Pediatr. 99:617, 1981.

235. Gross, S. J., Geller, J., and Tomarelli, R. M.: Composition of breast milk from mothers of preterm infants, Pediatrics 68:490, 1981.

236. Lemons, J. A., and others: Differences in the composition of preterm and term human milk during early lactation, Pediatr. Res. 16:113, 1982.

237. Anderson, G. H., Atkinson, S. A., and Bryan, M. H.: Energy and macronutrient content of human milk during early lactation from mothers giving birth prematurely and at term, Am. J. Clin. Nutr. 34:258, 1981.

238. Atkinson, S. A., Bryan, M. H., and Anderson, G. H.: Human milk: difference in nitrogen concentration in milk from mothers of term and premature infants, J. Pediatr. 93:69, 1978.

239. Gross, S.J., and others: Nutritional composition of milk produced by mothers delivering preterm, J. Pediatr. 96:641, 1980.

240. Moran, J. R., and others: Epidermal growth factor in human milk: daily production and diurnal variation

during early lactation in mothers delivering at term and at premature gestation, J. Pediatr. 103:403, 1983.

241. Read, L. C., and others: Changes in the growth-promoting activity of human milk during lactation. Pediatr. Res. 18:133, 1984.

242. Gaull, G. E., Wright, C. E., and Isaacs, C. E.: Significance of growth modulators in human milk. Pediatr. 75:142, 1985.

243. Reid, B., Smith, H., and Friedman, Z.: Prostaglandins in human milk, Pediatrics 66:870, 1980.

244. Lindberg, T., and Skuda, G.: Amylase in human milk, Pediatrics 70:235, 1982.

245. Gross, S. J., and others: Elevated IgA concentration in milk produced by mothers delivered of preterm infants, J. Pediatr. 99:389, 1981.

246. Goldman, A. S., and others: Effects of prematurity on the immunologic system in human milk, J. Pediatr. 101:901, 1982.

247. Goldman, A. S., and others: Immunologic factors in human milk during the first year of lactation, J. Pediatr. 100:563, 1982.

248. Yoshioka, H., Iseki, K., and Fujuta, K.: Development and differences of intestinal flora in the neonatal period in breast-fed and bottle-fed infants, Pediatrics 72:317, 1983.

249. Narayanan, I., Prakash, K., and Gujral, V. V.: The value of human milk in the prevention of infection in the high-risk low-birth-weight infant, J. Pediatr. 99:496, 1981.

250. Atkinson, S. A., Radde, I. C., and Anderson, G. H.: Macromineral balances in premature infants fed their own mothers' milk or formula, J. Pediatr. 102:99, 1983.

251. Chan, G. M.: Human milk calcium and phosphate levels of mothers delivering term and preterm infants, J. Pediatr. Gastroenterol. Nutr. 1:201, 1982.

252. Rowe, J., and others: Hypophosphatemia and hypercalciuria in small premature infants fed human milk: evidence for inadequate dietary phosphorus, J. Pediatr. 104:112, 1984.

253. Schanler, R. J., Garza, C., and Nichols, B. L.: Fortified mothers milk for very-low-birth-weight infants: results of growth and nutrient balance studies, J. Pediatr. 107:437, 1985.

254. Schanler, R. J., Garza, C. and Smith, E. O.: Fortified mothers milk for VLBW infants: Results of

macromineral balance studies, J. Pediatr. 107:767, 1985.

255. Ronnholm, K. A. R., and others: Supplementation with human milk protein improves growth of small premature infants fed human milk, Pediatrics 77:649, 1986.

256. Carey, D. E., and others: Growth and phosphorus metabolism in premature infants fed human milk, fortified human milk, or special premie formula, Am. J. Dis. Child. 141:511, 1987.

257. Karp, T., and others: Nondiluted formula well tolerated by VLBW infants on enteral feeding, Pediatr. News August:36, 1983.

258. Olson, M.: The benign effects on rabbit's lungs of the aspiration of water compared with 5% glucose or milk, Pediatrics 46:538, 1970.

259. Bergman, K. E., Ziegler, E. E., and Fomon, S. J.: Water and renal solute load. In Fomon, S. J., editor: infant nutrition, Philadelphia, 1974, W. B. Saunders, Co.

260. Dancis, J., O'Connell, J. R., and Holt, L. E.: A grid for recording the weight of premature infants, J. Pediatr. 33:570, 1948.

261. Lubchencho, L. O., and others: Intrauterine growth as estimated from liveborn birth-weight data at 24 to 42 weeks of gestation, Pediatrics 32:793, 1963.

262. Brosius, K. K., Ritter, D. A., and Kenny, J. D.: Postnatal growth curve of the infant with extremely low birth weight who was fed enterally, Pediatrics 74:778, 1984.

263. Babson, S. G.: Growth of low-birth-weight infants. J. Pediatr. 77:11, 1970.

264. Gairdner, D., and Pearson, J.: A growth chart for premature and other infants, Arch. Dis. Child. 46:783, 1971.

265. Horwood, S. P., and others: Mortality and morbidity of 500 to 1499 gram birthweight infants liveborn to residents of a defined geographic region before and after neonatal intensive care, Pediatrics 69:613, 1982.

266. Bennett, F. C.: Neurodevelopmental outcome of premature/low-birth-weight infants: The role of developmental intervention. In Guthrie, R. D.: Neonatal intensive care. New York, 1988, Churchill Livingstone, Inc.

13

Nutrition and Feeding of Children with Developmental Delay and Related Problems

Peggy L. Pipes
Robin Pritkin Glass

OBJECTIVES

After studying this chapter, the student should:

1. Be aware of the many physical and environmental factors which affect food and nutrient intake in handicapped children.

2. Be able to identify children at risk for nutritional problems for whom preventive intervention is appropriate.

3. Have knowledge of ways to secure anthropometric measurements for children with contractures.

4. Recognize factors that may modify the energy needs of handicapped children from those of normal children.

5. Be able to screen children with motor difficulties that affect eating and who need referral to a therapist.

6. Have knowledge of the many factors that must be assessed to design an intervention program for any nutritional and feeding problems that may be found in developmentally delayed children.

Approximately 3% of all infants and children are developmentally delayed. Often these children also have medical conditions (such as heart disease or seizure disorders) that may increase or modify their nutrient and energy needs. In addition, psychosocial factors, developmental issues, or motor dysfunction may create nutritional and feeding concerns.

Nutritional problems in this population range from severe undernutrition to gross obesity; activity patterns from immobility to hyperactivity. Often a nutritional problem has several etiologic factors. For example, children who are referred for failure to thrive and osteomalacia may be undernourished because of oral motor dysfunction and interactions with their parents while the osteomalacia may have been caused by the interaction of drugs used to control seizures and nutrients.

Commonly reported parental and professional concerns relating to handicapped children's food and nutrient intakes include the following:

1. Slow growth in length and lack of appropriate weight gain
2. Excessive weight gain in relation to gains in length
3. Obesity
4. Iron deficiency anemia
5. Refusal of the child to consume specific foods or groups of foods
6. Refusal of the child to progress in feeding behavior when developmentally ready
7. **Pica**
8. Bizarre feeding patterns
9. Lack of appetite
10. Excessive appetite
11. Gagging, vomiting, or rumination
12. Food allergies
13. Limited fluid intake
14. Constipation
15. Abnormal motor patterns that affect the child's ability to consume food
16. Inability or unwillingness of the child to finger-feed or self-feed
17. Limited attention span at mealtime
18. Disruptive behavior at mealtime

One diagnostic and evaluation center reported that the most frequent inadequacies of nutrient intake were of ascorbic acid, iron, fluoride, and high-quality protein. Another center found an incidence of 21.3% overweight, 15% underweight, 7.7% bizarre feeding habits, 13% inadequate nutrient intake, and 30.6% feeding problems in 500 patients.[1] Caliendo,

Booth, and Moser found that 31% of a population of 3.1- to 9-year-old developmentally delayed children consumed less than 70% of the recommended intake for iron from food.[2] However, when those who took supplemental iron were excluded, only 21% of the subjects consumed less than 70% of the 1980 RDA for iron. Most of the serum ferritin values were within the normal range. Older children with relatively good feeding skills, as assessed by the mother, were likely to have higher serum ferritin levels.

Difficulties in weight control are often clustered in specific syndromes. Obesity is commonly a problem in children with Down's syndrome, Prader-Willi syndrome, Carpenter's syndrome, Cohen's syndrome, and Laurence-Moone-Biedl syndrome. Underweight is frequently noted in children with athetoid cerebral palsy, hyperactivity, and behavior problems.

Underweight children with limited energy intakes commonly have limited intakes of several nutrients because of the limited volume of food they consume. Inadequate intakes of vitamins A, C, and D and folate are the most frequent problems.

NUTRITIONAL NEEDS OF THE DEVELOPMENTALLY DELAYED CHILD

Developmentally delayed children require the same nutrients as any individual. There are, however, no dietary standards applicable to groups of developmentally delayed children. Many of these children, although not all, are growth retarded because of a genetic or biological defect. Syndromes with which growth retardation is associated include Down's syndrome, Prader-Willi syndrome, trisomy 13 and 18, de Lange syndrome, Hurler's syndrome, Turner's syndrome, Russell–Silver syndrome, and Williams syndrome.

Early studies of the growth and nutrient intake of developmentally delayed children were conducted primarily in institutions on children with cerebral palsy. More recent studies have focused on children in the free-living population and on nutrition problems encountered in specific syndromes.

Measurements of Physically Handicapped Children

Evaluating the adequacy of a child's nutrient and energy intake includes assessment of their physical growth. This means the child must be accurately weighed and measured and the data plotted on growth charts (Chapter 1). However, difficulties may be encountered in securing and interpreting the data for children who have developmental delays.

Accurate measurements of linear growth may be impossible to secure for children who have contractures or cannot stand. Roche[3] suggests using crown rump length or sitting height. The measurements, however, cannot be considered accurate when a child's trunk or torso is affected. To estimate linear height Manenica and others[4] have investigated the applicability of measurements of arm span for children with spina bifida, and Gleason[5] has used tibia length for boys with Duchenne's muscular dystrophy.

Using a control group of normal children, Manenica and others[4] found a correlation of arm span to linear height. They found that a normal arm span to height ratio of 1:1 provides a simple approximation technique. Arm span measurements are made with an anthropometer, a stainless steel detachable rod approximately 7 feet long with etched gradations to 0.1 cm and one movable sleeve. The arm span has been defined as "the greatest distance between the outstretched fingers of the right and left hand with the arms and forearms extended horizontally sidewards and the back pressed against a flat surface."[6] To secure this measurement, the subject stands in the erect position with arms outstretched (Figure 13-1). The fixed end of the anthropometer is held by one individual at the tip of the subject's middle finger of one hand, while another individual positions the sleeve at the tip of the middle finger of the subject's other hand. The subject is then told to stretch his or her arms, and the movable sleeve is adjusted to the maximum arm span.[7] This method was developed by K. Manenica, nutritionist, and M. Hurlich, physical anthropologist.

Estimation of linear length and height using tibia length had higher standard errors because

Figure 13-1   Arm span is measured from the tip of one middle finger to the other.

of the dynamics of relative tibial length. Although less accurate than arm span, this measurement was believed to provide useful information for individuals who had contractures in the arms and had previously been mobile.[5]

Tibia length is defined as the distance between the medial tibial epicondyle to the medial malleolus.[8] To measure tibia length, subjects are seated with their feet resting as flat on the floor as possible. The top of the right tibia is located by palpating downward from the medial condyle of the femur to the zone of articulation between the femur and the tibia. This point is marked at the closest approximation to the highest point of the medial condyle of the tibia, which is buried. The tip of the medial malleolus is easily identified and marked. The distance between these two points is measured with a sliding anthropometer. Height is estimated from the equation[7]:

$$\text{Height (cm)} = 3.54 \times \text{tibial length} + 32.23.$$

This method was developed by C. Gleason, nutritionist, and M. Hurlich, physical anthropologist (Figure 13-2).

Though more data are needed on normal children to establish standards, arm span can be used to estimate linear height for children who cannot stand and tibia length can be used for children with contractures in their arms.

Some classifications of handicapped children show normal growth, whereas others with **congenital** or metabolic disorders are associated with significant growth deviation. Researchers realize that the growth standards for normal children are not applicable for individuals with some handicapping conditions and that there is a need for syndrome specific reference data. Growth curves have been developed for children with dysplasia congenita, pseudoachondroplasia, and Down's syndrome.[9,10] These growth grids should be used when measurements of these children are plotted. For other children who have developmental delays, monitoring the rates of gain in height and weight, weight for height percentiles, midarm circumference, and triceps fatfold measurements over time provides useful information. The professional interpreting this data should have knowledge of specific syndromes associated with growth retardation.

Energy Requirements

Culley and Middleton[11] have reported that institutionalized retarded children who are ambulatory have energy requirements similar to those of normal children if height is used as a standard for estimating calorie needs. Because many of the children in their study had short stature, their calorie requirements were less than those of other children the same age. Only

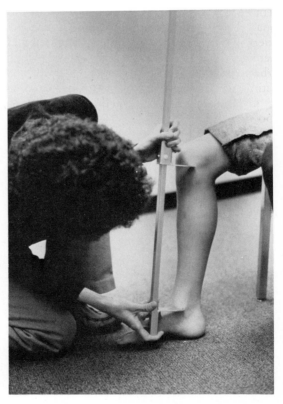

Figure 13-2   Tibia length measurement.

when motor dysfunction became severe enough to cause children to be nonambulatory did it reduce the calorie requirement per centimeter of height significantly. Pipes and Holm[12] have reported that children with Prader-Willi syndrome have reduced energy requirements per centimeter of height as compared with energy requirements of normal children. Mertz and others,[13] on the other hand, reported that a group of emaciated children in an institution for the mentally handicapped had energy requirements in excess of those of normal children. Even though such children consumed calorie intakes recommended for their ages, they remained emaciated.

Children with **spasticity** (**hypertonia**) frequently become overweight for their heights, consuming low-calorie intakes for their ages. Eddy, Nicholson, and Wheeler[14] studied one female with spasticity, an obese 16-year-old quadriplegic, and found her to have a basal energy expenditure of that of a person half her body weight. The girl was confined to a wheelchair; her total energy expenditure was estimated to be 1270 to 1370 kcal/day.

Children with athetosis (mixed pattern of too much and too little tone) consume greater numbers of calories than do those with spasticity and are less likely to become obese because they are able to engage in greater amounts of activity. Some children with athetosis expend energy constantly in involuntary movements. Researchers have found that basal energy expenditures of children with athetosis are similar to those of normal children and that the energy cost of activity depends on the child's capacity for muscular work. As levels of activity reach limits, activity becomes costly and uneconomical.[14]

Developmentally delayed children are often less active than their peers because of low muscle tone, immobility, or general disinterest in their environments. This inactivity limits their energy expenditures and therefore their energy requirements. Grogan and Ekvall[1] found levels of 7 kcal/cm of height necessary to produce weight reduction in children with myelomeningocele. Children with cerebral palsy who have decreased levels of activity have been noted to need 10 kcal/cm of height, whereas those with normal or increased levels of activity need 15 kcal/cm of height.

Recommendations for energy intakes of developmentally delayed children must be individualized. Because physical growth of handicapped children frequently deviates from the norm, kilocalories per kilometer of height may prove to be a more useful reference on which to base estimated needs than kilocalories per kilogram of body weight.

Cerebral Palsy

Children who are diagnosed as having cerebral palsy have abnormal motor patterns that range from hypotonia to hypertonia and include spasticity athetosis. Most studies have focused on those who have spasticity and athetosis. Body compositions of individuals with cerebral palsy may differ from those of normal children. Isaksson[15] found reduced body cell mass in children with both spasticity and athetosis caused by atrophy of skeletal muscles resulting from disease and low levels of physical activity. Reduced cell mass may reduce requirements for both essential nutrients and calories. On the other hand, a reduced cell mass may result from a lifetime of limited nutrient and energy intakes.

Children with cerebral palsy generally grow in both height and weight at rates less than average. Weight may be greater than that of normal children in children with spastic cerebral palsy and less than average in children with athetoid cerebral palsy. Oral motor involvement may be associated with growth retardation. Ruby and Matheny[16] found mouth area involvement closely associated with poor food intake and believed that the extent of mouth involvement and poor growth were generally parallel. Krick and Van Duyn found a relationship between oral motor involvement as defined by two or more of the following: weak suck, swallow, **tongue thrust,** tongue incoordination, tonic bite reflex, lip retraction, hypotonia of the tongue and lips, and growth retardation. Children with cerebral palsy who had oral motor problems were significantly thinner for their age and height than their age-matched counterparts who had cerebral palsy but no oral-motor impairment. They were also shorter, but this was of borderline significance.[17]

Bone age delays have been reported, indicating less than optimal intakes of nutrients. Hammond, Lewis, and Johnson[18] reported a range of 19 to 35 months delay, Leamy,[19] a range of 1.4 to 47.4 months delay, and Ruby and Matheny,[16] an average of 19.3 months delay in bone age.

Studies of free-living populations of children with cerebral palsy have shown acceptable intakes of nutrients other than iron.[20] Dietary intakes of less severely retarded children have been found to be markedly higher in all nutrients except vitamins A and C than intakes of the more severely delayed children. The energy value of the diets is influenced by the children's ability to self-feed. Children with motor involvements and mental retardation severe enough to interfere with their ability to feed themselves tend to consume fewer calories than do those who are able to self-feed.[18]

Prader-Willi Syndrome

Children with Prader-Willi syndrome (caused by the absence of minute portions of chromosome 15) have nutritional problems both in infancy and in older childhood.

This syndrome is characterized by hypotonia, hypogonadism, obesity, and learning disabilities. Infants are difficult to feed because of hypotonia and a weak suck. They often require tube feeding and may be diagnosed as failure to thrive. Between 2 and 4 years of age, these children become obese unless aggressive intervention is instituted before the rapid rate

of weight gain. An insatiable appetite will be noticed. Then food behaviors that include gorging, stealing, and hording food develop. They eat unusual food items such as raw hamburger and ornamental berries. One individual with Prader-Willi syndrome ate 12 pies at one sitting and 14 milkshakes at one time.

Most of these children gain excessive weight if permitted an energy intake recommended for normal children their age. Restriction of energy intakes to approximately two thirds that recommended is necessary to maintain a weight gain within the growth channel. However, the ranges of appropriate intake are wide at any age. A successful approach to management of weight control in children with this syndrome is as follows: Parents record (in household measures) all food offered and returned for 30 consecutive days. During this period individuals are weighed on a beam balance scale every two weeks. The energy value of the food consumed is calculated. The energy value of weight lost or gained is added to or subtracted from this energy value of that consumed (using the conversion figure of 7.7 kcal/gm of weight change). The individual's energy needs per centimeter of height are estimated and a diet plan to effect weight maintenance or loss is prescribed.[21]

Successful intervention requires control of the environment so that food is totally inaccessible to the child with the Prader-Willi syndrome. Refrigerators and cupboards must be locked. Food must be removed from the table as soon as a meal is finished. The children must be supervised at school so that they do not steal others' lunches or rummage in the garbage.

Down's Syndrome

Children with Down's syndrome (trisomy 21) often have problems of nutrient intake. Some have conditions that require nutrition therapy and/or can be prevented by anticipatory nutrition guidance. For example, there is a high incidence of cardiac anomalies among infants with Down's syndrome, which often make the children difficult to feed. Constipation secondary to hypotonia is not uncommon.

Overweight has been suggested as a characteristic of children with Down's syndrome from 2 to 3 years of age to adolescence. Some feel there is a constitutional but not inevitable tendency for individuals with this syndrome to be obese.

Limited intakes of nutrients may create concern. One study of 47 children with Down's syndrome ages 6-months-old to 6- to $6\frac{1}{2}$ years-old noted 16% to have low intakes of calcium; 14%, low intakes of iron; and 10%, low intakes of vitamin D and ascorbic acid.[22] Feeding problems were also identified. These children commonly refused to chew textured food when developmentally ready to do so. This resulted in the child accepting only a limited variety of foods. Social and emotional situations also resulted in feeding problems that compromised feeding and the children's nutrient intakes or developmental progress in feeding behavior or both.

Early individual or group intervention has proven effective in remediating these problems. Effective programs use an interdisciplinary approach including a nutritionist, an occupational or physical therapist, and a behaviorist. Counseling and therapy should focus on developmental readiness for the transition to appropriate textures of foods, the use of food to support developmental progress, parental feelings about and interaction with their children, physical growth, maintenance of normal weight for height, and foods that supply appropriate nutrients.[23]

Phenylketonuria

Infants born with metabolic disorders are at high risk for developmental disorders. Early detection, intervention, and surveillance are urgent. Of the many disorders identified, programs for the hyperphenylalanemias are the most comprehensive because mental retardation can be prevented if treatment is begun immediately after birth.

Currently, all states have newborn screening programs for children with phenylketonuria (PKU) and other disorders. Blood samples obtained by heel prick and applied to Guthrie filter paper are taken from every infant before he or she leaves the nursery. Infants who leave the hospital before 24 hours of age are screened again at 3 weeks of age.[24] Newborns with a positive screening test are tested again by both qualitative and quantitative methods. Criteria for the diagnosis of PKU are blood levels of phenylalanine consistently above 16 to 20 mg/dl, tyrosine levels less than 3 mg/dl, and the presence of 0-hydroxyphenylacetic acid in the urine.

Nutrition Therapy

Effective management of PKU requires special formulas, food products modified in their content of phenylalanine, and a cohesive team that includes the child, parent, nurse, social worker, psychologist and pediatrician.[25] Goals of nutrition therapy include both the provision of an adequate energy and nutrient intake and restriction of phenylalanine to maintain appropriate blood levels (between 2 and 10 mg/dl) so that normal growth and development proceed. To achieve these goals, blood levels are taken frequently and the diet is adjusted until the exact prescription for the individual child is developed.

Several low-phenylalanine or phenylalanine-free formulas supplemented with tyrosine are available. Most frequently, Lofenalac is used with infants and toddlers, and Phenyl-free with children and adolescents. In infancy and early childhood, Lofenalac should provide 90% of the protein and 80% of the calories. Foods with a low-phenylalanine content are introduced when it is developmentally appropriate for the child and in amounts to maintain the desired blood levels.

Phenyl-free is usually introduced between 3 and 6 years of age and allows greater flexibility in food choices. Blood levels continue to be monitored frequently and adjustments made in children's phenylalanine intake to support their changing needs as they grow larger.

Current recommendations are to continue the diet throughout adulthood. Discontinuation of the diet at ages 4 to 6 has resulted in learning difficulties, progressively decreasing IQ, poor attention span, and behavioral difficulties.

Other Nutrition Problems of Developmentally Delayed Children

Pica, an eating disorder commonly found in institutionalized retarded individuals but found also in the free-living population, has been shown to result in malabsorption of zinc and iron. Danford, Smith, and Huber[26] found individuals with pica had low plasma zinc levels and measures of iron status even though they received adequate dietary intake of minerals.

Socioculturally developmentally delayed school-age children have been shown to consume less protein, iron, thiamine, and fewer kilocalories than nonretarded children of the same age and sex from low-income families. Intakes of iron, calcium, and ascorbic acid were less than recommended in the developmentally delayed children.[27]

Drug and Nutrient Interrelationships

Anticonvulsant drugs prescribed to control seizures increase children's needs for vitamin D and alter their folate metabolism. Evidence of vitamin D deficiency has been found in both institutionalized patients and outpatients treated with anticonvulsant drugs for longer than 6 months for control of seizures. Serum calcium levels may be normal or low; serum parathyroid hormone concentrations, increased; serum phosphate levels, low; and serum alkaline phosphatase levels, elevated. Plasma 25 OHD levels have been found to be low. The degree of reduction of serum 25-OHD concentrations correlates with the relative decreases in serum calcium concentration, intestinal calcium absorption, and bone mass.[28]

Cases of rickets and osteomalacia confirmed by roentgenograms have been reported. All drugs commonly used to control seizures have been implicated. The incidence of abnormalities increases with duration of therapy. Multiple drug regimens cause the most problems. The abnormalities may result from an increase in hepatic microsomal catabolism or a biliary excretion of vitamins. The drugs may also have an inhibitory effect on calcium transport and bone metabolism. In addition, some feel that anticonvulsant drugs may effect the metabolism of vitamins D_2 and D_3 differently.[28]

Rickets and osteomalacia are most often diagnosed in nonambulatory individuals who have infrequent exposure to sunlight and receive a combination of anticonvulsant medications.[29]

Although many children consume anticonvulsants without biochemical or clinical evidence of rickets or osteomalacia, most of those who take the drugs have significant derangement of mineral metabolism. Serum 25-OHD levels have been found to be 40% to 70% lower than normal values and bone mass 10% to 30% lower than normal values.[30]

Amounts of vitamin D necessary to prevent deficiency and rickets in children receiving anticonvulsant therapy appear to vary depending on the number of anticonvulsant drugs, the dosage, the duration of therapy, the pattern of mobility, and the exposure to sunlight.[30] Hahn and colleagues administered 75,000 IU vitamin D_2 per week for 6 weeks to patients maintained on diphenylhydantoin and phenobarbital. This treatment normalized the serum levels of calcium and parathyroid hormone in seven of the twelve patients.[28]

Assessment of vitamin D status and appropriate intervention are important for children maintained on anticonvulsant therapy for more than 6 months. Such children should be monitored biochemically.

Folate

Drug-induced disturbances of folate metabolism have been found in a significant number of patients receiving anticonvulsants. Phenytoin is the drug of primary concern; however, therapy with phenobarbital, primidone, or carbamazepine is also associated with folate deficiency. Low-serum–folate levels accompanied by a fall in red cell folate and cerebrospinal folate levels have been reported in 27% to 91% of patients studied.[28] **Megaloblastic anemia** is reported to occur in less than 1% of patients.[29] The mechanism by which these drugs cause a fall in folate concentrations is not understood. Suggested hypothesis include the following:

1. Malabsorption of folate caused by an increased intraluminal pH effected by the drug
2. Inhibition of intestinal conjugases that split dietary polyglutamate forms of folate to the absorbable monoglutamate
3. Compromised transport of folate into the tissue
4. Depletion of folate due to its use as a cofactor in some metabolic process that is increased because of the drug's ability to induce liver enzymes.[31]

Administration of folate has been reported to precipitate seizures or to increase seizure frequency in some patients treated with anticonvulsants. In most patients no effect has been noted. At least eight different large controlled studies found no significant difference in seizure frequency between folate deficient patients treated with folate and those treated with placebo.[31] However, Chien and others[32] have suggested that there may be some folate-sensitive patients and some folate-insensitive patients and that folate should be administered with caution. They describe the effect of an intravenous infusion of folate on an 18-year-old girl treated with phenytoin and phenobarbital who showed electroencephalographic evidence of seizures followed by tonic and clonic seizures after the intravenous administration of 14.4 mg of folate. In the same study there were no reactions to the infusion of 75 mg of folic acid in seven other patients. Although the amounts infused seem large, individuals who receive megadoses of vitamins might ingest as much.

Long-term anticonvulsant therapy may be associated with other vitamin deficiency states. Clinical evidence of cardiac beriberi and subclinical ascorbic acid deficiency has been noted in a 28-month-old black girl who allegedly was receiving a full diet in a nursing home and was receiving phenobarbital, phenytoin sodium (Dilantin), and primidone (Mysoline).[33]

Megavitamin therapy

For many years there have been claims that megadoses of vitamins and minerals will increase the intelligence of children who are developmentally delayed.[34,35] Evidence supporting the claims has been scant and unconvincing. Not much attention has been focused on this therapy. However, Harrell and others[36] reported in 1981 that 16 developmentally delayed children experienced gains in IQ with **megavitamin therapy**. Children with Down's syndrome experienced the greatest gains. Attention was again focused on the use of nutrients. Many parents became very hopeful that help was available for their children and requested help in following the megavitamin regimen.

Replication of the Harrell study has been undertaken in several clinical settings using a double-blind control design to test the hypothesis. The studies were conducted on both school-age children and adults with Down's syndrome. In no instance has the vitamin supplement increased intelligence, motor performance, or communicative abilities of the individuals involved.[37,38] However, some who offer the supplements for sale continue to offer false hope at considerable expense to families of affected children.

FEEDING THE DEVELOPMENTALLY DELAYED CHILD

Planning for feeding developmentally delayed children implies that recommendations for intakes of energy, nutrients, and textures of food as well as expectations for the acquisition of self-feeding skills must be individualized for each child. Some children may have oral, fine, and gross motor, language, and personal/social development that is proceeding at a less than normal rate. Others may also have physical anomalies that imply the need for special equipment to sustain sitting posture to eat and adaptation of utensils to self-feed.

Many of the problems of nutrient intake in developmentally delayed children are preventable. Guidance and support for parents as they select nutritionally adequate foods for their children and as they create an environment in which children learn to consume foods in a manner appropriate for their developmental level are important. Parents may need instruction as to the appropriate stages at which to change the textures of food, to expect the child to feed himself or herself, and the degree of messiness to expect when a child is self-feeding.

Factors that Influence Food Intake

Because of the many factors that interact to determine the food available to and accepted by developmentally delayed children, concerns about food and nutrient intake and feeding rarely result from a single cause; many factors must be considered. An understanding of those factors that contribute to problems of food intake is important in planning for feeding of such children.

Developmentally delayed children experience the same responses to parental anxiety about their food intake as any child; they too can control their parents by their acceptance or rejection of food. Most normal preschoolers reduce their intakes of milk and vegetables, go on food jags, and have brittle, unpredictable appetites. It is not unreasonable to expect developmentally delayed children to present the same food-related behaviors. There may be, in addition, difficulties in feeding developmentally delayed children that are not encountered with normal children.

Developmental level

Delays in motor development may result directly or indirectly in an inappropriate nutrient intake. The development and sequence of acquisition of feeding behaviors of delayed children proceed in the same orderly predictable sequence as that of normal children. The chronological age at which the developmental stages occur, however, is not predictable, and wide ranges are seen both in the timing at which stages occur and in the ultimate developmental level of function of delayed children. Abnormal motor and behavioral patterns may interfere with the sequence of development and acquisition of feeding skills.

Parents who fail to recognize developmental readiness often fail to provide children with appropriate stimuli. If this happens, parents do not encourage their children to progress in the oral motor skills of eating and the gross and fine motor skills of self-feeding. For example, parents may offer their children strained foods when they are capable of masticating coarser foods or may feed children who have the ability to learn to feed themselves.

Readiness to accept solids is demonstrated blatantly in normal children and is difficult to ignore: they reach for food and bring it to their mouths. Handicapped children may give more subtle clues, and as a result the stage is often ignored. Some parents do not realize the importance of the introduction of solids at the proper time. When these parents finally decide it is time for children to learn to eat table food, conflicts often occur between children and their parents that may appreciably reduce the children's nutrient and caloric intakes. The children refuse to eat at all or skillfully spit out lumps while sucking and swallowing the soft, strained foods.[39]

Parents have reported restraining their children and forcing them to accept foods with texture. For example, one mother stated that it took four adults to hold her 10-year-old child who was developmentally 4 years of age when she attempted to make the transition from strained to table food. The child eventually accepted the foods but later accepted only small amounts of very soft food and lost weight.

Some children are hypersensitive in the oral area. It may be important for an occupational, physical, or speech therapist to institute a program to normalize sensation before presenting more textured foods to the child.

Children so delayed that they are unable to feed themselves depend on other people. Feeding the infant is a culturally defined maternal role, but feeding a handicapped child over a period of many years may become a tedious process that interferes with other activities several times a day. Some parents become so overwhelmed with such a schedule that they continue feeding soft foods that do not support developmental progress; others cease their efforts at feeding their children before the children consume sufficient food. Achieving self-feeding skills may appreciably increase the child's nutrient intake, self-confidence, and self-image. For example, Scales[40] describes an experience in teaching a 13-year-old severely retarded child to feed himself. The boy gained 9 lb in 6 weeks. A marked improvement in social behavior was noted.

Children whose delays in motor development impair their ability to learn to walk must be moved by their care givers. The more weight the children gain, the more difficult they become to lift, move, and care for. Parents and care givers of such children have expressed concern about the difficulties that may be created for them when children grow and gain weight; some have been known to limit inappropriately the amounts of food they feed. Obesity must be prevented, but children should have the advantage of nutrient and energy intakes that support the best possible growth and development for them. Parents may need information and counseling in methods of moving and caring for their children and in accepting their needs for increased amounts of nutrients and energy.

Abnormal oral-motor patterns and muscle tone

Problems in sucking, swallowing, and coordinating these functions with breathing can potentially be life threatening and may require that a child be fed in alternative ways such as **gavage** or gastrostomy feeding. In addition to demonstrating pathological oral motor patterns (i.e., oral patterns that are never observed as part of the normal developmental sequence), a child may show primitive oral patterns with the retention of primitive oral reflexes. These immature, primitive patterns can make the acquisition of mature feeding skills difficult. For example, a child who sucks reflexively when food is placed in the mouth cannot learn to chew until this reflexive behavior is integrated and more isolated movements of lips, tongue, and jaw are developed.

Abnormalities in overall muscle tone can exacerbate problems in oral control. Many pathological oral patterns are seen in association with specific types of abnormal muscle tone and are frequently exacerbated by the tonal abnormalities. A tongue thrust may be seen as part of increased **extensor** tone throughout the body. With **extension** of a child's head, the tongue thrust can be exaggerated. Poor lip closure and an open mouth position are frequently seen in the child with a hypotonic face and body. Asymmetry in the distribution of muscle tone can be observed in jaw deviation toward the more involved side during chewing or during opening of the mouth for spoon insertion.[41]

Abnormal oral motor patterns resulting in a lack of control of the tongue, lips, and cheeks or lack of coordination of swallowing and breathing can make eating a difficult and prolonged event requiring patience on the part of the child and the feeder. The amount of food lost from the mouth may be appreciable and may cause an inadequate intake of nutrients. Children so affected require the skills of occupational, speech, and physical therapists to achieve motor patterns necessary for feeding.

For some infants with abnormal muscle tone and abnormal oral patterns or for infants with structural defects, gavage feeding may be necessary to ensure adequate nutritional intake. Problems with increased **tactile sensitivity** in the oral area may become apparent when the transition from nonoral to oral feeding begins. Techniques can be used to prepare the child for oral feeding even while the child is predominantly fed by tubes. Oral intervention techniques used by occupational, physical, and speech therapists designed to maintain normal oral-tactile sensitivity should be continued during this period.[42]

The association between sensations in the mouth and sensations in the stomach can be maintained by using a pacifier during tube feedings.[43] For the toddler or older child who is receiving gastrostomy feedings, the hunger-satiation cycle may be established by normalizing the volume at each gastrostomy feeding to approximate the normal mealtime schedule. Thus, a gastrostomy-fed child who receives six equal-volume feedings per day might have the schedule changed to three larger gastrostomy "meals" and three smaller gastrostomy "snacks." This feeding schedule would approximate that of a normal child and would help the developmentally delayed child experience hunger and satiation while still maintaining the necessary caloric intake per day.

Termination of prolonged tube feeding is often followed by a difficult and sometimes

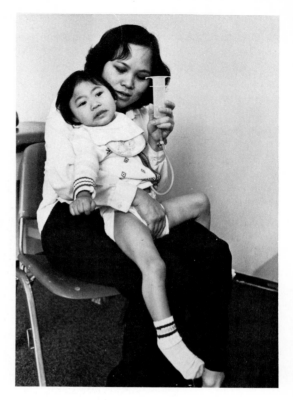

Figure **13-3** **A,** Oral motor problems in some children make gavage feeding necessary for normal growth and development.

lengthy adjustment period. A child who has been fed by tubes for a long period may have missed the critical or sensitive period for the introduction of solid foods.[39] Preparation before initiating oral feeding while the child is still being fed by tubes and the use of an interdisciplinary team of professionals to combat problems during the adjustment period may ease this transition.

Primitive oral reflexes. The full-term infant is normally born with a variety of well-established oral reflexes making the infant fully equipped to take in nourishment. Bosma[44] cites research showing that the human fetus can develop a functional swallow by 12.5 weeks

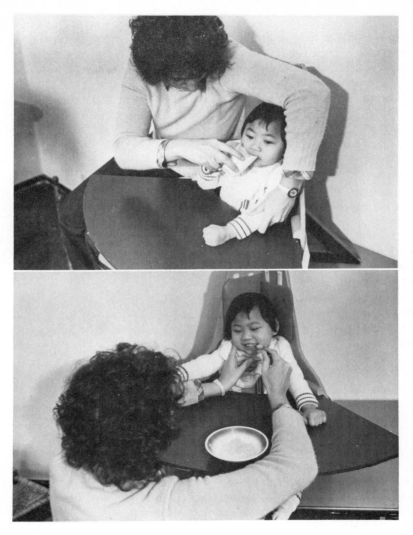

Figure 13-3 cont'd.   B and C, Even though gavage feeding is necessary, therapy is needed to foster the development of eating and drinking skills so normal eating patterns will be achieved in the future.

gestation and sucking behavior by 14 weeks gestation. Many premature babies have extremely weak, inefficient sucks at birth. With increasing maturation, strength of suck, endurance, and rhythmicity of sucking improves. Some premature babies, however, require intervention to establish more mature feeding behavior. Tactile and **proprioceptive facilitation** techniques used by occupational and physical therapists or nurses in special care nurseries have resulted in better weight gain, faster transition from nasogastric feedings to bottle feedings, and more sustained sucking ability in premature infants.[44,45]

In a child who has feeding difficulties, the evaluation of individual primitive oral reflexes may provide some insight into the nature of the feeding difficulty. Ingram,[46] however, believes that merely testing oral reflexes provides little information about the individual's feeding abilities other than the presence of basic reflex arcs. Rather, Ingram states that one needs to consider how the primitive reflexes are integrated with breathing, adaptive feeding behavior, and vocalizations to adequately assess a child's feeding problems.

Protective oral reflexes. The cough and gag reflexes are oral reflexes that do not become integrated with increasing maturation but remain as protective reflexes throughout an individual's life. These reflexes serve to open the air passage when it is blocked or is in danger of being blocked. A cough reflex is a violent expiratory effort preceded by a preliminary inspiration; the accessory muscles of expiration are brought into action as air is noisily expelled. When related to food, the stimulus is the presence of food or liquid in the laryngeal vestibule that must be expelled so that it does not enter the lungs. The *gag reflex* is an involuntary attempt to vomit to remove food from the oral cavity so that it does not travel into the airway. Gagging occurs when the soft palate is stroked or pressure is applied to the posterior wall of the pharynx or the posterior half of the tongue; there is an arching of the tongue, mouth opening, head extension, and facial grimacing.[47] Intense gagging may induce a vomit response.

In normal development, the gag reflex is frequently elicited when a baby puts a toy far into the mouth. Oral play helps the child to accommodate to a variety of sensations and aids in the normal reduction in the intensity of the gag reflex. Through oral exploration, the infant experiences a variety of textures, temperatures, shapes, and sizes that may lay the groundwork for future learning. Frequently, the parent of a child with feeding problems will report that the child never participated in this normal mouthing stage of development. This fact should alert the professional to a potential problem with a hyperreactive gag reflex.

Treatment for hypersensitivity to oral and tactile stimulation is a gradual, careful program of increasing the sensory experiences. The program is carefully graded according to the child's response because overstimulation could cause negative emotional and behavioral reactions or further increases in abnormal muscle tone that might interfere with feeding to a greater extent than the original problem. The therapeutic techniques used by occupational, physical, and speech therapists to normalize facial and oral sensitivity therefore are varied according to the individual child's reactions and needs.[48]

The gag reflex can also be inhibited or sensitized (increased) by physiological and psychological factors. A physiological sensitization may occur when a person is ill, dizzy, or emotionally upset. The normal reaction to these feelings is to avoid eating. If food were to be offered or forced, the reaction might well be a gag. Fear of choking resulting from a previous incident may cause a gag response at the sight of a particular food. This behavior usually receives attention from adults, who frequently do not persist in offering the undesirable food. Children with these sorts of behavioral responses often severely restrict the variety of food textures in their diet, resulting in further sensory deprivation and increased oral sensitivity. A graded oral tactile stimulation program under the direction of a pediatric occupational, physical, or speech therapist would be indicated.

Positioning of children. The position of the child during feeding is of prime importance.[42,48] Proper positioning considers the child as a whole—the relationship of the head position to the body, as well as the overall body position. Frequently a child's feeding difficulties can be greatly improved just by changes in the child's position during meals. Normalization of the child's muscle tone through positioning may minimize abnormal oral movement patterns and increase the child's voluntary oral control.

Head position is especially important for children who have swallowing difficulties or who do not have a normally responsive gag or cough response. The child should never be fed with the head or body tipped backwards in a position often referred to as a "bird-feeding" position. In this position normal swallowing and tongue control are impaired, and the child is in danger of aspirating food into the lungs or choking. Food in the lungs may lead to pneumonia or other respiratory difficulty. The head should be upright or slightly flexed forward 5° to 10°. The body should be upright or, if support is needed for head and trunk, within 30° of vertical.[49]

Children with feeding problems, especially those with abnormal muscle tone, are often difficult to position. It is essential that a pediatric occupational or physical therapist assess each child and recommend appropriate positioning. A consistent effort should be made to follow through with these techniques. Adapted positioning during mealtimes should be comfortable for both the child and the care giver and should enable communication and interaction.

Figure 13-4 demonstrates some feeding positions that may be prescribed by occupational and physical therapists. Each position incorporates basic principles of appropriate, therapeutic positioning.[42,29] The head is in good alignment with the body, and the mouth is in the midline. With the head aligned with the body or slightly **flexed** forward, abnormal head extension or pushing backward can be inhibited. In some children, pushing back with the head is not caused by increased extensor tone but is a compensatory behavior that reflects an inability to stabilize the head in an upright position. Proper head support can normalize abnormal tone or provide stability if needed.

The position of the arms is related to and influences head and trunk control. When the arms and shoulders pull backward, the head tends to tilt backward and overall muscle tone increases. Therefore the shoulders and arms should be held forward and oriented toward the midline of the body. This forward position of the arms can be achieved by the manner in which the child is held near the feeder's body or by rolled towels or cushions placed behind the child's shoulders in the child's chair. Some children learn to stabilize their arms forward by grasping the far end of the wheelchair tray or supporting themselves with both elbows on the table.

Trunk stability is essential because the trunk provides the base on which to achieve good head and arm control. If the child is unable to sit independently, support should be provided by the feeder or through the use of a back rest. If the child falls sideways, lateral supports can be provided through adaptations built into a wheelchair or through supportive cushions. Chest straps may be helpful for the child with minimal trunk control who falls forward. It would be preferable, however, to find a chair with a slight backward tilt to allow gravity to assist with trunk control.

The position of the hips and legs affects trunk control and thus influences the position of the rest of the body. Extension at the hips can increase tone throughout the body and cause extension of the head and mouth opening. Stiffness or spasticity in the legs can cause the legs to pull together, narrowing the child's sitting base and impairing the postural adjustments needed for sitting balance. A pommel placed between the child's legs to widen the base of support provides adequate leg separation.

The hips should be flexed to a 90° neutral position. If the hips tend to extend, causing the child's hips to slip forward in the chair, greater than 90° of hip flexion can be provided by adding a wedge to the child's chair, with the larger edge under the child's knees. Often just a seatbelt firmly fastened across the hips keeps the hips in a normal neutral position

Figure 13-4 **A,** A young infant or child can be fed while being held in someone's lap. The head is in line with the body, with the arms forward. With the left knee raised, hip flexion can be maintained. **B,** By using a firm wedge, a young child can be fed while facing the feeder. The legs are abducted and flexed, which inhibits extension. The feeder's hands are freed to assist with jaw control. **C,** Rolls can be inserted into a wheelchair to provide temporary trunk support and help keep the arms forward and toward the midline.

and provides a better base for trunk control. Finally, good stability at the feet can be achieved through a foot rest allowing the feet to be flat and flexed at the ankle.

Proper positioning during mealtime supports the child's highest level of oral motor control. The relationship between the child's gross motor level at rest and during eating must be considered. The ability to independently control head or trunk position may deteriorate when a child is asked to eat or self-feed. Mealtime should not be the time to make the child work on better head and trunk control. Rather, adapted positioning should reinforce the child's motor level while fostering better oral and feeding skills.

In addition to the type of static positioning used during meals, the environment and the placement of the food or spoon can influence the child's feeding skills. If the spoon and foods are presented above eye level, the child may tilt the head backward to orient toward the food and thus reinforce an extension pattern. Presenting the food in the middle, from a low angle, encourages slight head flexion and symmetry. Placing the container or plate of food at the side may encourage the child to turn sideways and increase asymmetry. By placing the food in front of the child, a symmetrical midline position can be encouraged. Withdrawal of the spoon can also influence head position. If the spoon is lifted up and scraped against the upper front teeth, the head will tend to tilt backward and lip control will be impaired.

Screening children to determine the primary concerns and the criteria for referral was discussed in Chapter 3. The foregoing information should prove useful in improving the quality of food intake when therapy services are not immediately available. It is important to use a problem-solving approach that includes ideas and feedback from the child and the care giver. The rationale for any suggestions should be thoroughly explained and expectations for fol-

low-through must be reasonable. Since it may take more time to feed a child in the desired position, especially at first, the new techniques should be used only toward the beginning of the meal for a short time, increasing the amount of time as both the child and the care giver become used to techniques. Consideration of the child's and the care giver's comfort, feelings, and opinions is likely to yield good results. Changes in motor control may be slow to develop, but the quality of the daily feeding experience has great impact on the ultimate skills that develop.

A few children who have abnormal oral motor patterns have difficulty ingesting fluids. As a result, their intakes of liquids are very limited and they remain at risk of dehydration. The fluid intakes of such children should be carefully monitored. Heavily salted foods, such as bouillon and commercially prepared soups, should be avoided, as should high intakes of other nutrients that obligate water.

Management of Feeding

The diversity of concerns about the food and nutrient intake of handicapped children and the many factors that affect children's level of function and food acceptance imply that the skills of several disciplines may be necessary to find solutions to the concerns and to set priorities for therapy for individual children. The occupational, physical, or speech therapist will be called on to provide therapy for children with abnormal motor tone. The dentist will correct dental caries and malocclusions. A professional proficient in behavior modification techniques may be required to change behavior. Correcting these concerns may solve nutrient intake concerns. Parents may, however, still need help in planning appropriate foods for their children.

Behaviors

Children may have inappropriate nutrient intakes and food habits because of learned behavior. Children learn from the model set for them by their parents, peers, and relatives. If examples of poor food habits are set, the children will imitate them.

Disruptive and inappropriate feeding behaviors such as throwing food and utensils, stuffing the mouth before swallowing, and refusing to eat generally attract parental attention. These behaviors often compromise a child's nutrient intake. Resolution of the problems requires a structured, well-defined behavior modification program (Chapter 15). Since, as a rule, behaviors get worse before they begin to get better, energy and nutrient intake should be monitored when the programs are implemented.

The behavior pattern and attention span of children affect their calorie and nutrient needs and consumption. Hypoactivity reduces energy expenditure and needs. Lack of planned activity and stimulation for such children often results in boredom, which leads to children spending their days seeking and consuming excessive amounts of food.

Hyperactive children never appear to be quiet and expend much energy in their numerous activities. The attention span of hyperactive children may be as limited at the dinner table as in other activities, resulting in very small intakes of food at one time. It may be important to offer hyperactive children frequent small feedings of high nutrient content.

Constipation

Constipation is a common problem in children with developmental delays, especially in those who are hypertonic or hypotonic. The infrequent passage of feces or the passage of unduly hard, dry fecal matter results from a variety of causes, such as lack of muscle tone in the intestine or duodenal wall, excessive fatigue, anxiety, inappropriate dietary intake, or failure to establish a routine bowel pattern. When children are constipated, they usually complain of stomachache, distention, swelling of the abdomen, discomfort, or pain.

Increasing the amount of fluid and roughage in the diet may be useful for treating children who are constipated. Parents should also observe for individual food stimuli. Some children may need to limit milk intake to 1 pint/day. Prunes and prune juice are also frequently helpful.

Appetite

Central nervous system damage causes a lack of appetite in some children. These children never express hunger, and some mothers of such children have stated that setting alarm clocks helps them remember to feed their children. Children so affected are rarely pleased by any food and limit the volume of food they consume. The children's unresponsiveness gives the parents no positive reinforcement for their efforts to feed the children. This lack of positive interplay between parent and child may cause dissatisfaction in each; the parents may lose motivation to continue helping the child consume food, and the children may lose motivation to consume appropriate energy and nutrient intakes.

Damage to or developmental defects of the hypothalamus can cause insatiable appetites in children. Children so affected sometimes gorge, steal food, or eat animal food. Extreme measures, such as locking refrigerators and kitchen cupboards, have been necessary to control obesity in such children. Food-related behaviors of such children cannot be altered by behavior modification methods.

Parental Expectations

Parents need to have realistic expectations about the child's potential for physical growth. It is not possible to increase a child's height beyond his or her genetic potential; it is possible to increase a child's weight for height. Parental concern about a child's slow rate of growth may create anxiety about the volume of food the child is consuming. Counseling about expectations and growth response to food intake is important.

The daily use of high-protein, high-calorie drinks that contain raw eggs should be discouraged. Sweetman and others[50] have described biotin deficiency in an 11-year-old mentally retarded male who consumed a drink with two raw eggs daily for 5 years. Clinical manifestations were alopecia totalis and an erythematous, **exfoliative** dermatosis.

People who take care of the handicapped are often overindulgent, giving such children large amounts of preferred high-carbohydrate, sweet foods frequently. As with anyone, it is difficult to design a food intake pattern that provides necessary amounts of essential nutrients and maintain weight gain in growth channel if many of the foods consumed supply only carbohydrate and fat and few other nutrients. It may be important to help parents find ways to express their affection other than with food. Parents should also be aware of why they offer the foods they do.

Identifying readiness to progress

Assessing children's developmental levels of function and their readiness to progress in eating and self-feeding is necessary to define reasonable expectations for parents and care givers. Parents often need help in accepting their children's handicaps and in recognizing their potential to progress.

Changes in food and feeding behavior should be effected when the children are developmentally 6 to 7 months of age, when they demonstrate readiness to self-feed and to use a cup. Table 13-1 defines important developmental landmarks and suggested food appropriate for changes in feeding behavior.

Early intervention programs can aid in preventing later problems of food and nutrient intake.

Assessment of problems and suggested solutions

Efforts to prevent problems of nutrient intake are not always successful. Frequently expressed concerns about food and nutrient intake of developmentally delayed children, factors that need to be assessed, and suggested solutions are provided in Table 13-2.

Developmentally delayed children frequently experience failure in their many efforts. It is therefore important that any plan to modify a child's food intake pattern be designed so that success is obtainable and the child and the parents are reinforced for each gain, however small. Adequate nutrition is important for every child to achieve his or her physical, mental, and emotional potential. Delayed and physically handicapped children should have the advantage of a nutrient intake that can support well-being, optimal growth, and development. Solutions to difficulties in attaining such goals may be complex and may require a multidisciplined approach.

Summary

Children who are developmentally delayed are vulnerable to the same problems of nutrient intake as other children. The incidence of feeding and nutrition problems appears to be greater than in the normal population, and they are often more severe. The causes of nutritional problems in developmentally delayed children often involve motor abnormalities or delays, infantilism, and lack of attention to critical periods of development. Therefore an interdisciplinary approach to intervention is appropriate. Specific syndromes are associated with undernutrition; others, with obesity.

SUGGESTED LEARNING ACTIVITIES

1. Describe factors that must be addressed in evaluating the nutrient intake of a 3-year-old child with athetoid cerebral palsy.
2. Describe syndromes associated with mental retardation also associated with growth failure.
3. Define the nutritionist's role in early intervention programs for developmentally delayed children.

Table 13-1   Developmental stages of readiness to progress in feeding behaviors

Developmental Landmarks	Change Indicated	Examples of Appropriate Foods
Tongue laterally transfers food in the mouth Voluntary and independent movements of the tongue and lips Sitting posture can be sustained Beginning of chewing movements (up and down movements of the jaw)	Introduction of soft, mashed table food	Tuna fish; mashed potatoes; well-cooked mashed vegetables; ground meats in gravy and sauces; soft diced fruit such as bananas, peaches, pears; liverwurst; flavored yogurt
Reaches for and grasps objects with scissor grasp Brings hand to mouth	Finger-feeding (large pieces of food)	Oven-dried toast, teething biscuits, cheese sticks, peeled Vienna sausage (food should be soluble in the mouth to prevent choking)
Voluntary release (refined digital grasp)	Finger-feeding (small pieces of food)	Bits of cottage cheese, dry cereal, peas, etc.
Rotary chewing pattern	Introduction of more textured food from family menu	Well-cooked chopped meats and casseroles, cooked vegetables and canned fruit (not mashed), toast, potatoes, macaroni, spaghetti, peeled ripe fruit
Approximate lips to rim of the cup	Introduction of cup	
Understands relationship of container and contained	Beginning self-feeding (messiness should be expected)	Food that when scooped will adhere to the spoon, such as applesauce, cooked cereal, mashed potatoes, cottage cheese
Increased rotary movement of the jaw Ulnar deviation of wrist develops	More skilled at cup and spoon feeding	Chopped fibrous meats such as roast and steak Raw vegetables and fruit (introduce gradually)
Walks alone	May seek food and get food independently	Food of high nutrient value should be available
Names food, expresses preferences; prefers unmixed foods Goes on food jags Appetite appears to decrease		Balanced food intake should be offered (child should be permitted to develop food preferences without parents being concerned that they will last forever)

Table 13-2 Assessment of concerns about foods and nutrients

Symptom	Assessment	Action and Counseling Suggestions
Lack of appetite	What is child's total food and nutrient intake?	Counsel with parents about child's needs and help them obtain needed food
	Is some essential nutrient consumed in insufficient amounts?	Provide only between-meal snacks of high-nutrient content at intervals that will not interfere with appetite at mealtime
	Is child receiving adequate amounts of food at other meals without having to eat large amounts?	Serve very small portions
	Is the food properly prepared?	Provide child with a quiet period before mealtime to prevent weariness
	Is child's rate of growth normal in spite of his or her apparent lack of appetite?	Reinforce child's acceptance of food with social reinforcement
	Is child reinforced?	Do not reinforce with food
	When he or she is eating? (appropriate)	Eat with child to provide a model
	When he or she is not eating? (inappropriate)	Refer the emotionally deprived child to the nurse or social worker
	Is child receiving too many snacks? (inappropriate)	
	Is child too weary to eat at mealtime?	
	Is child attending to eating or is his or her attention diverted at mealtime?	
	Is child psychologically deprived?	
Refuses specific groups of foods	Is food properly prepared?	Continue offering very small portions of foods refused
	Has child had previous experiences with the foods?	Reinforce foods accepted with foods child likes
	Does child have a model (parents, teacher, peers, etc.) who eats these foods?	Provide a model for child by eating the foods
		Provide guidance in food preparation for children
Inappropriate feeding behavior	What started the behavior?	All inappropriate behaviors should be ignored even if it is necessary to remove child from feeding situation
Throwing	What follows the behavior?	
Gorging	Is child reinforced?	
Stuffing food in the mouth	Is child punished?	All attempts at appropriate eating should be encouraged through social reinforcement and food the child likes
Will not sit at the table	Is child ignored?	

Continued.

Table 13-2 Assessment of concerns about foods and nutrients—*cont'd*

Symptom	Assessment	Action and Counseling Suggestions
Refuses to eat table food; insists on strained food	Has child had experience with table food? Has it been offered and refused? Has child eaten table food previously but refuses it currently? How is child positioned for feeding? Can he or she sit upright? Has a critical stage of development been ignored? Is child delayed so that strained foods are appropriate for his or her stage of motor development? Can child bite or chew? Is child hypersensitive in and/or around the mouth?	Consult with occupational, physical, or speech therapist regarding positioning, development, and hypersensitivity Seat child in upright sitting position (using props if necessary) If child demonstrates readiness: Choose a food the child enjoys and place it between back molars (watch your fingers) Offer crunchy foods such as arrowroot biscuits, melba toast, crackers (be careful of foods that splinter, such as graham crackers)
Will not bite	Does child have a hypersensitive gag reflex? Does child have dental caries or malocclusion? Can child close the mouth? Has child been offered foods that require biting? Can child breathe through the nose?	Offer easy-to-bite foods such as arrowroot biscuits and melba toast Manually assist child in closing the jaw Provide social reinforcement when child takes a bite
Does not chew with a rotary motion	Is child delayed so that only munching or sucking is appropriate? Can child lateralize the tongue? Has child been offered foods that require chewing? Is child hypersensitive or hyposensitive? Are foods offered that are too tough to chew?	Consult an occupational, physical, or speech therapist regarding lateralization of the tongue and sensitivity Model for child by demonstrating chewing Manually move the jaw in chewing motions Encourage chewing with social reinforcement and with foods child likes
Refuses harder-to-chew foods	Is hypertonia or hypotonia preventing development of oral motor skills? Does child have dental caries? Is child sufficiently delayed that hard-to-chew foods are inappropriate for him or her?	Consult with occupational, physical, or speech therapist about oral motor skills; stimulate area around the lips and mouth before feeding as directed Consult about dental caries

		Give small bites; encourage with social reinforcement and foods child likes
	Is there too much in child's mouth at one time for him or her to chew anything adequately?	
	Has child had experience with harder-to-chew foods?	
Lack of self-feeding	What cues of readiness to self-feed does child demonstrate?	If child is ready:
	Can child bring hand to mouth?	Use behavior modification (i.e., putting the child through the motions of feeding, phasing out assistance)
	Can child hold the spoon?	Reinforce child's attempts to
	Is child so delayed that self-feeding is inappropriate?	Hold spoon
	Can child sit either unsupported or propped in an upright position?	Put spoon in dish
	Do adults interrupt when child begins to make efforts to self-feed?	Bring spoon to the mouth
	Does child have behavior incompatible with self-feeding?	Close the lips around the spoon
	Physiologically, does child have any spasticity?	Return spoon to dish
	Behaviorally, does child throw food, utensils, etc?	
	Is child receiving attention by not feeding himself or herself?	
	Is child controlling parents by not feeding himself or herself?	
	Is child offered foods that will stick to the spoon?	
	Is child attending to eating, or is he or she distracted by others in the environment?	
Lean for height	Is child receiving sufficient amounts of food?	Family should keep a food record if there is concern about amounts of food and frequency of eating
Weight loss	Is child receiving sufficient calories?	Feed more frequently; small feedings
Failure to gain adequate weight	Is some essential nutrient consumed in inappropriate amounts?	Provide high-calorie snacks of high-nutrient value, such as milkshakes or peanut butter or fruit on crackers or bread
	How frequently is child given food?	Counsel with parents regarding appropriate feedings for the child
	At school?	Reinforce with activities, not with food
	At home?	
	Does child eat on a regular schedule?	
	What is the family body type?	
	Does child have an illness or disease contributing to the lack of weight gain?	

Continued.

Table 13-2 Assessment of concerns about foods and nutrients—*cont'd*

Symptom	Assessment	Action and Counseling Suggestions
	Vomiting or diarrhea? Other chronic illness? What is child's history of weight gain? Has child always been lean? Has child recently lost weight? Is there sufficient food available to child? Is food presented to child in a manner appropriate for his or her level of function and self-help skills?	
Overweight	What is child's activity pattern? What foods does child have available at home? How has child's pattern of overweight been achieved? Has child gained weight recently? Is child currently gaining weight in the same channel, and is overweight a result of earlier feeding experiences? How does the family feel about child's weight? Is child reinforced for eating? What is child's activity level? What is child's snacking pattern?	Offer nonfat milk instead of whole milk, unsweetened fruit instead of desserts Limit fried foods, gravies, and sauces Provide low-calorie snacks Feed child on a schedule; discourage indiscriminate snacking Limit the number of desserts, cookies, candy, and other sweets offered Increase portion size of vegetables, meat, and fresh fruits; decrease portion size and number of servings of breads, potatoes, cereals, and fatty foods Reinforce with activities, not with food Help the family find ways of increasing child's level of activity Direct efforts at a reduction in the rate of weight gain, not a weight loss
Obesity	Assess as above	Weight reduction diet planned to effect weight loss of no more than 2 lb/month Counsel with all who offer food to child in the weight reduction program Plan physical activities daily in any manner compatible with the child's level of function Provide continuing support for parents and children as the program progresses

4. How would you respond to parents of a developmentally delayed child who were considering megavitamin therapy?

5. How would you determine an appropriate energy intake for a 14-month-old girl with Down's syndrome?

6. Observe a school lunch program in a school for special education. What motor problems of feeding do you observe? What adaptive equipment is being used to facilitate self-feeding?

7. To experience the effect of head position on eating, try to chew or swallow semisolid foods with your head tilted backward, try to drink with your head tilted backward.

8. To experience the effects of the position of the body on the head and on feeding ability, try to eat with your hips slid forward in the chair without your feet touching the ground.

REFERENCES

1. Palmer, S., and Ekvall, S.: Pediatric nutrition in developmental disorders. Springfield, Ill., 1978, Charles C. Thomas, Publisher.

2. Caliendo, M. A., Booth, G., and Moser, P.: Iron intakes and serum ferritin levels in developmentally delayed children, J. Am. Diet. Assoc. 81:401, 1982.

3. Roche, A. F.: Growth assessment of handicapped children. Diet. Curr. 6:25, 1970.

4. Manenica, K., and others: Evaluating growth and obesity in the child with meningomyelocele. [Unpublished master's thesis. Seattle, 1981, University of Washington.]

5. Gleason, C.: Nutritional assessment of boys with Duchenne's muscular dystrophy, unpublished master's thesis, Seattle, 1982, University of Washington.

6. Berke, A. R., and Wilmore, J. H.: Evaluation and regulation of body build and composition, Englewood Cliffs, N.J., 1974, Prentice-Hall, Inc.

7. Zorab, P. A., Prime, F. J., and Harrison, A.: Estimation of height from tibia length; Lancet 1:195, 1963.

8. Horton, W. A., and others: Growth curves for height for diastrophic dysplasia, spondyloepiphyseal dysplasia congenita, and pseudoachondroplasia, Am. J. Dis. Child. 136:316, 1982.

9. Cronk, C. C., and others: Growth charts for children with Down syndrome: 1 month to 18 years of age, Pediatrics 81:102, 1988.

10. Culley, W. J., and others: Calorie intake of children with Down's syndrome (mongolism), J. Pediatr. 66:772, 1965.

11. Culley, W. J., and Middleton, T. O.: Calorie requirements of mentally retarded children with and without motor dysfunction, J. Pediatr. 75:380, 1969.

12. Pipes, P., and Holm, V.: Weight control of children with Prader-Willi syndrome, J. Am. Diet. Assoc. 62:520, 1973.

13. Mertz, E. T., and others: Protein malnutrition in mentally retarded children. In Food and Nutrition Board: Meeting protein needs of infants and children, Pub. No. 843, Washington, D.C., 1961, National Academy of Sciences, National Research Council.

14. Eddy, T. P., Nicholson, A. L., and Wheeler, E. F.: Energy expenditures and dietary intakes in cerebral palsy, Dev. Med. Child Neurol. 7:377, 1965.

15. Isaksson, B.: The nutritional needs of disabled children. In Blix, G., editor: Nutrition in preschool and school age, Symposium of the Swedish Nutrition Foundation, VII, Stockholm, 1969, Almqvist & Wiksell Forlag A.B.

16. Ruby, D. O., and Matheny, W. D.: Comments on growth of cerebral-palsied children, J. Am. Diet. Assoc. 40:525, 1962.

17. Krick, J., and Van Duyn, M.A.S.: The relationship between oral motor involvement and growth: a pilot study in a pediatric population with cerebral palsy, J. Amer. Diet. Assoc. 84:555, 1984.

18. Hammond, M. I., Lewis, M. N., and Johnson, E. W.: A nutritional study of cerebral palsied children, J. Am. Diet. Assoc. 49:196, 1966.

19. Leamy, C. M.: A study of the food intake of a group of children with cerebral palsy in the Lakeville Sanitorium, Am. J. Public Health 43:1310, 1953.

20. Karle, I. P., Blehler, R. E., and Ohlson, M. A.: Nutritional status of cerebral-palsied children, J. Am. Diet. Assoc. 38:22, 1961.

21. Pipes, P.: Nutritional management of children with Prader-Willi Syndrome. In Holm, V., Sulzbacher, S. and Pipes, P.: The Prader-Willi Syndrome, Baltimore, University Park Press, 1980.

22. Pipes, P. L.: Feeding children with Down's syndrome, J. Am. Diet. Assoc. 77:277, 1980.

23. Pipes, P. L.: Nutrition and feeding of children with Down Syndrome. In Dmitriev, V. ed.: Advances in Down Syndrome, Seattle, Wash., 1988, Special Child Publications.

24. American Academy of Pediatrics, Committee on Genetics. New issues in newborn screening for phenylketonuria and congenital hypothyroidism, Pediatrics 69:104, 1982.

25. Trahms, C. M.: Long-term nutrition intervention model: the treatment of phenylketonuria, Top. Clin. Nutr. 1:62, 1986.

26. Danford, D. E., Smith, J. C., and Huber, A. M.: Pica and mineral status in the mentally retarded, Am. J. Clin. Nutr. 35:958, 1982.

27. Wilton, K. M., and Irvine, J.: Nutritional intakes of socioculturally mentally retarded children vs. children of low and average socioeconomic status, Am. J. Ment. Defic. 8:79, 1983.

28. Hahn, T. J., Shires, R., and Halstead, L. R.: Serum dihydroxyvitamin D metabolite concentrations in patients on chronic anticonvulsant therapy: response to pharmacologic doses of vitamin D_2, Metab. Bone Dis. Relat. Res. 5:1, 1983.

29. Silver, J., and others: Prevalence and treatment of vitamin D deficiency in children on anticonvulsant drugs, Arch. Dis. Child. 49:344, 1974.

30. Hahn, T. J.: Bone complications of anticonvulsants, Drugs 12:201, 1976.

31. Rivey, M. P., Schottelius, D. D., and Berg, M. J.: Phenytoin - folic acid: A review, Drug Intell. Clin. Pharm. 18:292, 1984.

32. Chien, L. F., and others: Harmful effect of megadoses of vitamins: electroencephalogram abnormalities and seizures induced by intravenous folate in drug treated epileptics, Am. J. Clin. Nutr. 28:51, 1975.

33. Klein, G. L., and others: Multiple vitamin deficiencies in association with chronic anticonvulsant therapy, Pediatrics 60:767, 1977.

34. Turkel, H.: Medical amelioration of cytogenic anomalies, Brooklyn, N.Y., 1971, Copen Press.

35. Williams, R. J.: Let's pursue nutrition to heal and prevent, Fam. Week. p. 4, April 25, 1976.

36. Harrell, R. J., and others: Can nutritional supplements help mentally retarded children, Proc. Natl. Acad. Sci. 78:574, 1981.

37. Ellis, N. R., and Tomporowski, R. D.: Vitamin/mineral supplements and intelligence of institutionalized mentally retarded adults, Am. J. Ment. Defic. 88:211, 1983.

38. Bennett, F. C., and others: Vitamin and mineral supplements in Down's syndrome, Pediatrics 72:707, 1983.

39. Illingworth, R. S., and Lister, J.: The critical or sensitive period with special reference to certain feeding problems in infants and children. J. Pediatr. 65:839, 1964.

40. Scales, H. E.: The application of operant conditioning to establish self-help feeding patterns in two mentally retarded children, unpublished Master of Nursing thesis, Seattle, 1966, University of Washington.

41. Connor, F. P., Williamson, G. G., and Siepp, J. M., editors: Program guide for infants and toddlers with neuromotor and other developmental disabilities, New York, 1978, Teachers College Press.

42. Morris, S. E.: The normal acquisition of oral feeding skills: implications for assessment and treatment, New York, 1982, Therapeutic Media, Inc.

43. Measel, C. P., and Anderson, G. C.: Nonnutritive sucking during tube feedings: effect on clinical course in premature infants, J. Obstet. Gynecol. Neonatal Nurs. 8(15):265, 1979.

44. Bosma, J. F.: Structure and function of the infant oral and pharyngeal mechanisms. In Wilson, J., editor: Oral motor function and dysfunction in children, Chapel Hill, N.C., 1977, University of North Carolina, Division of Physical Therapy.

45. Leonard, E. L., Trukowski, L., and Kirkpatrick, B. V.: Nutritive sucking in high-risk neonates after perioral stimulation, Phys. Ther. 60:299, 1980.

46. Ingram, T. T. S.: Clinical significance of infantile feeding reflexes, Dev. Med. Child Neurol. 4:159, 1962.

47. Radtke, S.: Feeding reflexes and neural control. In Wilson, J., editor: Oral motor function and dysfunction in children, Chapel Hill, N. C., 1977, University of North Carolina, Division of Physical Therapy.

48. Mueller, H.: Facilitating feeding and prespeech. In Pearson, P. H., and Williams, C. E., editors: Physical therapy services in the developmental disabilities, Springfield, Ill., 1972, Charles C. Thomas, Publisher.

49. Mueller, H.: Feeding. In Finnie, N. R.: Handling the young cerebral palsied child at home, New York, 1975, E. P. Dutton & Co., Inc.

50. Sweetman, L., and others: Clinical and metabolic abnormalities in a boy with dietary deficiency of biotin, Pediatrics 68:553, 1981.

14

Diet and Behavior

Betty Lucas

OBJECTIVES

After studying this chapter, the student should:

1. Be familiar with possible effects of diet on behavior.

2. Be aware of the effect of omitting breakfast on learning.

3. Know the symptoms of hyperactivity (attention deficit disorder).

4. Be aware of the effect of stimulant medication prescribed for control of hyperactivity on appetite, food intake, and growth.

5. Be aware of the limitations of an additive-free diet on the treatment of hyperactivity.

6. Be aware of the theories and studies about megavitamins and hyperactivity.

7. Be familiar with the many theories about sugar and behavior and the results of well-designed studies on the issue.

Does sugar make a child "hyper"? Does skipping breakfast really make any difference in school performance? Are food additives or allergies a cause of behavior problems in children? These and similar questions are often asked by parents, teachers, and health care workers. A good deal of information on diet and behavior is available, but some of it is myth, some is controversial, and some is based on sound scientific research. This chapter attempts to clarify the issues of diet's effect on the behavior of children, including diet and cognitive development, stimulant medication and hyperactivity, and the behavioral effects of food additives, sugar, megavitamins, and allergies.

NUTRITION AND COGNITIVE DEVELOPMENT

Dozens of studies over the last few decades have documented the negative effect of malnourishment on children's intellectual development. (See Chapter 1 for a thorough discussion.) A more gray area of any diet-cognitive connection is whether "marginal" malnutrition or skipping meals affects behavior or school performance. A review of nutrition and school performance studies over several decades suggests that children who go to school without breakfast are likely to be more inattentive, lethargic, and irritable, but there has been no strong documentation to support this association.[1] A study of 9- to 11-year-old children in a laboratory setting measured problem solving, memory, and attentiveness after the children had eaten or not eaten breakfast. Although blood glucose levels were not significantly different between children fed or not fed, other biochemical parameters suggested a metabolic stress on those without breakfast. The children who had fasted made more errors on the problem-solving task but performed better on short-term memory recall.[2]

A similar study assessed these same cognitive abilities throughout the morning in same-age children who received or did not receive breakfast. The fasting children made more errors and had a more variable performance on a continuous performance task over the course of the morning than the children who had had breakfast.[3] Although these results show that brief fasting has an impact on cognitive function, the degree to which skipping breakfast alone affects behavior or school performance remains unclear.

Iron deficiency, the most common nutrient deficiency in children, has long been implicated in negative changes in behavior and performance. Iron is involved in the functioning of many molecules in the brain and nervous system, and these systems are sensitive to lowered iron levels long before overt anemia is diagnosed. In a recent review, Pollit and associates[4] concluded that, compared with controls, iron-deficient infants with and without anemia tend to score lower on standard scales of mental development. They also found

that, compared with controls, preschool children with iron deficiency with or without anemia are less likely to pay attention to relevant cues in problem-solving situations. This information has clinical implications in terms of assessing the overall nutrient quality of the diet of a "behavior problem" child, as well as implications for public policy in addressing the nutrition needs of low-income, high-risk children.

A relatively new research focus has been the relationships between nutrition, the brain, and behavior. Studies have addressed the influence of dietary components on the synthesis of brain neurotransmitters, which in turn affect behaviors such as appetite, mood, and depression.[5] Results support the hypothesis that mental alertness is lower and lethargy and sleepiness increased after a high-carbohydrate rather than a high-protein lunch.[6] The carbohydrate-rich meal appears to enhance **serotonin** production, which effects the mental changes. Although most of this research has been done with adults, Yogman and Zeisel[7] reported on a study that examined the relationship between diet and sleep behavior in newborns. The infants fed a tryptophan-carbohydrate formula entered active and quiet sleep sooner than infants fed a valine–low-carbohydrate formula. These and other studies have demonstrated a general relationship between diet, brain chemistry, and behavior, but research will be needed to reveal the significance of individual variability, and to discern clinical implications for children.

HYPERACTIVITY

Over the last several decades the terms hyperactivity, **hyperkinesis,** and learning disability have become commonly used in American homes, in classrooms, in electronic media, and in print media. Although hyperactivity is ill defined and poorly understood, it has been identified as one of the most common problems among school-age children in the United States.

An estimated 3% to 5% of schoolchildren are believed to be affected by hyperactivity.[8] Boys are affected more often than girls; reported ratios range from 3:1 to 9:1.

A multitude of diagnostic terms have been used to describe the behavior and learning problems seen in these children: hyperkinetic syndrome, minimal brain dysfunction, learning disability, and others. The current preferred term is attention deficit disorder (ADD) with hyperactivity.[9] This difficulty with labels indicates the uncertainty regarding etiology and the tendency to emphasize symptoms rather than the overall problem. It may be that the hyperactive child syndrome is really a group of varying disorders with different causes.

According to the diagnostic criteria of the American Psychiatric Association,[9] a child with this disorder would display inappropriate inattention, impulsivity, and hyperactivity for his mental and chronological age. Signs must be observed by adults in the child's environment. Specific criteria for diagnosis include the following:

1. Inattention
2. Impulsivity
3. Hyperactivity
4. Onset before 7 years of age
5. Duration of at least 6 months
6. Not a result of **schizophrenia,** affective disorder, or mental retardation

Although a true diagnosis of hyperactivity is a result of assessment by medical or educational specialists, many children are labeled hyperactive by less formal measures of behavior in the school or home. Regardless of the looseness of the diagnosis, the main focus of those involved with the child becomes treatment and management.

Etiologic Factors

A variety of causes of ADD have been proposed over the years, yet the etiology remains relatively unknown. Possibly there are various causes, with hyperactivity and its associated behaviors being the common expression.

Perinatal complications such as **anoxia,** toxemia, prematurity, and infection have long been suggested as causes, as have insults during the early years, including head injuries, seizures, toxic agents, or infections. The greater incidence of a family history of hyperactivity and learning disabilities in the identified children suggests a genetic component.[10] Some studies have suggested a biochemical basis for ADD, but any mechanism in the disorder remains unclear.

Dietary factors have also been implicated as causes of hyperactivity. One of the best-known theories is that proposed by Feingold,[11] who identifies salicylate compounds and food additives as causes. Some experts also suggest that food allergy is highly correlated to the incidence of the syndrome, with basic foods such as milk, wheat, and egg being common culprits.[12] Sugar is currently the most often pinpointed of any foodstuff as a cause of hyperactivity and behavior disturbances, primarily in the popular media.

Other environmental factors that have been suggested in the etiology include exposure to fluorescent lights and heavy metals, such as lead. An unstable home environment or poor emotional relationships can also cause a child to exhibit some of the symptoms of hyperactivity.

In general, the etiology of hyperactivity continues to be a puzzle. Some of the proposed causes are mere associations without supportive data. Further investigations are needed to increase our understanding of the etiology of hyperactivity.

Treatment

The most widely used and accepted forms of therapy for ADD are medication, behavioral management, and special education. Stimulant medication has been used for more than 40 years, and its effectiveness is well accepted.

Methylphenidate (Ritalin) is the most widely used and accepted medication, with dextroamphetamine (Dexedrine) and pemoline (Cylert) used less frequently. Although the exact mechanism by which these medications work is not fully understood, hyperactive children respond to them with reduction in such undesirable behaviors as motor restlessness, short attention span, and irritability. Many people assume that, when the child is calmed down and paying more attention, academic performance improves. Some evidence, however, suggests that stimulant medications do not necessarily improve school learning and that long-term outcomes are no different from those of children who have no medication.[8,13]

For a long time it was believed that children responded to stimulant medication paradoxically; that is, hyperactive children were thought to be calmed by the medication, and nonhyperactive children were thought to be stimulated. Newer studies, however, have demonstrated that both hyperactive and nonhyperactive children respond to stimulant medication similarly, with decreased activity and improved cognitive performance.[14] Some specialists believe that long-term treatment of hyperactivity should emphasize behavior modification, parental counseling, and special school programs. Yet stimulant medication continues to be the most common therapy.

Dietary treatments of ADD have become more popular in the last decade. Included in this group are megavitamin therapy and diets that eliminate certain constituents (e.g., food additives, specific foods, salicylate compounds, sugar). Megavitamin therapy and these diets are discussed in depth later.

Stimulant medication and its effect on growth

One of the appeals of stimulant medication is its immediate dramatic effect with few toxic side effects. Anorexia is often noted as a side effect, but most authorities believe that this disappears, or at least diminishes, after a few weeks. Some initial weight loss is also reported, but generally it is believed to be transient. These assumptions have been supported by evidence that persons treated for obesity with stimulant medications develop tolerance for the drugs.

Safer, Allen, and Barr[15] first reported in 1972 on the negative effects of stimulant medication on physical growth. They found that hyperactive children receiving dextroamphetamine and methylphenidate had suppressed weight gain and height increase as compared with established norms. A later study showed that long-term use of dextroamphetamine resulted in a highly significant suppression of growth in weight and height. Methylphenidate caused a less striking growth suppression and only when the dosage was 20 mg/day or more. Safer and Allen[16] reported that tolerance developed to the weight-suppressant effects of dextroamphetamine after 3 years, but tolerance to its inhibition of height growth did not develop.

In a subsequent report, Safer, Allen, and Barr[17] presented data demonstrating a growth rebound in children who discontinued medication during the summer. The growth rates were 15% to 68% above the expected increment for the age groups. These findings suggested that in general, the degree of growth rebound is proportional to the degree of original medication suppression. Depending on the medication and dosage, however, a child may not be able to compensate completely in the summer for the growth suppression incurred during the school year.

Other reports have resulted in inconsistent findings.[18] Although most investigations have dealt mainly with dextroamphetamine and methylphenidate, pemoline seems to have the same growth-suppressing effect.[19] Many of these studies had methodological problems such as inexact methods for growth measurements, inadequate controls, and outdated growth norms.

Mattes and Gittelman[20] reported on the growth of 86 hyperactive children who received methylphenidate for up to 4 years. Height was significantly decreased after 2 to 4 years of treatment but not after 1 year. Significant weight loss occurred from the first year of treatment. There was a significant relationship between dosage and decreased growth, and larger children had greater growth decrements. Although the magnitude of the medication's effect was only about 2% of the variance in final height, the authors believed that growth should be monitored in children receiving stimulant medication, and dosage reductions should be considered individually.

The mechanism by which stimulant medication inhibits growth is unclear. Theories that have been postulated include (1) decreased energy intake resulting from anorexia, (2) inhibition of growth hormone secretion, (3) decreased production of **somatomedin**, (4) direct effect on bone and cartilage development, and (5) depressed blood prolactin levels.[18,21] For many of these proposed mechanisms, the data are conflicting and sketchy.

Two clinical case studies have documented the effect of stimulant medications on nutrient and energy intakes.[22] Both boys, who were followed for 12 months, had lower energy intakes when receiving medication, significantly so at higher levels. Methylphenidate appeared to have a less severe effect on energy intake than did dextroamphetamine. Increasing the dosage resulted in decreased kilocalorie levels (Figure 14-1). This suggests that actual reduced food consumption and subsequent low energy intakes may explain the growth retardation in these children. However, a combination of reduced energy intake and medication-induced endocrine abnormalities may be involved.

Hyperactive children receiving stimulant medication present a variety of feeding problems. Families and school personnel often report pickiness, dawdling at mealtime, school lunches refused or returned home, and disinterest in food. Some children have been observed to consume large amounts of concentrated carbohydrates and other low-nutrient foods because parents are concerned that the child eat something. Because of their children's poor appetites and slow growth, families frequently resort to bribery, indulgence, and threats to induce them to eat. It is easy to understand how a preoccupation with food and eating can lead to frustration for parents and children, resulting in inappropriate behaviors and interactions at mealtimes. When the children discontinue medication during vacations, their parents often note dramatic increases in appetite and food consumption.

Since it has been estimated that approximately 300,000 children in the United States are receiving stimulant medication,[21] it is reasonable to assume that a significant number of them are at risk of suppression of optimal physical growth. The efficacy of the medication should be assessed periodically using standard double-blind procedures. Since stimulant medications result in a moderate suppression of growth in weight and a minor suppression of growth in height, frequent measurement of weight and height is essential to monitor longitudinal changes in growth.

As for practical dietary management, it is important to know the type of medication, dosage, and time of administration. Since it takes about 30 minutes for the medication's effect to be clinically manifested, the medication should be given before or with meals to take advantage of optimal appetite. The medication's effect is usually minimal or absent after 4 to 6 hours, and energy-producing foods of high nutrient density should be offered at that time. Each child should be evaluated individually with regard to medication administration, meal and snack routine, and appetite response. Coordinating the child's daily schedule is essential to provide optimal nutrition status and

*Standard deviation

Figure 14-1 Calorie intake of one subject during baseline and drug therapy periods. (From Lucas B. and Sells, C.J.: Nutrient intake and stimulant drugs in hyperactive children, J. Am. Diet. Assoc. 70:373, 1977.)

physical growth. Some families benefit from counseling regarding specific feeding problems.

Food additives

In recent years the idea that chemicals added to food can cause children to exhibit a variety of behavior patterns such as restlessness, irritability, and short attention span has become popular. One of the best-known proponents of this idea was Benjamin Feingold, an allergist who in 1974 wrote a popular book on the subject of diet and hyperactivity.[11] He proposed that hyperactivity is related to the intake of artificial colors and flavors. He correlated the increased incidence of hyperactivity and learning disabilities with increased use of these substances in our food supply over the past few decades.

Feingold developed this theory as an outcome of his clinical work with allergy patients.

Many patients were sensitive to aspirin, which contains salicylate. This led Feingold to eliminate natural foods containing salicylate from their diet. Since many of these individuals were also allergic to tartrazine (a yellow dye), all artificial flavors and colors became suspect and were also eliminated.

Artificial colors and flavors are widespread in our food supply. Of some 2800 intentional additives used in foods, approximately 2100 are flavorings and 33 are colors, most of which are synthetic. Most concerns regarding additives center on safety issues and potential carcinogenicity. Two specific substances, however, cause adverse physical reactions in susceptible individuals. These are monosodium glutamate, which precipitates the Chinese restaurant syndrome, and tartrazine, which causes an allergic response in persons who are also sensitive to aspirin.[23,24]

Feingold diet

The Feingold diet is based on eliminating all foods containing natural salicylates (box below), all artificial colors and flavors, and the preservatives butylated hydroxyanisole (BHA) and butylated hydroxytoluene (BHT). Besides foods, items also excluded are aspirin, toothpaste, cough syrup, vitamins, and most medications for children. The entire family is encouraged to follow the diet, rather than isolating the child. After the child responds positively to the Feingold diet for approximately 4 to 6 weeks, the natural fruits and vegetables are gradually reintroduced to the child's diet as tolerated. This is commonly referred to as the modified Feingold diet. Recent data on the salicylate content of 333 food items show that the foods restricted on the Feingold diet do not make a complete list.[25]

Feingold reported a response rate of approximately 48%, but he was criticized because of the primarily subjective data, lack

---

Food Containing Natural Salicylates

Almonds	Mint leaves
Apples	Nectarines
Cider and cider vinegars	Oranges
Apricots	Peaches
Blackberries	Prunes and plums
Cherries	Raspberries
Cloves	Strawberries
Cucumbers and pickles	Tea, all kinds
Currants	Tomatoes
Gooseberries	Oil of wintergreen
Grapes and raisins	
Wine and wine vinegars	

From Feingold, B.F.:Hyperkinesis and learning disabilities linked to artificial food flavors and colors. Copyright 1975, American Journal of Nursing Company. Reproduced with permission from the American Journal of Nursing, May 1975, vol. 75, no. 5.

---

of control studies, and failure to report findings in reputed journals. Despite these criticisms, the diet became popular with the public. The National Advisory Committee on Hyperkinesis and Food Additives was formed to deal with the issue. Their report criticized the lack of double-blind controlled experiments on Feingold's theory, and it established guidelines for experimental studies to test the Feingold hypothesis.[26]

Experiments on the Feingold diet. One of the first double-blind controlled studies on the Feingold diet was conducted by Conners and others[27] using two diets (the Feingold diet and a control diet). Some improvements in behavior were noted while the children were on the Feingold diet, but there was difficulty in disguising the different diets from the families, and there were inconsistencies in the findings when the diet order was changed. The same investigators later reported on 16 hyperactive children who showed a minimum 25% improvement in behavior while on the Feingold diet. The children completed an 8-week double-blind challenge period in which they continued on the diet but were given specially prepared chocolate cookies with or without artificial color additives. The results showed no difference in behavioral parameters between challenge and placebo periods. However, younger children seem to be more susceptible to the challenge, and a greater number of performance deficits were noted when measured 1 to 2 hours after ingestion of the cookies with the additives.[28] An Australian group found similar results.[29]

Harley and others[30] conducted a study with 36 school-age boys and 10 preschool boys by using the Feingold diet and a control diet. When evaluated by neurological, psychological, and behavioral parameters, the results showed no significant improvement in the school-age boys. Ratings of the preschoolers showed a positive response to the diet, but the sample size was small and only parents reported. In a subsequent phase of the study, nine of the original children who had shown some positive response to the diet were put through a challenge regimen for 9 weeks. This consisted of maintaining the Feingold diet and adding cookies or candy bars with or without the food color additives. No significant differences were noted between challenge and placebo, but one child did appear to respond with alterations in behaviors.[31]

In another study, the effect of the Feingold diet was compared to the effect of stimulant medication.[32] Four different treatments were used for a week at a time: medication or placebo plus the diet with or without the additives. The ratings indicated some improvement with the Feingold diet, but stimulant medication was more effective than diet in decreasing hyperactive behaviors. On the other hand, teacher ratings suggested that the behavior was worse when the children were receiving placebo medication plus the additives.

Weiss and others[33] studied 22 children $2\frac{1}{2}$ to 7 years of age whose parents thought they were "super responders" to the Feingold regimen but who had not been diagnosed as hyperactive. In a double-blind trial, the children continued on the diet for 11 weeks but were challenged eight times with a carbonated beverage containing food color additives, receiving a placebo beverage the other days. Two children responded adversely to the additives when rated by parents and observers, one dramatically.

One of the criticisms of the controlled challenge study design is that the dose of additives has not been large enough to produce a response. Most of the studies have used 27 to 35 mg/day of mixed artificial colors in their challenge material—an amount that is supposed to represent an average intake for American children. Canadian researchers have suggested that the reaction to the additives may be related to dosage. Using a hospital clinical research unit, they challenged 40 children with 100 to 150 mg of the artificial colors and then measured response by a laboratory learning test rather than ratings.[34] The children's performance was significantly worse after receiving the challenge than after receiving the placebo, supporting the dose-response relationship. On the other hand, this information does not support Feingold's contention that even a single minor infraction of the diet causes a dramatic change in behavior. This study also suggests that laboratory learning tests may be a more sensitive measure of additive response than the behavior rating scales.

A nutritional assessment of the Feingold diet found that the diet produced poorer nutrient intakes than the control diet but that it still met the recommended dietary allowances.[27] Intakes of ascorbic acid were particularly low because of the exclusion of the natural salicylate–containing foods, many of which are excellent sources of this vitamin. In a later report the modified Feingold diet (eliminating only artificial colors and flavors) was analyzed for nutrient adequacy.[35] Mean intakes compared favorably with the recommended dietary allowances, and nutrient intakes did not change significantly while the subjects were on the Feingold regimen. Some people might assume that the overall nutrient quality of the modified Feingold diet is better than a control diet, since many foods containing the artificial flavors and colors are low nutrient-density items. A market survey in this study, however, showed that in each category of foods there were foods free of the additives that were of comparable nutritional quality to those foods excluded.

Overall, the controlled double-blind studies have not supported the Feingold diet as an effective therapy for hyperactivity.[36,37] The positive response that has been reported in uncontrolled studies and open trials is believed to be a placebo effect or the result of a significant change in the socioemotional environment of the child. It is certainly understandable that a family with a hyperactive child might expect a positive outcome from a diet that is relatively simple and without side effects. In addition, the focus on the dietary regimen may change the family setting by bringing the family together on a mutual project, giving positive attention to the hyperactive child, and lessening blame—changes that could result in a decrease in behaviors. The findings by one researcher that parents of children on the Feingold regimen were more rigid and controlling suggest that family structure and interaction may be critical in the use and success of the diet.[38]

On the other hand, evidence does exist that a small subgroup of hyperactive children benefit significantly from the diet. The research data suggest that the Feingold diet is effective for approximately 1 out of every 50 hyperactive children.[39] Although this calculated incidence of 2% is far from the 50% success rate reported by Feingold, it remains that some hyperactive children, perhaps 5% to 10%, will be dramatically improved on the regimen. The summary of a National Institutes of Health symposium on defined diets and hyperactivity states, "The Panel believes the defined diets should not be universally used in the treatment of childhood hyperactivity at this time. However, the Panel recognizes that initiation of a trial of dietary treatment or continuation of a diet in patients whose families and physicians perceive benefits, may be warranted."[36]

Many unknowns remain regarding food additives and behavior in children. Although there is little need to replicate the previously cited studies, future investigations may shed more light on the issue. Areas deserving more research include whether preschool children are more susceptible, whether there is an immediate pharmacological-related response, and whether there is an additive dose-behavior relationship. Current interest and research in behavioral **toxicology** may provide new information.

The clinician should make a comprehensive assessment of the individual child and discuss the various management options with the parents. For those parents who wish to use the Feingold diet and believe that it works, the reality of improvement cannot and should not be denied regardless of the source of that improvement. In addition, the modified Feingold diet, as long as it includes a wide variety of foods, can be quite adequate nutritionally. However, health professionals should take care to counsel the family not to disregard the potential help provided by special education, behavioral management, and other therapies that can combine appropriately with the diet.

Megavitamin therapy

The use of large doses of certain vitamins to treat hyperactivity and minimal brain dysfunction has become increasingly popular in recent years. Originating primarily from the popular press, lay groups, and some professionals, megavitamin therapy is loosely defined and varies a great deal in practice from individual to individual. It is also a component of "orthomolecular psychiatry," which is defined by Pauling[40] as "the achievement and preservation of mental health by varying the concentrations in the human body of substances that are normally present, such as the vitamins." The basis of megavitamin therapy is that children with ADD or learning problems have biochemical imbalances and that these disturbances can be eliminated by the consumption of large amounts of certain vitamins.

Megavitamin therapy was first used to treat schizophrenia, using nicotinic acid.[41] Currently, proponents of this treatment recommend its use for a variety of disorders including hyperactivity, autism, mental retardation, and degenerative diseases. Suspecting vitamin deficiency as a cause of mental and behavioral problems is a result of existing nutritional knowledge on deficiency states. Classic examples are the neurological and mental changes noted in persons with niacin deficiency (pellagra) and thiamine deficiency (beriberi).

Most commonly, megavitamin therapy includes niacin, ascorbic acid, pyridoxine, and calcium pantothenate. On the other hand, personal clinical experience has indicated that children receiving megavitamin therapy may be taking a wide assortment of vitamin and/or mineral supplements with or without expert guidance.

Generally, established medical professionals have not supported the megavitamin theory of treatment. A task force report of the American Psychiatric Association concluded that the claims of megavitamin advocates have not been confirmed by well-controlled studies and that most of the data are anecdotal.[41] Similarly, a statement by the American Academy of Pediatrics[42] reported that "megavitamin therapy as a treatment for learning disabilities and psychoses in children, including autism, is not justified on the basis of documented clinical trials."[42]

A few studies have tested megavitamin therapy using double-blind controlled studies. Arnold and others[43] reported on 31 children with minimal brain dysfunction who received either placebos or megavitamins during a 2-week trial. The megavitamin regimen was that advocated by Cott—1 gm of niacin, 1 gm of ascorbic acid, 100 mg of pyridoxine, 200 mg of pantothenate calcium, and 500 mg of glutamic acid, all twice daily. Parent and teacher behavior ratings taken before and after the trial showed no significant difference in the two groups. Only two children responded so well that stimulant medication was not considered necessary; they were both in the placebo group.

In an investigation by Kershner and Hawke,[44] 20 children with learning disabilities were put on a low-carbohydrate, high-protein diet and then given either megavitamins or placebos for 6 months. They were evaluated before and after this period with a combina-tion of intellectual, school achievement, perceptual, and behavioral measures. Results showed no difference between the two groups and thus failed to support the claim that megavitamins are helpful to children with learning disabilities. Most of the children, regardless of their group, showed behavioral progress; this may be a result of the diet alone, or it may be a placebo effect.

In a recent report, behavior and classroom performance of children with ADD actually worsened following megavitamin therapy, while the behavior of those receiving a placebo improved.[45] These studies were unable to support the theories advocated by the proponents of megavitamin therapy.

Although the literature is not extensive and reports on children are relatively few, potential dangers do exist from consuming large doses of vitamins. Toxicity from excess fat-soluble vitamins (A and D) has been documented.[46] These vitamins are not included in the standard megavitamin treatment, yet clinical experience reveals that some practitioners commonly recommend vitamins A and D, or that families may, on their own initiative, include them in their regimen. Other biochemical complications that have been reported are the destruction of vitamin B_{12} by large amounts of ascorbic acid, hyperbilirubinemia and liver damage by large doses of nicotinic acid, and liver damage by large doses of vitamin B_6.[47,48] A case of severe vitamin A intoxication has been reported for a 4-year-old child who was receiving megavitamins for minimal brain dysfunction. In another case, an 11-year boy who had been taking megavitamins for 4 years developed **cholelithiasis,** hepatitis, and thyroid dysfunction; he became well after a cholecystectomy and discontinuation of megavitamins.[50] Megavitamin therapy as an unfounded treatment for mental retardation is discussed in Chapter 13.

It is easy to understand why a family with a troubled child would respond to the appeal of megavitamin therapy. But too often it plays on the false hopes and guilt of the parents or provides a subject for blame. Some families can spend considerable money on vitamins and yet not deal with the basic problem related to the child's behavior.

There is no sound data to support the use of megavitamins with hyperactive children, yet the concept that some individuals may have increased needs for certain nutrients cannot be ignored. From a practical standpoint, the nutritional status of each child should be assessed and appropriate dietary intervention should be planned. In working with parents who choose to use megavitamins for their child, one needs to help them to recognize the practice as helpful, neutral, or harmful and to provide accurate information. At times counseling may be indicated to help families recognize and consider other treatment options.

SUGAR

Sugar (sucrose) has been implicated, mainly in popular books and anecdotal reports, as a causative factor in a multitude of diseases and disorders. Included in this group of disorders are diabetes, obesity, heart disease, and hypoglycemia, as well as mental and behavioral disorders such as hyperactivity, depression, and psychoses. Some practitioners believe that sugar is the most common food substance causing adverse behavior reactions in children. In addition, parents, teachers, and school nurses report dramatic negative changes in some children after receiving a load of sugar. Anecdotal stories describe children "climbing the walls" the day after Halloween. All these reports, however, are subjective and are not based on controlled studies.

One theory is that undesirable behavior is the result of low or fluctuating blood glucose levels in some individuals. In 1978 Langseth and Dowd[51] reported that nearly 75% of 261 hyperkinetic children had abnormal glucose tolerance curves following a 5-hour glucose

tolerance test. Lack of a control comparison group and controversy regarding glucose tolerance standards in children, however, make this data less conclusive. Other studies have not found abnormal glucose curves.[52]

A report by Prinz, Roberts, and Hantman[53] suggested that there was a positive correlation between sugar consumption and destructive-aggressive behavior in 4- to 7-year-old hyperactive children. This kind of correlation, however, does not imply a causative role for sugar in behavior problems of children. Other factors may be involved, such as a permissive home environment or a child who demands foods high in sucrose.

Compared to correlational studies, sucrose challenge studies have failed to detect significant negative behavioral effects of sucrose. Behar and associates studied sugar and behavior in 21 boys who, according to their parents, respond adversely to sugar.[54] Behavior ratings, motor activity, memory, and blood levels were monitored for 5 hours after a double-blind challenge of glucose, sucrose, or saccharin. These researchers found no significant effect of sugar on any of the behavioral measures in these children. Contrary to popular belief, the children who consumed sugar were less active and quieter after than those given the placebo. These results may support the theory that a high carbohydrate intake facilitates production of serotonin, or the results may derive from other unknown factors.

In another study, hyperactive boys were challenged with a sucrose or aspartame drink and then evaluated by measures of behavior, motor activity, and cognitive performance.[55] No significant differences were found between the sucrose and aspartame challenges for any of the tests. Similar studies, including those with preschool children, have reached the same conclusion.[52,56] One study of children hospitalized for severe behavioral disorders found a significant increase in movement and a decrease in appropriate behavior following a sucrose challenge.[3] Although measurable, the change in behavior was so subtle that teachers and nurses could not detect it. Also, these hospitalized children were not representative of the population at large.

At this time the only direct cause-effect relationship between sugar and disease is the role of sugar in dental caries (no such relationship exists with other diseases), but this does not preclude the possibility that an individual child might be responsive to a large sucrose load. More well-designed investigations of the relationship between sugar intake and behavior may help clarify the issue.

Americans consume large amounts of sugar, more than 100 lb per capita per year. It has been estimated that sugar represents approximately 24% of the average energy intake. Many foodstuffs that are high in sugar are low in nutrients, and thus they dilute the nutrient quality of the diet. Indeed, reducing or eliminating sugar in the diet serves to improve the overall nutritional and dental health of both child and family. These positive changes in families' diets have been observed in personal clinical experience. The professional can reinforce the dietary changes while stressing the lack of data supporting a sugar-behavior association.

ALLERGY

Food allergies are known to produce respiratory, gastrointestinal, and skin manifestations in the susceptible individual. Some experts also believe that they cause behaviors commonly found in hyperactive children—excessive activity, lack of attention, and irritability.[12] True allergies are a result of the production of antibodies against specific proteins in the foods that the child eats. The most common food allergies are the proteins of milk, egg, wheat, nuts, and soy.

There have been reports indicating that hyperactive children have a higher incidence of food allergies and that they respond pos-

itively to an elimination diet, thus supporting a causal relationship between food allergies and hyperactivity.[12,57,58] One report suggests that a 7-day fast supplemented with an elemental formula can be a useful diagnostic procedure in determining those hyperactive children who are food hypersensitive by measuring an improved behavior response.[59] Some of these reports are subjective, however, and controversy exists regarding the validity and interpretation of the allergy tests used.

In cases in which food allergy is suspected, it is appropriate to obtain a thorough diagnosis by an expert clinician, including a double-blind food challenge.[60] However, there is no guarantee that behavioral symptoms will improve. Currently, no strong evidence is available to support a direct relationship between food allergy and hyperactivity, but the possibility that some children have adverse behavior reactions to food, whether they be immunological reactions or not, cannot be ruled out.

For a further discussion of food allergies, see Chapter 11.

Summary

There seem to be more questions than answers about the role of diet in behavior. Although no sound data have definitively implicated dietary factors as causes or shown dramatic improvement as a result of diet treatment, not all the evidence is clear-cut. Studies of free-living populations have their design and control limitations; other investigations remain to be done.

The various proposed dietary treatments for hyperactivity or other behavioral disorders have not been supported by documentation. It appears that a small percentage of children, however, may be susceptible to certain food additives, and it cannot be ruled out that some children might react to large amounts of commonly consumed foods. On the other hand, it remains difficult to ascertain the environmental and emotional aspects that may affect a child's behavior.

It is important that an objective and comprehensive assessment and diagnosis be done initially. Children using stimulant medication should have their physical growth monitored frequently, and nutritional counseling should be available as needed.

When working with families who are using some of the dietary approaches (e.g., Feingold diet, megavitamins, sugar-free diet), remaining open minded and objective is critical. In that way rapport can be maintained, and the professional continues to be a resource. For the individual child, the actual dietary practices should be assessed as to adequacy and rationale. Obviously, positive changes in the diet should be reinforced, such as decreasing sugar consumption or using more nutrient-dense foods. Practices that are undesirable or potentially harmful (such as some megavitamin doses) can be discussed with the family on a factual level and incorporated in any decisions to change. Lecturing or emotional appeals are usually not productive.

Children with ADD or other behavior difficulties tend to be difficult to manage and hard to live with. Their families deserve great credit for handling the symptoms and subsequent problems as well as they do. It is certainly a relief to them when a dietary treatment decreases the negative behaviors and makes their child more enjoyable and less stress-producing for the family. Despite whatever components were involved in the change, their success is real and should not be denied.

The years to come will no doubt bring more information and definitive answers to the questions posed by this topic.

SUGGESTED LEARNING ACTIVITIES

1. Prepare a talk for a parent group on the relationship of diet and hyperactivity.
2. Check a drug store or a health food store for vitamin and mineral supplements for children. Compare the nutrient dosage levels and the costs of the supplements.
3. Assess the nutritional status of a child who has been on long-term stimulant medication. What is the growth pattern? Is the appetite and nutrient intake appropriate?
4. Obtain a 3-day food record for a 7- to 9-year-old child. Modify the menus to fit the Feingold diet, making substitutions for food items eliminated. Determine nutrient adequacy of the modified diet.
5. Plan a list of snacks representing all food groups that would contain no sucrose but that would be acceptable to school-age children.

REFERENCES

1. Pollitt, E., Gersovitz, M., and Gargiulo, M.: Educational benefits of the United States' school feeding program: a critical review of the literature, Am. J. Public Health 68:477, 1978.
2. Pollitt, E., Leibel, R. L., and Greenfield, D.: Brief fasting, stress, and cognition in children, Am. J. Clin. Nutr. 34:1526, 1981.
3. Conners, C. K., and Blouin, A. G.: Nutritional effects on behavior of children, J. Psychiatr. Res. 17:193, 1982/1983.
4. Pollitt, E., and others: Iron deficiency and behavioral development in infants and pre-school children, Am. J. Clin. Nutr. 43:555, 1986.
5. Wurtman, R. J.: Ways that foods affect the brain, Nutr. Rev. 44(suppl):2, 1986.
6. Spring, B. J., and others: Effects of carbohydrates on mood and behavior, Nutr. Rev. 44(suppl):51, 1986.
7. Yogman, M. W., and Zeisel, S.: Diet and sleep patterns in newborn infants, N. Engl. J. Med. 309:1147, 1983.
8. Varley, C. K.: Attention deficit disorder (the hyperactivity syndrome): a review of selected issues, Dev. Behav. Pediatr. 5:254, 1984.
9. American Psychiatric Association task force on nomenclature and statistics: Diagnostic and statistical manual of mental disorders, ed. 3, Washington, D.C., 1980, The Association.
10. Millichap., J. G.: The hyperactive child with minimal brain dysfunction, Chicago, 1975, Year Book Medical Publishers, Inc.
11. Feingold, B.F.: Why your child is hyperactive, New York, 1974, Random House, Inc.
12. Crook, W. G.: Food allergy—the great masquerader, Pediatr. Clin. North Am. 22:227, 1975.

13. Kolata, G. B.: Childhood hyperactivity: a new look at treatment and causes, Science 199:515, 1978.

14. Weingartner, H., and others: Cognitive processes in normal and hyperactive children and their response to amphetamine treatment, J. Abnorm. Psychol. 89:25, 1980.

15. Safer, D. J., Allen, R. P., and Barr, E.: Depression of growth in hyperactive children on stimulant drugs, N. Engl. J. Med. 287:217, 1972.

16. Safer, D. J., and Allen, R. P.: Factors influencing the suppressant effects of two stimulant drugs on the growth of hyperactive children, Pediatrics 51:660, 1973.

17. Safer, D. J., Allen, R. P., and Barr, E.: Growth rebound after termination of stimulant drugs, J. Pediatr. 86:113, 1975.

18. Roche, A. E., and others: The effects of stimulant medication on the growth of hyperkinetic children, Pediatrics 63:847, 1979.

19. Friedmann, N., and others: Effect on growth in pemoline-treated children with attention deficit disorder, Am. J. Dis. Child. 135:329, 1981.

20. Mattes, J. A., and Gittelman, R.: Growth of hyperactive children on maintenance regimen of methylphenidate, Arch. Gen. Psychiatry 40:317, 1983.

21. Shaywitz, S. E., and others; Psychopharmacology of attention deficit disorder: pharmacokinetic, neuroendocrine, and behavioral measures following acute and chronic treatment with methylphenidate, Pediatrics 69:688, 1982.

22. Lucas, B., and Sells, C. J.: Nutrient intake and stimulant drugs in hyperactive children, J. Am. Diet. Assoc. 70:373, 1977.

23. Nagy, M.: Monosodium glutamate and the "Chinese restaurant syndrome," J.A.M.A. 225:1665, 1973.

24. Zlotlow, M. J., and Settipane, G. A.: Allergic potential of food additives: a report of a case of tartrazine sensitivity without aspirin intolerance, Am. J. Clin. Nutr. 30:1023, 1977.

25. Swain, A. R., Dutton, S. P., and Truswell, A. S.: Salicylates in foods, J. Am. Diet. Assoc. 85:950, 1985.

26. The National Advisory Committee on Hyperkinesis and Food Additives: Report to the Nutrition Foundation, New York, 1975, The Nutrition Foundation, Inc.

27. Conners, C. K., and others: Food additives and hyperkinesis: a controlled double-blind experiment, Pediatrics 58:154, 1976.

28. Goyette, C. H., and others: Effects of artificial colors on hyperactive children: a double-blind challenge study, Psychopharmacol. Bull. 14(2):39, 1978.

29. Levy, F., and others: Hyperkinesis and diet: a double-blind crossover trial with a tartrazine challenge, Med. J. Aust. 1:61, 1978.

30. Harley, J. P., and others: Hyperkinesis and food additives: testing the Feingold hypothesis, Pediatrics 61:818, 1978.

31. Harley, J. P., Mathews, C. G., and Eichman, P.: Synthetic food colors and hyperactivity in children: a double-blind challenge experiment, Pediatrics 62:975, 1978.

32. Williams, J. I., and others: Relative effects of drugs and diet on hyperactive behaviors: an experimental study, Pediatrics 61:811, 1978.

33. Weiss, B., and others: Behavioral responses to artificial food colors, Science 207:1487, 1980.

34. Swanson, J. M., and Kinsbourne, M: Food dyes impair performance of hyperactive children on a laboratory learning test, Science 207:1485, 1980.

35. Harper, P. H., Goyette, C. H., and Conners, C. K.: Nutrient intakes of children on the hyperkinesis diet, J. Am. Diet. Assoc. 73:515, 1978.

36. National Institutes of Health Consensus Development Conference Summary: Defined diets and childhood hyperactivity, vol. 4, no. 3, Washington, D.C., 1982, The Institutes.

37. Wender, E. H., and Lipton, M. A., Chairmen, National Advisory Committee on Hyperkinesis and Food Additives: Final report to the Nutrition Foundation, New York, 1980, The Nutrition Foundation, Inc.

38. Feingold families found to be "rigid" in discipline, Nutrition Week, No. 20, Washington, D.C., May 19, 1983, Community Nutrition Institute.

39. Lipton, M. A., and Mayo, J. P.: Diet and hyperkinesis—an update, J. Am. Diet. Assoc. 83:132, 1983.

40. Pauling, L.: On the orthomolecular environment of the mind: orthomolecular therapy, Am. J. Psychiatry 131:1251, 1974.

41. American Psychiatric Association task force on vitamin therapy: Megavitamins and orthomolecular therapy in psychiatry, Nutr. Rev. 1(suppl):44, 1974.

42. Committee on Nutrition, American Academy of Pediatrics: Megavitamin therapy for childhood psychoses and learning disabilities, Pediatrics 58:910, 1976.

43. Arnold, L. E., and others: Megavitamins for minimal brain dysfunction: a placebo-controlled study, J.A.M.A. 240:2642, 1978.

44. Kershner, J., and Hawke, W.: Megavitamins and learning disorders: a controlled double-blind experiment, J. Nutr. 109:819, 1979.

45. Haslam, R. H. A., Dalby, J. T., and Rademaker, A. W.: Effects of megavitamin therapy on children with attention deficit disorders, Pediatrics 74:103, 1984.

46. Committee on Safety, Toxicity, and Misuse of Vitamins and Trace Minerals, National Nutrition Consortium: Vitamin-mineral safety, toxicity, and misuse, Chicago, 1978, American Dietetic Association.

47. White, P. L.: Megavitamin this and megavitamin that, J.A.M.A. 233:538, 1975.
48. Winter, S. L., and Boyer, J. L.: Hepatic toxicity from large doses of vitamin B$_3$ (nicotinamide), N. Engl. J. Med. 289:1180, 1973.
49. Shaywitz, B. A.: Megavitamins for minimal brain dysfunction: a potentially dangerous therapy, J.A.M.A. 238:1749, 1977.
50. Wright, K.: Personal communication, 1978.
51. Langseth, L., and Dowd, J.: Glucose tolerance and hyperkinesis, Food Cosmet. Toxicol. 16:129, 1978.
52. Rapoport, J. L.: Diet and hyperactivity, Nutr. Rev. 44(suppl):158, 1986.
53. Prinz, R. J., Roberts, W. A., and Hantman, E.: Dietary correlates of hyperactive behavior in children, J. Consult. Clin. Psychol. 48:760, 1980.
54. Behar, D., and others: Sugar challenge testing with children considered behaviorally "sugar reactive," Nutr. Behav. 1:277, 1984.
55. Wolraich, M., and others: Effects of sucrose ingestion on the behavior of hyperactive boys, J. Pediatr. 106:675, 1985.
56. Ferguson, H. B., Stoddart, C., and Simeon, J. G.: Double-blind challenge studies of behavioral and cognitive effects of sucrose-aspartame ingestion in normal children, Nutr. Rev. 44(suppl):144, 1986.
57. Tryphonas, H., and Trites, R.: Food allergy in children with hyperactivity, learning disabilities and/or minimal brain dysfunction, Ann. Allergy 42:22, 1979.
58. Rapp, D. J.: Does diet effect hyperactivity? J. Learning Disabilities 11:56, 1978.
59. Hughes, E. C., and others: Food sensitivity in attention deficit disorder with hyperactivity (ADD/HA): a procedure for differential diagnosis, Ann. Allergy 49:276, 1982.
60. Hypersensitivity to food. In Committee on Nutrition, American Academy of Pediatrics: Pediatric nutrition handbook, 2nd ed., Elk Grove Village, Ill., 1985, American Academy of Pediatrics.

15

Management
of Mealtime Behaviors

OBJECTIVES

After studying this chapter, the student should:

1. Be aware of behavior management as a therapeutic approach to changing food patterns of children.

2. Understand one approach to the analysis of behavior.

3. Recognize the need to individualize reinforcers.

4. Understand when it is appropriate to use food as a reinforcer.

5. Be aware of methods used to teach children self-feeding.

Parent-child interactions are important determinants of children's acceptance of food and attitudes toward eating. They often are responsible for difficulties presented to health professionals. Parents, anxious about their children's nutrient intakes, sometimes urge, nag, or pressure children to eat, and children often assume control of the feeding environment. The battle for control may become so intense that the children's nutrient intakes may be compromised. The conflict may result in a variety of problems including failure to thrive, overweight, and obesity.

Parent-child interaction is a complex reciprocal process in which each response to an action can become the cause of future behaviors and in which both parents and children learn new behaviors. This interaction continuum includes parents' expressions of attitudes, values, interests, beliefs, and their caregiving behavior, as well as children's individual growth patterns, learning potential, and ability to incorporate increasingly complex experiences into their current stages of thinking and functioning. Behavior is both the cause and effect of other behaviors. All parent-child interactions are both elicited by the child and influence the child. For instance, the cries of an infant who is hungry can become the stimulus for the mother to respond by feeding the infant.

Behavior modification is a therapeutic tool often employed to extinguish socially unacceptable feeding behaviors (such as throwing food), to increase a child's acceptance of a variety of foods, or to teach self-feeding. Sometimes nutritionists and dietitians work jointly with behaviorists in establishing and monitoring such programs. Often, nutritionists and dietitians apply behavior management concepts themselves. Concepts and methods of behavior modification are presented in this chapter.

BASIC CONCEPTS IN BEHAVIOR ASSESSMENT AND MANAGEMENT

Behaviorists have determined that behaviors are increased, maintained, or decreased by the consequences that immediately follow them.[1] These consequences can be reinforcing or punishing. Since *reinforcers* and *punishers* are defined from an individual's point of view, what may be reinforcing to one person may not be to someone else; the determination of what is reinforcing or punishing depends on the effect of a particular consequence on the behavior that preceded it. To be a reinforcer, a consequence must increase the behavior that it follows.

Reinforcers are of two types: positive and negative. Positive reinforcement is a consequence in which something desirable to the subject is added or applied to his or her environment as a result of a specific behavior. A smile, a hug, praise, food, and money are examples of positive reinforcers. Negative reinforcement, on the other hand, is a consequence in which something unpleasant is removed or terminated. For example, a person who is annoyed by loud static on the radio may turn down the volume or turn off the radio. The silence, or absence of static, is a negative reinforcer for turning off the sound, and the person is likely to do it again if static recurs. All reinforcers must increase the behavior that they follow. The important distinction between these two concepts is that in positive reinforcement something pleasant is added as a consequence and in negative reinforcement something unpleasant is removed as a consequence.

Punishers decrease the behaviors that they follow. They are defined operationally in two ways. *Punishment* involves consequences in which something averse is added or applied, such as a spanking. *Extinction* involves those consequences in which a positive reinforcer is removed. For example, the withholding of adult attention (ignoring) during a child's temper tantrum or withholding eye contact when someone else is talking should decrease negative behaviors.

Interaction Processes Between Positive and Negative Reinforcement and Punishment

To examine positive and negative reinforcement and punishment as interactive processes, it is important to analyze the various parts of interaction. Peterson has suggested that one way to do this effectively is to consider interaction in terms of *A* (antecedent events), *B* (behavior), and *C* (consequences).[2] Consider the following example in which the ABC analysis is used. A mother takes her preschool son into a grocery store. The child immediately begins to ask for candy, then whines and cries when the mother refuses to give him any. After several minutes of loud crying and repeated looks from other shoppers, the mother gives the child a piece of candy. The child immediately stops crying. A diagrammatic analysis of this situation is presented below.

A (antecedent)	B (child's behavior)	C (consequence)
1. Entering grocery store	2. Asks for candy	3. Mother refuses
	4. Cries and yells	5. Mother gives candy
	6. Stops crying	

In giving her child candy the mother reinforced her child for crying. Also, because he was reinforced, it is highly likely that the child will repeat this behavior during future trips to the grocery store. The mother received negative reinforcement because the crying ceased after the mother gave the child the candy. By giving candy, she terminated something that was aversive to her—the child's crying. In this interaction both mother and child were reinforced for their behaviors. The child was positively reinforced (candy was added) for crying, and the mother was negatively reinforced (crying was removed) for giving the candy. Both are likely to repeat their behaviors next time.

What if, in a similar situation, the mother decided to ignore the child? What would the mother's consequences be if ignoring stopped the crying? As before, she is negatively reinforced if she successfully stops the crying. Because the mother will be negatively reinforced for whatever she does that stops the crying, she may be reinforced for being inconsistent: giving candy one time, ignoring the child the next, and perhaps spanking another time.

It is easy for parents to become trapped in their responses to their children's behaviors and thus become unable to see those aspects of their interactions that are ineffective for both of them. It becomes important for parents to consider how they would like to respond most consistently to their child in the light of the behaviors they would like their child to learn. Parents have to consider their child's stage of development and reinforcers that fit his or her particular stage and personality. In addition, they have to be aware of the effects of the child's behavior on themselves. This is no small task, and it seems to become especially important around mealtimes. Since nutrition, socialization, and intense family interactions converge in this event, it is no wonder that so many clinical issues arise around mealtime behaviors.

Assessment of Mealtime Behaviors

Initial assessment consists of identifying the patterns of parent-child mealtime behaviors. The observation checklist on page 406 is a useful recording guide that pinpoints both problem behavior and desirable behavior. This tool can be used by professionals who are recording their direct observations or by parents who are recording the mealtime behaviors of themselves and their children. Behaviors can be tallied for each meal.

Once problem behaviors are identified, the most frequent eating and noneating behaviors and their consequences can be identified in ABC sequences. Parents are helped to identify those child behaviors that they wish to change as well as the appropriate eating behaviors that they wish to foster in their children. The next step is to determine appropriate consequences for all the behavior categories.

As I noted earlier, parents generally behave toward their children (reinforce, punish, or ignore) in certain ways because of the reinforcement they receive from their children. For instance, they may reinforce a crying child with a cookie because they know this will stop the crying. Thus the parent is negatively reinforced for giving the child the cookie. Frequently, to help parents change the consequences they provide their children, it is necessary to look at the reinforcers parents are getting for their own behavior. One way to do this is to help them identify the subsequent child behavior step to the ABC pattern. For parents to alter their antecedent cues to the child, they must be aware of these behaviors and their part in the entire ABC pattern.

The brief case studies that follow illustrate a variety of parent-child ABC patterns that relate to mealtimes.

1 Laura refuses to drink milk.

A (mother)	B (child)	C (mother)
1. Pours milk into glass	2. Starts crying 4. Cries 6. Stops crying and drinks soda	3. "Drink your milk." 5. Removes milk and gives child soda

In this instance the mother was negatively reinforced. She successfully terminated the crying by giving the child soda, which, in turn, positively reinforced the child's crying when milk was presented to her.

2 Billy, a toddler, writes his own menu.

A (mother)	B (child)	C (mother)
1. Presents applesauce to toddler in highchair	2. Cries and whines, points to the refrigerator 4. Cries, points to cupboard 6. Cries, points to cupboard and refrigerator 8. Cries, points to refrigerator 10. Child screams 12. Stops crying	3. "What do you want?" 5. "Do you want a cracker?" Gives him a cracker 7. "What do you want? Here is some cereal." 9. "No you can't have ice cream." 11. "OK, here is some ice cream."

In this situation the child keeps his mother going in circles in an effort to stop his crying. A management plan was developed with her in which she would leave the room and when the child would stop crying she would return and praise him for eating so nicely. The ABC looked like this:

A (mother)	B (child)	C (mother)
1. Presents applesauce to toddler in highchair	2. Cries, points to cupboard 4. Slowly stops crying, starts eating applesauce 6. Child laughs and keeps on eating	3. Leaves room (can see child but he can't see her) 5. Returns and says "My, what a big boy!"

3 John, a school-age child who has a hearing impairment, wanders at mealtimes.

A (parents)	B (child)	C (parents)
1. Announce dinner	2. Sits at table with parents 4. Gets up and wanders around house 6. Approaches dining room 8. Wanders away from dining room 10. John sits and looks at food 12. John leaves table	3. Talk to each other, ignore child 5. Yell, "Come back here, John." 7. Ignore John 9. "Come here, John," Father goes and leads him to table 11. Ignore John

Child Behaviors at Mealtime

Meals Observed

Noneating behaviors	1	2	3	4	5	6
Arguing						
Complaining						
Crying						
Hitting						
Noncomplying						
Not sitting at table						
Teasing						
Yelling						
Pouting						
Whining						
Moving hands nonpurposefully						
Talking back						
Throwing food or utensils						
Spitting						
Gagging						
Refusing certain foods						

Eating behaviors	1	2	3	4	5	6
Using fingers for finger foods						
Using utensils appropriately						
Sitting at table						
Accepting variety of foods						
Socializing as appropriate						
Complying to requests						

Parent Behaviors at Mealtime

Meals Observed

Antecedents to child behaviors	1	2	3	4	5	6
Commanding						
Requesting						
Questioning						
Prompting verbally						
Physically assisting						
Interrupting						
Positioning child appropriately						
Presenting food appropriately						
Presenting appropriate utensils						

Consequences of child behaviors	1	2	3	4	5	6
Commenting positively						
Commenting negatively						
Ignoring						
Touching						
Spanking						
Yelling						
Arguing						
Laughing						
Using same tone of voice						
Talking irrelevantly						

In discussing this ABC with John's parents they decided that they had been reinforced by John's absence at the table since, before that time, he had had tantrum behavior at the table. They believed that he should eat with them, but it was more comfortable to eat without him and to feed him later. A management program was developed with them in which they agreed to reinforce him for sitting at the table, using signing as well as verbal praise, and to try to include him in the general conversation. A subsequent ABC looked like this:

A (parents)	B (child)	C (parents)
1. Announce dinner	2. John sits at table, starts eating	3. Talk and sign to John
	4. Leaves table	5. Ignore John
	6. Approaches table	7. Talk and sign to John, discussing day's events
	8. Sits down, starts to eat	9. Eat, yet continue to socialize with John
	10. John talks, signs, eats, and remains seated during meal	

The importance of antecedents

Although consequences are important in maintaining behaviors, the antecedent events frequently tell a child or parent that certain behaviors will be reinforced. As discriminative stimuli, antecedents set the occasion for reinforcers. For example, when the mother in case 1 poured the milk, the child knew that if she cried at that time she would be likely to get soda instead.

Frequently, in an attempt to get control of such a situation this parent may have suggested as she poured the milk, "You have to drink milk, you will not get soda this time." However, the child cries anyway, even louder and longer than before. To terminate the crying the parent generally gives in and replaces the milk with soda. Instead of discouraging the child, the parent has only made the discriminative stimulus even stronger by adding the verbal reminder when pouring the milk.

Another example of important antecedents is demonstrated in case 4.

4 Suzi, a preschooler, uses cues supplied by her mother to control her mother's behavior.

A (mother)	B (child)	C (mother)
Meal 1		
1. Presents food	2. Eats	3. Sits with book, does not talk to child
Meal 2		
1. Presents food	2. Gags and spits up food	3. Attends, cleans up child, then finishes feeding her the meal

In assessing this situation, it was found that Suzi did not vomit every meal. Yet somehow she was getting cues as to when to vomit. In an attempt to further identify these cues, the mother's meal preparation was observed as part of the antecedent behavior. Surprisingly, the typical ABC pattern for vomiting and nonvomiting meals looked like this:

A (mother)	B (child)	C (mother)
Vomiting meal		
1. Preparing lunch, mother says, "Suzi, you have carrots today. I hope you don't vomit them."	2. Starts eating, then gags and vomits carrots	3. Attends, cleans her up, and feeds her the rest of the meal
Nonvomiting meal		
1. Preparing lunch, mother says, "Oh good, Suzi, you have macaroni today."	2. Eating well	3. Sitting with book, ignoring Suzi

For the vomiting meal, mother was cuing Suzi to the fact that if she vomited she would get attention, be cleaned up, and be fed her lunch. For the nonvomiting meal no such cue was given, so Suzi ate her lunch as expected. These ABC patterns were discussed with the mother, and a strategy was developed in which she would not read at mealtime, would reinforce Suzi for eating by talking with her at mealtime, and would only provide antecedent verbal cues such as in the nonvomiting meal. A later ABC pattern looked like this:

A (mother)	B (child)	C (mother)
1. "Suzi, we have egg sandwiches today."	2. Eats, smiles, and talks to mother	3. Attends to Suzi by smiling and conversing

ADDITIONAL CONCEPTS IN BEHAVIOR MANAGEMENT

There is no doubt about the importance of food as an effective reinforcer for most people. Since it meets a basic biological need, it is considered to be a primary reinforcer. Secondary reinforcers such as affection, praise, and touch derive their reinforcing qualities from having been paired with food during the early infant period. Later, money becomes reinforcing when used to buy a wide variety of reinforcers such as food, shelter, clothing, and other desirable items. Food is a potential reinforcer for a wide variety of activities; it is frequently paired with or follows attendance at outings, movies, sports, and social events.

The decision to use food as a reinforcer is made after a careful assessment process in which a variety of reinforcers are tried. Reinforcers are individualized, as discussed earlier. What may be reinforcing for one individual may not be for another, depending on biophysiological factors within an individual and his or her history of experiences.

For some children social praise may be reinforcing, for others food may be reinforcing. For still others neither social praise nor food is reinforcing, and parents must seek other kinds of reinforcer. Children who have developmental delays may not be able to use the usual things that most children find reinforcing. Because of sensory deficits or problems in neuromuscular development or because experiences have been limited, these children may need specialized reinforcers such as vibration, flickering lights, or even music. Therefore an effort must be made to determine what kind of reinforcer is effective for any given individual. In some instances food is the only reinforcer with which a child can learn appropriate behaviors. If this is the case, food should be used and other reinforcers (e.g., affection and praise) can be paired with it until they also become reinforcing for this particular individual and food no longer needs to be used.

When it has been determined that food will be the most effective reinforcer for a particular child, several considerations are important. The first factor is the kind of food to use. Again, this should be individualized according to the child's tastes, and care should be taken to use food with high-nutrient value whenever possible. In many instances potato chips and candy are used when raisins or cheese might be just as effective. Any food reinforcement should be considered as part of the total nutrient and caloric intake for the child.

Another factor to consider is the timing of food reinforcers. If one is concerned that the child eat adequate meals, training programs that use food reinforcers should not immediately precede a meal. Likewise, if success in the training program is important, a program using food reinforcers should not directly follow a meal. Any individual may become satiated by food unless adequate time has elapsed between intervals of food intake.

Satiation can also occur when too much of the same food is given to ensure maximum effectiveness of the reinforcer, particular foods used during a training program should not be available to the child at any other time of the day. For instance, a child may be given a dish of ice cream daily at home. If a decision is made to use a dish of ice cream in a program at school, the ice cream should no longer be available at home.

Another factor to consider when using food reinforcement is the pairing of another potential reinforcer with food. Because it is important for the child to be able to use other reinforcers, it is necessary to provide reinforcers such as praise at the same time that food is given. After it is determined that the combination of food and praise is reinforcing to the child, the food can be given less frequently, whereas praise will still be provided every time the desired behavior occurs. The food is gradually eliminated, and praise will have become a reinforcer for the child.

Consistency is also important when applying reinforcers. As children learn an increasing variety of behaviors, they learn about new and different reinforcers. Food and feeding habits may be incorporated into behavioral repertoires designed to gain adult attention. Throwing utensils or food may cause a variety of interesting adult reactions. A parent may laugh at one such incident, respond with anger at another, and at a third may feed the child in exasperation. In the effort to keep up with the child, parents may respond inconsistently, depending on their mood at the time. Consistency means that desirable behaviors generally are reinforced, whereas undesirable behaviors are not reinforced and may even be punished. The child should know what desirable behaviors are expected by his or her parents and, in turn, what consequences can be expected for certain behaviors.

Experience has indicated that reinforcers other than food are more effective for managing feeding behaviors. For instance, if a child must be on a special diet for a biological reason such as allergy, parents and professionals usually become concerned that the child may not eat adequate amount of acceptable foods. In this instance the child receives mixed messages if he or she is reinforced with food yet perceives that the parents will not allow certain other foods. The child quickly learns that by refusing foods that are allowed he or she can gain a great deal of attention and may even receive the forbidden foods as parents become upset by the child's refusal to eat. The use of nonedible reinforcers such as outings, toys, and games following meals generally helps to refocus the parents' and child's attention to other activities.

TEACHING SELF-FEEDING BEHAVIORS

In addition to the use of reinforcement, *shaping* and *fading* techniques are useful for teaching new behaviors and skills. Both of these procedures are used by parents and professionals for teaching feeding behaviors.

Shaping is the reinforcement of successive approximations to a desired behavior. In this procedure the behavior is broken down into its component steps. The types and number of steps are determined by the task to be learned. The first step is reinforced; when that step is learned, the next step is added and the reinforcement is shifted to the second step in the chain of responses that lead to the desired behavior.

Teaching spoon-feeding by shaping

1. Desired behavior: independent spoon-feeding
2. Changing steps in child responses:
   a. Child looks at spoon
   b. Child moves hand toward spoon
   c. Child touches spoon
   d. Child picks up spoon
   e. Child puts spoon in dish
   f. Child scoops food
   g. Child brings food to mouth
   h. Child takes food off spoon
   i. Child returns spoon to dish
3. Reinforcement: bites of food or other reinforcers as each step is accomplished

Fading is a different procedure in that the entire behavior is used each time for reinforcement. Instead of requiring the child's responses to proceed through several steps, the trainer's cues are changed as the child's skill develops. For example, the trainer holds the child's hand around the spoon and puts the child through the motions of scooping food onto the spoon, bringing the spoon to the mouth, and returning the spoon to the dish. As the child gradually assumes independent movement, physical assistance is decreased and the trainer only provides assistance as needed to complete the task. The number and type of trainer cues needed depends on the task to be learned and the abilities of the child.

Teaching spoon-feeding by fading

1. Desired behavior: independent spoon-feeding
2. Steps:
   a. Holding child's hand around spoon, scoop food, bring arm, hand, and spoon *to* mouth. Allow child to take food off spoon in mouth, then (still holding child's hand around spoon) return spoon to dish.
   b. Holding child's hand around spoon, bring it *toward* mouth and allow child to complete movement to mouth if possible. Assist through rest of cycle.
   c. Assist child in holding spoon and scooping food. By touching arm slightly, provide cues that assist child in completing movement to mouth. Also by touches, assist child in returning spoon to dish.
   d. Provide only as much assistance as child needs to pick up spoon, scoop food, move spoon to mouth, and return to dish.

The actual number of steps delineated for any given individual depends on the developmental level and skill that the individual possesses before using either of these procedures.

GENERAL CONSIDERATIONS IN THE USE OF BEHAVIOR MANAGEMENT TECHNIQUES

Behavior modification is generally easy to use as a method of therapeutic intervention. The difficulties lie in the behavioral analysis, which is necessary to pinpoint specific behaviors and their consequences. Frequently, the relationships between behaviors and their consequences (particularly when two or more persons are involved) are difficult to discover, and care must be taken to delineate them with accuracy and reliability. Behavior is never simple and becomes increasingly complex when viewed within a framework of human interaction. Yet to try to remedy behaviors in isolation is to treat them outside the context of their everyday occurrence. This, in turn, leads to unsuccessful programs.

The preceding examples have been assessed by direct observation of mealtime behaviors, yet there are more complex situations that would preclude direct observation or that would be greatly altered by the presence of an observer. In-home videotaped recordings frequently work well for these situations. Parents are usually quite willing to allow several meals to be videotaped to pinpoint difficulties. These tapes are analyzed according to their ABC patterns. Important segments of tape are then played back to the parents, who frequently are able to discover the problems themselves. Frequently, this is an impetus for them to discuss their feelings and concerns about the situations and to generate alternative ways of behaving with their children.

Professionals must consider all the possible effects of the techniques before implementing them and should secure assistance while learning the procedures involved. Collaboration of nutritionists, nurses, and professionals from other disciplines helps continually refine observation and recording techniques and management procedures. The role of each discipline in the analysis, program design, and implementation must be well defined to make the program successful.

During nutrition and feeding evaluation, observations of parental and child behaviors by professionals from two or more disciplines help to identify more reliably the cause of a specific problem. Programs should be designed jointly with parents by one team member who is skilled in behavior management. Changes in physical growth, nutrient intake, and behavior should be monitored on an interdisciplinary basis to direct attention to both psychosocial (behavioral) and physical parameters.

Summary

Feeding and nutrition problems during childhood may result from inappropriate parent-child interactions. Behavior management programs when adequately implemented can resolve these problems. Observations of parent-child interactions give clues as to the antecedent to the behavior and the reinforcers that cause it to continue. Reinforcers used in behavior management programs must be individualized for each client. If food is used as a reinforcer, the program and nutrient intake should be carefully monitored to ensure that it does not compromise the child's nutritional status.

SUGGESTED LEARNING ACTIVITIES

1. Observe a child eating a family meal. What cues do parents give the child to eat? Identify positive and negative reinforcers parents consciously or unconsciously use.
2. How would you identify appropriate foods and reinforcers for a child who needs a behavior management program?
3. Describe feeding problem behaviors for which a behavior management program would be appropriate.
4. Define factors that should be monitored to ensure that a child's nutritional status is not compromised when a behavioral management program is planned to change a child's feeding behavior.
5. Design a behavior management program to effect an increase in textures of food acceptable to a developmentally delayed child.

REFERENCES

1. Cooper, J. O., Heron, T. E., and Heward, W. L.: Applied behavior analysis, Columbus, Ohio, 1987, Merrill Publishing Co.
2. Peterson, L. W.: Operant approach to observation and recording, Nurs. Outlook 15:28, 1967.

GLOSSARY

acidosis   Pathological condition resulting from accumulation of acid or depletion of alkaline reserves

allergen   Substance that causes an altered response of cells and, as a result, symptoms of allergy

allergy   Hypersensitive state caused by the interaction of an allergen with an antibody

alopecia totalis   Complete loss of hair

amenorrhea   Absence or abnormal stoppage of the menses

amylase   Enzyme that catalyzes the hydrolysis of starch to glucose

anaerobic   Occurring in the absence of oxygen

anorexia   Lack of appetite

anoxia   Lack of oxygen in the tissues or body

antibody   Protein synthesized in response to an antigenic stimulus

antigen   Any substance that produces an immune response as a result of contact with the tissue: hypersensitivity may result

asphyxiation   Suffocation

aspiration   Inhaling

assessment   Critical analysis on the status or quality of a condition

asymmetry   Dissimilarity in corresponding parts or organs on opposite sides of the body that are normally alike

atonic   Lacking normal tone or strength

bioavailability   Degree of availability of a substance to an organism

"bird-feeding"   Feeding an individual with his or her head thrown back

bonding   Development of a close emotional tie to another individual or to a newborn infant

bone density   Compactness of the bone

botulism   Food poisoning caused by the toxin produced by *Clostridium* organisms botulinum

bronchopulmonary dysplasia   Disorder characterized by hypoxia, hypercardia, and oxygen dependency; a computation of hyaline membrane disease

bulimia   Gorging and vomiting

calcitonin   Hormone secreted by the thyroid gland that is concerned with the regulation of calcium ions in the blood

casein   Principal protein of milk

celiac disease   Malabsorption syndrome in which the child or adult cannot tolerate gluten

cell differentiation   Diversification of cells

cephalocaudal   From head to toe; the sequence in which a normal developmental pattern occurs

cerebrum   Main portion of the brain

cholelithiasis   Stones or calculi in the gall bladder or bile duct

cholestatic jaundice   Jaundice caused by arrest of the flow of bile

cm   Abbreviation for centimeter

colic   Acute abdominal pain

colostrum   First milk secreted by the mammary gland after parturition

congenital   Existing at, and usually before, birth

creatinine   Anhydride of creatine, formed largely in the muscles by irreversible and nonenzymatic removal of water from creatine phosphate; the amount excreted in the urine is an index of muscle mass and may be used as a measure of basal heat production

digital grasp   Grasp of objects with the thumb and fingers

diuresis   Increased excretion of urine

Down's syndrome   Congenital condition caused by trisomy 21, a chromosomal abnormality; characterized by a small, anteroposteriorly flattened skull, short flat-bridged nose, epicanthus, short phalanges, widened space between the first and second digits of hands and feet, and moderate to severe mental retardation

enteral   By way of the intestine

epiglottis   Structure that covers the entrance to the larynx

epilepsy   Condition characterized by paroxysmally recurring impairment or loss of consciousness, involuntary excess or cessation of muscle movements, psychic or sensory disturbances, and perturbation of the autonomic nervous system

epiphyseal closure   Final calcification of the ends of the long bones causing cessation of growth

erythematous   Redness of the skin caused by congestion of the capillaries

erythropoiesis   Production of red blood cells

evaluation   Judgment of the value of that which is being assessed

exfoliative   Falling off in scales or layers

extension   Movement that brings the members of a limb into or toward a straight condition

extensor   Any muscle that extends a joint

ferritin   One of the chief forms of iron stored in the body—an iron-apoferritin complex

flexed   Bent or put into a state of being bent

gag reflex   Elevation of the soft palate and retching elicited by touching the back of the tongue or the wall of the pharynx

gastroschisis   Congenital fissure of the abdominal wall

gavage   Feeding by insertion of a stomach tube through the mouth into the stomach

gestational age   Age of the infant calculated from the beginning of conception, often used with low birth weight infants

glia   Supporting tissue of brain and spinal cord

HANES   Abbreviation for Health and Nutrition Examination Survey, a nutritional status survey of the United States' population, conducted on a 2-year cycle

Heimlich maneuver   Technique for removing foreign matter from the trachea of a choking victim

hematocrit   Volume percentage of red blood cells in the blood

hemoglobin   Oxygen-carrying pigment of the erythrocytes

heparin   Anticoagulant; inhibits coagulation by preventing conversion of prothrombin to thrombin

hydroxyproline   Proline to which a hydroxyl group has been added; found in the structural protein collagen

hyperactivity   Abnormally increased activity

hyperbilirubinemia   Excess bilirubin in the blood that may lead to jaundice

hyperkinesis   Abnormally increased mobility or activity

hyperplasia   Increase in cell number; increase in the number of normal cells

hypersensitivity   Abnormally increased sensitivity

hypertension   Elevation of blood pressure above normal

hypertonia   Condition of excessive tone, tension, or activity

hypertrophy   Increase in cell size

hypocalcemia   Reduction of blood calcium below normal

hypochromic   Abnormal decrease in hemoglobin content of red blood cells

hyponatremia   Deficiency of sodium in the blood

hypotonia   Conditions of abnormally diminished tone, tension, or activity

immunity   Protection against invasion by infectious agents because of the presence of antibody or reactivity of antibody–forming cells and of phagocytic cells

insensible water loss   Loss of water nonperceptible to the senses

intestinal atresia   Complete occlusion of the intestinal tract

ketones   Compounds derived from the oxidation of a secondary alcohol

kg   Abbreviation for kilogram

kilocalorie   Amount of heat required to raise the temperature of 1 kg of water 1°C

kwashiorkor   Protein deficiency disease occurring in children

laryngeal   Of or pertaining to the larynx—the muscular and cartilaginous structure at the top of the trachea and below the root of the tongue and the hyoid bone

lateralization   Moving from one side to the other

linoleic acid   Essential fatty acid; a polyunsaturated fatty acid with 2 double bonds and 18 carbon atoms

marasmus   Form of extreme undernutrition

maturation   Stage of process of becoming fully developed

mechanical ventilation   Mechanically supplying oxygen through the lungs

megaloblastic anemia   Type of anemia characterized by an increased level of megaloblasts, which are primitive nucleated red blood cells much larger than the mature erythrocytes

megavitamin therapy   Treatment of disease with massive doses of vitamins

menarche   Beginning of the menstrual function

methemoglobemia   Presence of methemoglobin, a compound formed after poisoning by some substance in the blood

microcytic   Abnormally small red blood cell

myelin   Fatty substance forming a sheath around certain nerve fibers

myelinization   Taking on of myelin by nerve cells

myoglobin   Iron-protein complex in muscle that acts as a store of oxygen

neonatal   Pertaining to the newborn

neuronal   Pertaining to one or more nerve cells

neurotransmitters   A substance released on excitation that either inhibits or excites the target cell

neutrophil   Cell that stains easily with neutral dye

occiput   Back part of the head

omphalocele   Hernia of the navel

osteomalacia   Inadequate mineralization of the organic matrix of the bones, resulting in skeletal deformities and fractures

osteopenia   Insufficiency of bone resulting from reduced production or increased breakdown of bone

palmar grasp   Grasp of objects with the palm of the hand

parenteral   Injection of substances into the body through any route other than the alimentary tract

patent ductus arteriosus   Open lumen in the ductus arteriosus after birth causing recirculation of arterial blood through the lungs

pharynx   Muscular and membranous tube extending from the oral cavity to the esophagus

photon absorption   Absorption of a particle of radiant energy

phytate   A compound that forms insoluble compounds that reduce the coefficient of utilization of certain minerals

pica   Abnormal craving to consume unusual articles such as clay, chalk, laundry starch, and dirt

pincer grasp   Grasp of small objects with the thumb and index finger

Prader-Willi syndrome   Syndrome characterized by small genitals, mental retardation, and obesity; affected individuals have an abnormal craving for food

prehension   Act of seizing or grasping

prenatal   Before birth

proprioceptive facilitation   Promotion or hastening of receiving stimulations within the tissues of the body

prothrombin   Protein in blood plasma needed for blood clotting

raking grasp   Grasp of objects by raking with palm of the hand

reflex   Sum total of any particular involuntary activity

reflux   Backward or return flow

roentgenographic studies   Study of x-ray films

rooting   Food-seeking movement that occurs in response to stimulation of the lips or cheeks characterized by the head turning toward the stimulus and the mouth opening

schizophrenia   Mental disorder characterized by delusions, hallucinations, and withdrawn, bizarre, or regressive behavior

self-esteem   Satisfaction in oneself

sepsis   Infection in the blood stream

seratonin   A tryptophan derivative that is a powerful vasoconstrictor and plays a role in brain and nerve function, gastric secretion and intestinal peristalsis

slough   Dead tissue in or separated from living tissue

solute   Substance dissolved in a solution

somatomedin   Group of peptides that mediate the effect of growth hormone

spasticity   State of increase over the normal tension of a muscle, resulting in continuous increase of resistance to stretching

supraorbital   Situation above the bone cavity that contains the eyeball

tactile   Pertaining to the sense of touch

tactile sensitivity   State or quality of being unusually responsive to touch

tetany   Syndrome characterized by muscle twitchings, cramps, and convulsions

tongue thrust   Moving the tongue through the lips when swallowing, normally associated with suckling in infants less than 4 months of age; an abnormal reflex in some individuals with motor coordination difficulties

tonic neck pattern   When the head is turned forcibly to one side, the arm and leg on that side extend while the opposite arm and leg are flexed; described as the fencing position

toxemia   Spread of bacterial products in the blood stream

toxicity   Quality of being poisonous

toxicology   Study of poisons

tracheoesophageal fistula   Abnormal tube-like passage in the esophagus often connecting the trachea and distal esophagus

transferrin   Serum B-globulin that binds and transports iron

vegan   Vegetarian who excludes all animal protein from the diet

volvulus   Intestinal obstruction caused by twisting of the bowel

whey   Residue of milk remaining after the curd and cream have been removed

Index

Page numbers in *italics* indicate boxes and illustrations.
Page numbers followed by *t* indicate tables.